AF335549

The Lactoperoxidase System

IMMUNOLOGY SERIES
NOEL R. ROSE

Professor and Chairman
Department of Immunology and
* Infectious Diseases*
The Johns Hopkins University
School of Hygiene and Public Health
Baltimore, Maryland

Other Volumes in Preparation

The Lactoperoxidase System
Chemistry and Biological Significance

Edited by

Kenneth M. Pruitt
The University of Alabama at Birmingham
Birmingham, Alabama

Jorma O. Tenovuo
Institute of Dentistry
University of Turku
Turku, Finland

MARCEL DEKKER INC.   New York and Basel

Library of Congress Cataloging in Publication Data
Main entry under title:

The Lactoperoxidase system: chemistry and biological
    significance

    (Immunology series ; v.27)
    Includes bibliographical references and index.
    1. Peroxidase. 2. Immunity. 3. Saliva. I. Pruitt,
Kenneth M.   II. Tenovuo, Jorma O. III. Series
[DNLM: 1. Peroxidases. 2. Saliva--enzymology.
W1 IM53K v.28 / QU 140 L151]
QP603.P4L33 1985   612'.313   84-26040
ISBN 0-8247-7298-9

MARCEL DEKKER, INC.
270 Madison Avenue, New York, New York 10016

Current printing (last digit):
10 9 8 7 6 5 4 3 2 1

PRINTED IN THE UNITED STATES OF AMERICA

Preface

Secretory proteins play an important role in protecting mucosal surfaces
from infection. These proteins include secretory antibodies as well as
other proteins whose antimicrobial properties do not depend upon prior
exposure to an antigen.

The nonantibody or innate proteins provide defense mechanisms to
the infant during the critical period prior to maturation of the antibody
system. In the adult, they augment the antimicrobial effectiveness of
the specific antibody-dependent immune response.

The best characterized innate antimicrobial proteins include animal
lectins, lysozyme, lactoferrin, and secretory peroxidase. The most
widely studied of the secretory peroxidases are the bovine milk enzyme
(lactoperoxidase) and human salivary peroxidase. Although the latter
has come to be known as "lactoperoxidase" because of similarities to
bovine milk peroxidase, recent work has shown that there are significant differences in the properties of these enzymes.

Peroxidase enzymes are widely distributed in animals. These enzymes, together with appropriate cofactors, have a remarkable range of
antimicrobial activity against viruses, mycoplasmas, bacteria, parasites,
and tumor cells. Excellent review articles* have been published on the
myeloperoxidase system of phagocytes, but there have been no comparable summaries of the state of knowledge with respect to secretory peroxidases. This book will review the major biochemical and biological
properties of the lactoperoxidase system including both the bovine milk
and human salivary enzymes. Chapter topics range from the basic chemistry of peroxidase-catalyzed reactions to clinical applications of peroxide system antimicrobial effects.

---

*R. A. Clark: Extracellular effects of the myeloperoxidase-hydrogen
peroxide-halide system. Adv. Inflam. Res. 5, 107, 1983
S. J. Klebanoff: Antimicrobial mechanisms in neutrophilic polymorphonuclear leukocytes. Semin. Hematol. 12, 117, 1975
S. J. Klebanoff and R. A. Clark: The Neutrophil: Function and Clinical Disorders. North-Holland Publishing Co., Amsterdam, 1978

There is a definite need for a compilation and critical review of the many published studies of the lactoperoxidase system. The system has been of interest to investigators with varied professional backgrounds. As a consequence of the diversity of training and interests of these research workers, their numerous publications have been widely scattered in the scientific literature and are not easily collected.

In order to provide the reader with an appropriate perspective of the lactoperoxidase system, this book begins with a general review of human nonimmunoglobulin defense mechanisms (Chapter 1). The remainder of the book is addressed to a mixed audience.

Chapters 2–5 will appeal to those readers whose primary interests are in the biochemical aspects of peroxidase systems. Chapter 2 covers the structure of lactoperoxidase. Chapter 3 reviews the chemistry of peroxidase-catalyzed oxidation and halogenation reactions, while the steady state kinetics of these reactions are discussed in Chapter 4. Chapter 5 deals with the genetic polymorphism of human salivary peroxidase.

Chapters 6–9 will be of interest to readers concerned with the biology of the lactoperoxidase system. This section of the book describes peroxidase systems in human secretions (Chapter 6), the lactoperoxidase system in bovine milk (Chapter 7), the biochemistry of antimicrobial actions of peroxidase systems (Chapter 8), and hydrogen peroxide production by bacteria (Chapter 9).

The final chapters focus on topics that should appeal to readers with interests in clinical applications. The effects of sugar diets on salivary peroxidase are discussed in Chapter 10, while clinical studies of the activation of salivary peroxidase systems are described in Chapter 11. The book concludes with a discussion of antibody targeting of peroxidase-catalyzed reactions (Chapter 12).

The role of the specific immune response in biological defense is a dominant theme in the current rapid advances in cellular and noncellular immunology and in immunochemistry. We hope that this book will stimulate further research on the peroxidase sytems as well as the other proteins that comprise the nonantibody defense system. The observations of synergistic interactions among the various defense systems seem to offer especially fertile areas for future studies.

The editors wish to acknowledge the substantial contributions of Dr. Bruno Reiter to this book. In addition to his authorship (Chapter 7) and coauthorship (Chapter 8) of important chapters, he carefully reviewed other chapters and made valuable suggestions. Also, he gave us significant help in writing the preface. The final version reflects several of his ideas.

We also acknowledge the skilled technical assistance of Ms. Nancy Hawkins and Ms. Paivi Vainio in typing the manuscripts. Ms. Hawkins also provided invaluable assistance with the routine editing chores.

Kenneth M. Pruitt
Jorma O. Tenovuo

Contents

Index 243

Contributors

Roland R. Arnold, Ph.D.   Chairman and Professor, Department of Oral Biology, Emory University School of Dentistry, Atlanta, Georgia

Edwin A. Azen, M.D.   Professor, Departments of Medicine and Medical Genetics, University of Wisconsin, Madison, Wisconsin

William G. Bardsley   Senior Lecturer, Department of Biochemistry, The University of Manchester and Department of Obstetrics and Gynecology, St. Mary's Hospital, Manchester, England

Solon A. Ellison, D.D.S., Ph.D.   Professor of Dentistry, School of Dental and Oral Surgery, Columbia University, New York, New York

Henk Hoogendoorn   Senior Research Scientist, Akzo Consumenten Produkten bv, The Hague, The Netherlands

Kauko K. Mäkinen, Ph.D.*   Professor of Biochemistry, Department of Biochemistry, Institute of Dentistry, University of Turku, Turku, Finland

Irwin D. Mandel, D.D.S.†   Professor of Dentistry, School of Dental and Oral Surgery, Columbia University, New York, New York

Per-Ingvar Ohlsson, Dr. Med. Sci.   Research Engineer, Department of Physiological Chemistry, University of Umeå, Umeå, Sweden

---

Current affiliations:
*Professor of Biochemistry, Department of Oral Biology, School of Dentistry, The University of Michigan, Ann Arbor, Michigan
†Director, Center for Clinical Research in Dentistry, School of Dental and Oral Surgery, Columbia University, New York, New York

Karl-Gustav Paul, M.D.   Professor, Department of Physiological Chemistry, University of Umeå, Umeå, Sweden

Kenneth M. Pruitt, Ph.D.   Professor of Biochemistry and Biomathematics, Biochemistry Department, The University of Alabama at Birmingham, Birmingham, Alabama

Bruno Reiter, Ph.D., D.Sc. Honary Research Fellow, University of Oxford, John Radcliffe Hospital, Headington, Oxford and National Institute for Research in Dairying,* Shinfield, Reading, England

Jorma O. Tenovuo, D. Odont.   Docent of Dental Biochemistry, Departments of Dental Biochemistry and Periodontology, Institute of Dentistry University of Turku, Turku, Finland

Edwin L. Thomas, Ph.D.   Associate Member, Department of Biochemistry, St. Jude Children's Research Hospital, Memphis, Tennessee

---

*Retired

The Lactoperoxidase System

1

The Biological Significance of the Nonimmunoglobulin Defense Factors

IRWIN D. MANDEL and SOLON A. ELLISON / *School of Dental and Oral Surgery, Columbia University, New York, New York*

I. INTRODUCTION

In the competition among species for a secure niche the ability to resist infectious disease has been a major attribute. Long before the advent of antibiotics, the evolutionary development of a multiplicity of protective mechanisms provided humans with a rich inheritance. Both the diversity and the orchestration of these protective instruments are becoming increasingly apparent as investigators clarify the nature of the various systems.

In a division of labor characteristic of most successful enterprises, protection of the mucosal surfaces is largely the responsibility of the exocrine glands and their secretions. The attention given to the secretory immune system since its identification has tended to overshadow exciting developments in our knowledge of the nature and function of a variety of nonimmunoglobulin secretory products that are also effective defenders of mucosal integrity. The latter are varied in nature and function, having distinct actions, but with less restrictive specificities than are characteristic of the immune factors. Although individual factors have limited activities, their total impact appears to be most effective. Interactions of the protective proteins with other secretory components, with each other, and with the immunoglobulins can amplify the antibacterial potential of the mucosal secretions. These defense systems can (a) prevent establishment of specific organisms; (b) limit multiplication; (c) inhibit spread within the host; and (d) create an environment in which pathogenic mechanisms are inhibited or made ineffective.

Although each of the mucous membrane surfaces (eye, nose, mouth, intestines, and so on) has special functions and specific defense mechanisms, all of the exocrine gland secretions share an assortment of nonimmunoglobulin antibacterial systems. The best known of these antibacterial systems, involving lysozyme, lactoferrin, and lactoperoxidase, are similar to antibacterial mechanisms characteristic of the phagolysosomes of the polymorphonuclear leukocyte (41). In addition to direct antibacterial activities, the exocrine secretions interfere with bacterial adherence and thus help clear bacteria from the tissues they bathe. A number of mechanical and chemical processes are involved, some common to all secretions, others, variations on a theme. This chapter will deal primarily with our current view of the operation of these direct and indirect antibacterial systems in saliva, tears, milk, and intestinal secretions.

II. BACTERIAL CLEARANCE

Colonization of tissue surfaces, adherence, is a critical event for survival of many bacteria, and interference with this process by mechanical, immunological, and nonimmunological means is a major host defense capability (9,19,39). In the past decade, exploration of the nature of the game has been an active research area, and the ground rules are becoming clearer.

A. Debridement/Lavage

The physical movement of exocrine gland secretions augmented by muscle activity mechanically entraps and effectively removes a large number of potentially harmful bacteria from mucosal surfaces. Comparable systems exist in all areas: (a) tearing and blinking the eye; (b) blowing and mucociliary movement in the nose; (c) coughing, expectoration, and ciliary movement in the lungs and in the tracheobronchial tree; (d) salivary flow and lip and tongue movement in the mouth; and (e) intestinal motility and the mucin film in the intestinal tract. The differential effects of peristalsis in the small and large intestine provide a dramatic example of the importance of mechanical factors in containing the bacterial population. In the small intestine peristalsis is vigorous and frequent, and bacterial growth is limited. In the large intestine, where peristalsis is episodic with long periods of stagnation, there is extensive proliferation of the bacterial flora. Clinical situations that involve decreased peristalsis in the small intestine result in extensive proliferation of bacteria in this area. Walker (67) aptly pointed out that "bacteria, viruses and macromolecules within succus entericus or loosely attached to the intestinal surface can be readily dislodged by peristaltic movement. Without attachment to an epithelial surface, organisms cannot proliferate and macromolecules (antigens) cannot be engulfed by enterocytes."

The extensive formation of dental plaque with associated rampant caries and the irritations and infections of the oral soft tissues that accompany loss of salivary gland functions (xerostomia) are all too common examples of the deleterious effects of inadequate exocrine gland secretion. Beachey (9) has suggested that "pathogenic organisms are able to gain a foothold only by taking advantage of impaired local defenses."

B. Aggregation

In addition to physical entrapment and flushing mechanisms, the exocrine secretions interfere with adherence by more direct means that depend on molecular interactions. The ability to inhibit bacterial attachment is a major property of the secretory IgA immune system and has been the subject of numerous publications (26). In addition to these made-to-order antibodies, however, there is a variety of ready-to-wear macromolecules in exocrine gland fluids, some very specific in action, which mask bacterial adhesins or compete with them for attachment sites on tissues. Alternatively, they may clump or aggregate bacteria so that they lose their capability of effectively adhering to tissue surfaces. These carbohydrate recognition molecules of mammalian origin markedly amplify the ability of secretory fluids to cope with variable numbers and types of bacterial antigens.

Formation of bacterial aggregates by secretory components other than sIgA is now a well-described phenomenon in vitro (20,23). It is not clear how closely the aggregates resemble antibody-agglutinated bacteria. It is highly probable, however, that the specificities of the reactants may be more flexible than in the case of the bacterial antigen-antibody interaction, and in the case of large molecules such as mucin, they have multiple specificities involving different organisms. The oral cavity, a site particularly susceptible to bacterial influx (except perhaps in tight-lipped individuals), has been the focus of considerable research in recent years on both adherence and aggregation and the potential competition between the two phenomena. It remains

to be established to what extent the in vitro observations based on
model systems with carefully controlled concentrations of cells and
reactant molecules can be applied in vivo. The studies do, however,
provide a means of at least measuring the potential capability of the
protective components.

A quantitative sense of the degree of effectiveness of the salivary-
bacterial interaction was provided by Clark and Gibbons (16) with
their findings that when *Streptoccocus mutans* cells are first suspended
in saliva and then exposed to hydroxyapatite disks, adsorption to the
disks is reduced more than 30-fold when compared with untreated
bacterium. That investigation also provided evidence that high molecular weight molecules from saliva were involved, most probably
blood group-reactive salivary glycoproteins. Further support for the
role of a high molecular weight aggregation factor was supplied by
Kashket and Guilmette (33) in studies with *S. sanguis* and *S. mutans*
and by Levine et al. (36) in their studies of the interaction of purified
salivary glycoproteins with *S. sanguis* and *S. mutans*. The latter
study provided insight into the nature of specificity in the interaction
by demonstrating that removal of terminal sialic acid from mucin-glyco-
protein results in loss of agglutinating activity for *S. sanguis* but not
for *S. mutans*. The role of sialic acid in saliva-induced aggregation
has also been noted by others (38). Preliminary data indicate that
S. mutans agglutination can be abolished by α-galactosidase treatment
of the mucin-glycoproteins (36).

Although several secretory proteins contribute to bacterial
aggregation in vitro or interfere with tissue adherence, most attention
has been given to the high molecular weight mucins. The presence of
multiple complex oligosaccharide side chains provides a variety of combinations for interactions (63). The microheterogeneity characteristic
of these highly glycosylated proteins provides an additional range of
possibilities for interactions. Mucosal glands do not possess the responsiveness provided by clonal expansion in the immune system, but
the state of readiness provided by the complex side chains and the
microheterogeneity is a valuable alternative defense feature.

Studies using the rabbit urinary bladder as a model system support
the concept that surface mucins are major antibacterial factors. Parsons and coworkers (51,54) have shown that disruption of the surface
mucin layer and acid treatment resulted in as much as a 10-fold increase
in bacterial adherence. This was equally true for the three kinds of
bacteria examined (*Escherichia coli*, *Staphylococcus aureus*, and
Klebsiella pneumoniae). An antibacterial effect could be restored by
intravesical instillation of the synthetic sulfonated glycosaminoglycan,
heparin, and with sodium pentosanpolysulfate, a similar polysaccharide
that lacks significant anticoagulant activity (53,54).

The hypothesis advanced by Parsons et al. (54) is that the glycos-
aminoglycans, because of their extreme hydrophilic nature, provide a
water barrier between the surface of the epithelial cells and the exter-

nal environment and "thus mask highly charged moieties on the cell
surfaces. The barrier would serve to interfere with electrochemical
reactions, thereby impairing bacterial binding."

In addition to interfering with electostatic adherence, as suggested
by Parsons et al., and the direct interaction of oligosaccharide side
chains and complementary bacterial surface molecules, mucin can provide a network that mechanically traps bacterial cells and then aids in
their physical removal. This mucin entrapment, however, may be
more than a mechanical snare. Mucin can complex with a variety of
secretory proteins, including IgA (61), lysozyme (17), and peroxidase
(see Chap. 6). Such combinations can thus provide mucus secretions
with a capacity that resembles the activities within a phagolysosome.
It may be a propos that the minor salivary glands of the mouth (e.g.,
labial glands), which provide products for protecting the oral mucous
membranes, are mucous glands whose secretions are rich in both IgA
and lysozyme. The combination of IgA and mucin is found in many
secretions. In the gastrointestinal tract, for instance, secretory antibodies are retained within the mucous coat on the surface of epithelial
cells by the interaction with cysteine residues in the mucin present
within the glycocalyx. This combination has been called an "antiseptic
paint" (11). Lysozyme and mucin have also been noted as coexisting
in a variety of cells that generate products that coat membrane surfaces (17). A cooperative effect has been inferred.

C. Other Protective Properties of Mucin

1. Antiviral Activity

Mucins are protective against viruses as well as bacteria. Salivary
mucins by virtue of their nonreducing terminal sialic acid (the N-
acetylneuraminic, not the N-glycolylneuraminic acid) can interact with
surface components of the influenza virus and block viral attachment
to host cells (25). Saliva (presumably the mucin) can also play a protective role against herpes simplex virus. Heineman and Greenberg
(28) demonstrated that human amnion cell cultures incubated with
saliva were protected against subsequent destruction by the virus.
The effect appeared to be specific in that the protection against herpes
simplex was considerably greater than that against vaccinia or vesicu-
lar stromatitis viruses.

2. Mucous Barrier Function

A variety of studies has established that the presence of a mucous
coating is essential for the protection of mucous membranes against
penetration of potentially hazardous substances such as toxins, hy-
drolytic enzymes, acids, and carcinogens. Gibson et al. (21) demonstrated increased permeability of the intestinal mucosa following removal
of its mucous coat by flushing with sodium bicarbonate. Lukie (37)

noted an inverse relationship between the rate of water penetration
and the concentrations of mucus on the rat intestinal surface. Adams
(2) examined the oral mucosa and found that treating it with mucolytic
agents increased dye permeability. He also reported increased pene-
trability of the oral mucosa when salivation was markedly decreased
through the use of antisialogogues (1). It has also been found that
inducing a state of dryness results in an increased incidence of malig-
nant change when chemical carcinogens are painted on oral tissue surfaces (68).

III. LYSOZYME

Lysozyme is widely distributed among organs, glands, and tissues
(30), including most of the human exocrine glands, where at least
part of the lysozyme is synthesized locally. The traditional view of
lysozyme function is that lysis is based on its ability to cleave the
specific linkage between N-acetylmuramic acid and N-acetylglucosamine.
In most bacteria the acetylmuramic acid residues are substituted; hence,
only organisms such as *Micrococcus lysodeikticus*, in which the specific
residues are exposed, are particularly sensitive to lysozyme. Lysozyme,
however, is not without allies and with help is capable of a broader
range of activity. Over the past 15 years, several investigators have
demonstrated that the interaction of IgA antibodies, the alternate
pathway of complement and lysozyme, can result in lysis of gram-negative
bacteria (3). A similar softening-up process can be accomplished by
hydrogen peroxide and ascorbic acid (49). It has also been noted that
oral streptococci could be lysed when lysozyme treatment was followed
by such agents as sodium lauryl sulfate (13).

Although tears are the richest source of lysozyme (with a concentration exceeding 100 mg%), most of the recent work on its mechanism
of action has involved the salivary system. Pollock and colleagues
(56,66) have gone beyond the traditional examination of the cleavage of
the sensitive linkages in the peptidoglycan of the cell wall to study
binding to lipoteichoic acids of *S. mutans* and the disruption of the
cell membrane of *Veillonella*. Especially exciting has been their demon-
stration that anions of low-charge density (chaotropic ions) can promote
gross lysis of *S. mutans* (BHT) once lysozyme has bound to the cell
surface (22). The order of efficacy in producing lysis is thiocyanate,
perchlorate, iodide, bromide, nitrate, chloride, and fluoride. Chloride
is present in saliva at levels comparable with those employed by Pollock et al. in the in vitro system. Thiocyanate in smokers may approach the high level required. Fluoride can reach appropriate levels
when introduced in dental preparations. Pollock et al. (56) have shown
also that bicarbonate promotes bacterial lysis by lysozyme after initial
binding of the enzyme. Stimulated saliva contains an appreciable concentration of bicarbonate. In tears, the thiocyanate concentration is

very low, but chloride and bicarbonate are high. The potential role
of thiocyanate is of special interest since it is also central to the action
of the lactoperoxidase system. It has been suggested that the combination of lysozyme and hypothiocyanite ion (formed as a result of lacto-
peroxidase-catalyzed oxidation of thiocyanate by hydrogen peroxide)
might be even more effective than thiocyanate with lysozyme. Bicarbonate is also interesting since it stabilizes the iron-binding site of
lactoferrin (26). The interaction of the various members of the salivary
antibacterial community is a fascinating example of communal living.

In more recent experiments with lysozyme, breakdown of the semi-
permeable character of the bacterial membrane is measured by efflux
of [14C]nicotinamide from *S. mutans* and cell lysis quantitated by the
liberation of deoxyribonucleic acid (DNA) as [14C]thymidine. The concept being advanced is that lysozyme binds to the bacterial membrane,
enlarges the pores, and irreversibly destroys the membrane's semiper-
meable character. The chaotropic anions disorder water and in the
process weaken hydrophobic interaction, leading to destabilization of
the membranes and biological macromolecules (55). Electron micro-
scopy has also been used effectively to assess lytic damage of bacterial
cells (66).

It has also been suggested (29) that the lysozyme binding to the
lipoteichoic acid of gram-positive bacteria (such as *S. mutans*) may result in lysis via another mechanism. In a number of bacterial species,
lipoteichoic acids have been shown to strongly inhibit autolysin activity
(70). Binding to lipoteichoic acid by lysozyme could result in a de-
regulation of autolysin activity that would affect cell division and
cause an alteration of the highly organized membrane system.

In addition to its role in bacterial lysis in phagocytic cells and
exocrine gland secretions, lysozyme appears to have other biological
properties of importance to host defense. Gordon et al. (23) found
that lysozyme was able to significantly dampen several responses of
neutrophils to inflammatory stimuli. This modulation of neutrophil
function, a means of modifying an overexuberant response with potential damaging to host tisuses, was expressed by decreasing the
chemotactic response and quenching superoxide generation. Lysozyme
can apparently function in a negative feedback system to help in
the regulation of polymorphonuclear leucocyte (PMN) activity.

Another intriguing role for lysozyme is that of immunomodulator
(31,50). Through its action on some bacteria cell walls it can give
rise to products (muramyl-peptides) that belong to a group of naturally
occurring substances known to possess adjuvant or immunostimulating
properties. The actual performance in vivo has not as yet been
shown, but the analogy to substances commonly employed as adjuvants
makes this a very likely prospect. The close association of lysozyme
and secretory IgA in many secretory fluids may not be a random
event. Lysozyme, however, can function independently of IgA. Indeed, lysozyme concentration has been shown to be significantly in-

creased in immunodeficient subjects (37). We have found that the
lysozyme content of saliva from 4- to 10-week-old infants is often severalfold higher than in older children (unpublished findings). During this
neonatal period, the secretory IgA system is already functional, but
IgA quantities are low.

A variety of experiments attest to the potential of lysozyme as an
important participant in host-defense systems. What is still lacking,
however, are model systems that can provide an assessment of its
actual importance in vivo.

IV. LACTOPEROXIDASE AND MYELOPEROXIDASE

There has been an appreciation of the antibacterial potential of perodi-
dase systems since Agner isolated what he called verdoperoxidase (4)
from leukocytes and then demonstrated that it would inactivate diphtheria toxins. Many studies have subsequently demonstrated that
the myeloperoxidase- (MPO) hydrogen peroxide-halide system is remarkably bactericidal in vitro against a variety of bacteria and yeasts
(35). Chloride is considered to be the halide most probably involved
as an electron donor in vivo, and the interaction with MPO-hydrogen
peroxide generates hypochlorite, an effective oxidant of sulfhydryl
groups in bacterial cells. Hypochlorite will also react with bacterial
cell amines and amides (58). These reactions lead to fragmentation of
bacterial proteins and cell death. It has been shown recently, however, that the thiocyanite ion can also serve as an electron donor for MPO-
hydrogen peroxide and in vitro can act bactericidally on *S. mutans*
at low pH (34). At neutral pH, viability was unaffected but glycolysis
was inhibited. There is good indirect evidence that MPO and hydrogen
peroxide do interact in the phagolysosome and that the peroxidase
system is an important part of the oxygen-dependent antibacterial
activity of the polymorphonuclear leukocyte (58).

Substantial indirect evidence that the lactoperoxidase-hydrogen
peroxide-mediated system is in many respects comparable with the
myeloperoxidase-halide system is offered in subsequent chapters.
Lactoperoxidase contributes to the antibacterial activities of a number
of mammalian exocrine gland secretions (see Chaps. 6-8) that help
protect a variety of mucosal surfaces. The effect on bacterial growth
and activity (see Chap. 8) provides a special benefit for hard tissues
of the oral cavity because a reduction in bacterial acid production is
an immediate consequence of interference with glycolysis and/or the
phosphotransferase system. Enamel demineralization and caries can
result from in situ acid production in the bacterial colonies attached
to the tooth surfaces.

Developing data from clinical studies (see Chap. 11) indicate that
augmentation of the lactoperoxidase system by appropriate levels of
additional hydrogen peroxide may result in reduced caries and can help

in protection of the oral mucous membranes against recurrent aphthous stomatitis and may reduce gingivitis.

In bovine milk (Chap. 7), activation of the lactoperoxidase (LP) system in vivo can result in bactericidal activity against *E. coli* without killing lactobacilli (57). LP does not appear to be present in human milk (see Chap. 6), and its peroxidase activity is derived from milk leukocytes. LP and thiocyanate, however, are present in saliva of the newborn (24), indeed at a relatively high level and, on swallowing, could contribute to the defense of the intestinal mucosa (43). The clinical significance of a combined LP-MPO system remains to be established.

A new dimension to LP activity has recently been revealed by the elegant study of Tenovuo et al. (65) on the interaction of LP and sIgA (but not IgG or IgM). The LP-sIgA combination significantly enhanced the antimicrobial effect of LP against *S. mutans* . No doubt numerous other examples of interactions will become apparent with further exploration and should help explain the function of the antibacterial systems when viewed as an integrated whole.

V. LACTOFERRIN

Lactoferrin (LF) is one of several iron-binding proteins, the others being transferrin and ferritin. Using an immunoperoxidase staining technique, Mason and Taylor (44) determined that the distribution of each in human tissue was distinctive. Lactoferrin was detected particularly in exocrine cells (e.g., mammary acinar cells, gastric mucous neck cells, and bronchial glandular cells). Gillette and Allansmith (18) used immunofluorescent staining to confirm its presence in acinar epithelial cells of main and accessory lacrimal glands, where it is essentially restricted to acinar epithelial cells. It is also present in the cytoplasm of neutrophil cells (47). Malmquist et al. (40) note that, although the several reports of radioimmune assay of plasma levels are in modest disagreement, it is quite clear that it is a minor component. the reported concentrations ranging between 13 and 220 μg/dl. This is in contrast to its concentration in colostrum (200 mg/dl), milk (100 mg/dl) (46), and saliva (1-2 mg/dl) (64).

Variation in plasma levels occurs, that is, there may be elevation in chronic myeloid leukemia in relapse (10-fold increase) and decrease in bone marrow-depressed persons (10). In inflammatory salivary gland disease, 10-fold or greater increase has been observed, with restoration of normal levels coincident with recovery. It has been suggested that such variations result in part from increased release from neutrophils and possibly from increased salivary synthesis (42). Characteristically, there is also an increase in the level of lactoferrin in milk in bovine mastitis (27) and in other inflammatory situations (64). In tears, in keratoconjunctivitis sicca, although the basal secretion is essentially normal in lactoferrin levels, the reflex secretions do not show the increase in concentration exhibited by normal subjects (62) when secretion is stimulated.

The essentiality of iron (Fe^{3+}) for bacterial growth and pathogenicity has been reviewed (15,69). Bullen et al. (15) point out that the amount of free iron in equilibrium with transferrin and ferritin is about 10^{-18} M normally, and that bacteria require iron-chelating agents with association constants similar to those of transferrin and lactoferrin in order to grow in normal tissue. *Neisseria* species, both commensal and pathogenic, can obtain necessary iron from hemin or hemoglobin. Pathogenic species can scavenge iron from 25% saturated transferrin, whereas commensals cannot. This activity seems specific, since partially saturated conalbumins cannot be substituted (48). In diseased tissues, with iron being released from injured cells, these proteins become saturated and are no longer able to make their metal unavailable.

Most studies of LF inhibition of bacterial growth describe the effect as reversible by iron, and more particularly as being a property of apo-lactoferrin and not of the iron-saturated protein. Strains of a given species are not uniformly sensitive. Arnold et al. (5) suggest that this could indicate difference in accessibility of the target.

A lactoferrin effect not reversed by supplemental iron, inhibited by secretory IgA with specificity for the test organism, and apparently initially requiring binding of lactoferrin to the cell surface has recently been described by Arnold et al. (8). Preincubation of *S. mutans* with apo-lactoferrin inhibited acid production from glucose even at a concentration (4 µM) too low to produce killing. At a 100-fold lower bacterial concentration, direct kill by LF (2 µM) was observed. Kill was greatest with early log-phase cultures incubated at 37°C at acid pH (pH 5). in glycine buffer. Ferric or ferrous iron or ferritin did not alter the effect. The explanation for this effect is uncertain (7).

Harmon, in reviewing the bactericidal properties of bovine milk (26) pointed out the importance of the bicarbonate ion for lactoferrin inhibition of *Klebsiella* spp. and *Staphyloccocus aureus*. Particularly, the report that bicarbonate is required for the chelation of iron by lactoferrin seems germane (45). Apparently, bicarbonate ion, an important buffer in secretions and in dental plaque, may stabilize the protein under conditions where lowered pH might otherwise diminish its activity.

Evidence that neutrophil lactoferrin is required for bacterial killing in phagocytosis was provided by Bullen and Armstrong (14). When PMNs phagocytose ferritin-antiferritin complexes, their cytoplasmic lactoferrin becomes iron saturated. This reduces cell bactericidal power, as evidenced by finding that phagocytosed bacteria survive and destroy the cell.

Although Spik et al. (60) reported an enhanced antibacterial effect for lactoferrin when specific sIgA antibody was present, Samson et al. (59) were not able to show increased kill of an *E. coli* strain when

specific sIgA antibody was added to sIgA-deficient colostrum. The
lactoferrin-sIgA interaction requires further clarification.

VI. SUMMARY

Based on a rapidly developing body of data from in vitro experiments,
it is becoming apparent that nonimmunoglobulin defense factors have
considerable potential and flexibility in protecting the mucosal surfaces
against a variety of pathogens and irritants. There are an ever-in-
creasing number of examples of cooperative arrangements among the
members of the nonimmunoglobulin team, as well as interactions with
the immunoglobulins. Although full characterization of all the individual components and delineation of their properties is of primary importance, it is clear that they do not function in isolated but rather in
a supportive and regulated fashion. The research in this area is now
poised for the leap from laboratory to clinical situations.

REFERENCES

1.   Adams, D., *Arch. Oral Biol. 19:* 505 (1974).
2.   Adams, D., *J. Dent. Res. 54:* B19 (1975).
3.   Adinolfi, M., Glynn, A. H., Lindsay, M., and Milne, C. M.,
     Immunology 10: 517 (1966).
4.   Agner, K., *Acta Physiol. Scand. 2:* 1 (1941).
5.   Arnold, R. R., Brewer, M., and Gauthier, J. J., *Infect.
     Immun. 28:* 893 (1980).
6.   Arnold, R. R., Prince, S. J., Mestecky, J., Lynch, D., Lynch,
     M., and McGhee, J., *Adv. Exp. Med. Biol. 107:* 401 (1978).
7.   Arnold, R. R., Russell, J. E., Champion, W. J., Brewer, M.,
     and Gauthier, J. J., *Infect. Immun. 35:* 792 (1982).
8.   Arnold, R. R., Russell, J. E., Champion, W. J., and Gauthier,
     J. J., *Infect. Immun. 32:* 655 (1981).
9.   Beachey, E. H., *J. Infect. Dis. 143:* 325 (1981).
10. Bennet, R. M., and Mohla, C. J., *J. Lab. Clin. Med. 88:* 156
     (1976).
11. Bienenstock, J., *Am. J. Vet. Res. 36:* 488 (1975).
12. Bienenstock, J., and Befus, A. D., *Immunology 41:* 249 (1980).
13. Bleiweis, A. S., Craig, R. A., Coleman, S. E., and Van De
     Rijn, I., *J. Dent. Res. 50:*1118 (1971).
14. Bullen, J. J., and Armstrong, J. A., *Immunology 36:* 781
     (1979).
15. Bullen, J. J., Rogers, H. J., and Griffiths, E., *Curr. Top.
     Microbiol. Immunol. 80:* 1 (1978).
16. Clark, W. B., and Gibbons, R. J., *Infect. Immun. 18:* 514
     (1977).

17. Crecth, J. M., Bridge, J. L. N., and Horton, J. R., *Biochem. J. 181*: 717 (1979).
18. Gillette, T., and Allansmith, M. R., *Am. J. Ophthalmol. 90*: 30 (1980).
19. Gibbons, R. J., in *Microbiology*, Schlessinger, D. (Ed.), American Society for Microbiology, Washington, D.C., pp. 395-406 (1977).
20. Gibbons, R. J., and Qureshi, J. V., *Infect. Immun. 22*: 665 (1979).
21. Gibson, L. E., Mattews, W. J., Minihan, P. T., and Patti, J. A., *Pediatrics 48*: 695 (1971).
22. Goodman, H., Pollock, J. J., Katona, L. I., Iacono, V. J., Cho, M., and Thomas, E., *J. Bacteriol. 146*: 764 (1981).
23. Gordon, L. I., Douglas, S. D., Kay, N. E., Yamada, O., Osserman, E. F., and Jacobs, H. S., *J. Clin. Invest. 64*: 226 (1979).
24. Gothefors, L., and Marklund, S., *Infect. Immun. 11*: 1210 (1975).
25. Gottschalk, A., Bhargava, A. S., and Murty, V. L. N., in *Glycoproteins: Their Composition, Structure and Function*, Gottschalk, A., (Ed.), Elsevier, Amsterdam, p. 810 (1972).
26. Harmon, R. J., in *Saliva and Dental Caries*, Kleinberg, I., Ellison, S. A., and Mandel, I. D. (Eds.), Sp. Suppl. Microbiol. Abst., Information Retrieval, Inc., New York, N.Y., p. 413 (1979).
27. Harmon, R. J. Schanbacher, F. L. Ferguson, L. C., and Smith, K. L., *Am. J. Vet. Res. 36*: 1001 (1975).
28. Heineman, H. S., and Greenberg, M. S., *Archs. Oral Biol. 25*: 257 (1980).
29. Iacono, V. J. MacKay, B. J. Pollock, J. J., Bolot, P. R., Ladenheim, S., Grossbard, B. L., and Rochon, M. L., in *Proceedings, Host Bacterial Interactions in Periodontal Disease*, Genco, R. J., and Mergenhagen, S. E. (Eds.), Am. Soc. Microbiol. Press, Washington, D.C., pp. 318-342 (1982).
30. Jolles, P., in *Lysozyme*, Osserman, E. F., Canfield, R. E., and Beychok, S. (Eds.), Academic Press, New York, N.Y., pp. 31-54 (1974).
31. Jolles, P., *Biomedicine 25*: 275 (1976).
32. Kashket, S., and Donaldson, C. G., *J. Bacteriol. 112*: 1127 (1972).
33. Kashket, S., and Guillmette, K. M., *Caries Res. 12*: 170 (1978).
34. Kersten, H. W., Moorer, W. R., and Wever, R., *J. Dent. Res. 60*: 831 (1981).
35. Klebanoff, S. J., *J. Bacteriol. 95*: 2131 (1968).
36. Levine, M. J., Herzberg, M. C., Levine, M. S., Ellison, S. A., Stinson, M. W., Li, H. C., and Van Dyke, T., *Infect. Immun. 19*: 107 (1978).

37. Lukie, B. E., *Mod. Prob. Pediatr. 19*: 46 (1977).
38. McBride, B. C., and Gisslow, M. T., *Infect. Immun. 18*: 35 (1977).
39. McNabb, P. C., and Tomasi, T. B., *Ann. Rev. Microbiol. 35*: 477 (1981).
40. Malmquist, J., Hansen, N. E., and Karle, H., *Scand. J. Haematol. 21*: 5 (1978).
41. Mandel, I. D., *J. Dent. Res. 55*: C22 (1976).
42. Mandel, I. D., in *Saliva and Dental Caries*, Kleinberg, I., Ellison, S. A., and Mandel, I. D., (Eds.), Sp. Suppl. Microbiol. Abst., Information Retrieval, Inc., New York, N.Y., p. 473 (1979).
43. Mandel, I. D., Turett, H., and Alvarez, J., *J. Dent. Res. 62*: (Abstracts) 217 (1983).
44. Mason, D. Y., and Taylor, C. R., *J. Clin. Pathol. 31*: 316 (1978).
45. Masson, P. L., and Heremans, J. F., *Eur. J. Biochem. 6*: 579 (1968).
46. Masson, P. L., and Heremans, J. F., *Comp. Biochem. Physiol. 39*: 119 (1971).
47. Masson, P. L., Heremans, J. F., and Schonne, E., *J. Exp. Med. 130*: 643 (1969).
48. Michelson, P. A., and Aparling, P. F., *Infect. Immun. 33*: 55 (1981).
49. Miller, T. E., *J. Bacteriol. 98*: 949 (1969).
50. Namba, Y., Hidaka, Y., Taki, K., and Morimoto, T., *Infect. Immunol. 31*: 580 (1981).
51. Parsons, C. L., and Mulholland, S. G., *Am. J. Pathol. 93*: 423 (1978).
52. Parsons, C. L., Mulholland, S. G., and Anwar, H., *Infect. Immun. 24*: 552 (1979).
53. Parsons, C. L., Pollen, J. J., Anwar, H., Stauffer, C., and Schmidt, J. D., *Infect. Immunol. 27*: 876 (1980).
54. Parsons, C. L., Stauffer, C., and Schmidt, J. D., *Science 208*: 605 (1980).
55. Pollock, J. J., Goodman Bicker, G., Katona, L. I., Cho, M. I., and Iacono, V. J., in *Saliva and Dental Caries*, Kleinberg, I., Ellison, S. A., and Mandel, I. D. (Eds.), Sp. Suppl. Microbiol. Abst., Information Retrieval, Inc., New York, N.Y., p. 429 (1979).
56. Pollock, J. J., Katona, L. I., Goodman, H., Cho, M. I., and Iacono, V. J., *Archs, Oral Biol. 26*: 722 (1981).
57. Reiter, B., Marshall, V. M. E., and Philips. S. M., *Res. Vet. Sci. 28*: 116 (1980).
58. Rosen, H., and Klebanoff, S. J., *J. Biol. Chem. 252*: 4803 (1977).

59. Samson, R. R., Mirtle, C., and McClelland, D. B. L., *Immunology 38*: 367 (1979).
60. Spik, G., Cheron, A., Montreuil, J., and Dolby, J., *Immunology 35*: 663 (1978).
61. Spohn, M., and McColl, I., *Biochem. Biophys. Res. Commun. 79*: 837 (1977).
62. Stuchell, R. N., Farris, R. L., and Mandel, I. D., *Ophthalmology 88*, 858 (1981).
63. Tabak, L., Levine, M. J., Mandel, I. D., and Ellison, S. A., *J. Oral Pathol. 11*: 1 (1982).
64. Tabak, L., Mandel, I. D., Karlan, D., and Baurmash, H., *J. Dent. Res. 57*: 43 (1978).
65. Tenovuo, J., Moldoveanu, Z., Mestecky, J., Pruitt, K. M., and Mansson-Rahemtulla, B., *J. Immunol. 128*: 726 (1982).
66. Tortosa, M., Cho, M., Wilkens, T. J., Iacono, V. J., and Pollock, J., *Infect. Immun. 32*: 1261 (1981).
67. Walker, W. A., *Pediatrics 57*: 901 (1976).
68. Wallenius, R., *Acta Pathol. Microbiol. Scand. (Supple.) 180*: 1 (1966).
69. Weinberg, E. D., *Microbiol. Rev. 42*: 45 (1978).
70. Westmacott, D., and Perkins, H. R., *J. Gen. Microbiol. 115*: 1 (1979).

2

The Chemical Structure of Lactoperoxidase

KARL-GUSTAV PAUL and PER-INGVAR OHLSSON / *University of Umeå, Umeå, Sweden*

I. INTRODUCTION

In 1941, Agner (1) succeeded in isolating in a pure form the first mammalian peroxidase. Several hundred milliliters of *empyema* from patients with pulmonary tuberculosis were shaken with water, ether, and ammonium sulfate in a flask, stoppered with a rubber bung. Centrifugation of the emulsion formed an interphase disc, which contained the activity. After several fractionations, and electrophoresis the peroxidase was obtained as a green solution. It was named verdoperoxidase by Agner, but later on renamed myeloperoxidase by Theorell (42) when lactoperoxidase (LP) too, was found to be greenish.

The peroxidase in milk was separated from oxidase activity by Thurlow (47) by means of ammonium sulfate fractionation. She demon-

strated a coupled oxidation in the system O_2-xanthine-xanthine oxi-
dase-peroxidase-guaiacol or nitrite, and identified the autooxidation
of several low molecular compounds as a source of hydrogen peroxide.
Elliot (11) was probably the first to get an indication of the chemical
nature of lactoperoxidase when he noticed that active preparations
from milk always had a brownish tint. He also observed a pyridine
hemochrome spectrum. An essentially correct lactoperoxidase spectrum
was given by Yakushiji (49). In 1943 Theorell and Åkeson (46) crystal-
lized lactoperoxidase after an elaborate isolation procedure: ammonium
sulfate fractionation, heating, dialysis, fractionations with basic lead
acetate and acetone, and finally electrophoresis with an overall yield
of "2% in successful cases" (43), a procedure characteristic of the
prechromatographic days. The technical difficulties were fully confirmed (22). Sedimentation and diffusion determinations together with
iron analyses indicated one heme group per molecule (45). The iron
content, 0.07%, would have given the correct molecular weight of
78,000, whereas the physicochemical data gave 93,000. The absorbance
of the Soret band, on the basis of dry weight determinations, was
given as $\varepsilon_{412} = 111.3$ mM^{-1} cm^{-1}, in good agreement with today's 112.3
(52).

The precipitation of casein by means of rennet (34) and the adsorption of lactoperoxidase from whey by an ion exchanger (24) enormously
facilitated the isolation of the enzyme. This batchwise adsorption technique had originally been introduced for the isolation of cytochrome C
from heart muscle extracts (29).

II. THE ISOLATION OF LACTOPEROXIDASE

Several authors have contributed to the present procedure for the isolation of LP from milk. Polis and Shmukler (34) introduced coagulation
of casein by rennin. They also separated LP into two fractions, A and
B, by means of displacement chromatography on calcium phosphate
and free electrophoresis. Fraction A was more acidic than fraction B,
the mobilities being $V_A = 3.94 \times 10^{-5}$ and $V_B = 2.85 \times 10^{-5}$ cm$^2 \times$ V $\times$
s^{-1} in 0.1 mM acetate pH 5. From a practical point of view the adsorp-
tion of LP onto the resin directly from the whey was a very important
step (24,25). Chromatography on the same resin confirmed the heterogeneity of LP (24). A first indication of the mechanism behind the
heterogeneity was obtained by Carlström, who found that LP, prepur-
ified to homogeneity on the cation exchanger CM-W cellulose, gave rise
to four fractions on DEAE-Sephadex (3). Disk electrophoresis revealed
five fractions, called LP 1-5 from the cathodal side (4). Moving
boundary electrophoresis subsequently confirmed this result (5,8).
Isoelectric focusing separated six fractions of which two, LP 2-I and
2-II, migrated together in disk electrophoresis (8). With improved
techniques both disk and free electrophoresis disclosed an even more

cathodal (negative) group of four components. This could be identified
with LP A of Polis and Shmukler, whereas the six previously observed
fractions contributed LP B. Thus, a total of 10 fractions of LP were
identified and named LP A 1-4 and B 1, B 2-I, B 2-II, B 3-5 (5). There
was no significant difference in activity between the LP fractions from
isoelectric focusing, using guaiacol-H_2O_2, on the basis of A_{412} (8).

The heterogeneity might have been the result of a partial hydrolysis of a peptide chain in LP by rennin, or it might express genetic
differences among cows (24,25). Both possibilities could be rejected
when heterogeneity was seen also with LP prepared without rennin (3,
25) or from a single cow (3,5). Thus, the fractions must exist in milk
in situ or very easily be formed. Eventually Carlström managed to
transform the various B components unidirectionally into each other,
and likewise LP B into LP A (5).

A simplified isolation procedure has recently been reported (33).
The number of dialyses is minimized by the use of alternating high
and low ionic strengths, and the harmful exposure to strong potassium
phosphate is avoided. Unpasteurized skim milk is coagulated by means
of rennin (2 mg/L), and the whey is cooled with ice and stirred for 3
h with the ion exchanger CG-50-NH_4, 20 g/L. The resin, which
carries LP, is washed two times with water and three times with 50 mM
sodium acetate. It is then transferred to a column and allowed to settle
in 50 mM sodium acetate under cautious stirring to prevent channeling.
LP is eluted with 2 M sodium acetate. Solid sodium acetate, to compen-
sate for the water in the resin, is added to the eluate until a drop of
2 M sodium acetate gives no Schlieren formation. The solution is directly transferred to a small column of phenyl-Sepharose in 2 M sodium
acetate. Washing with this solution removes much inert material, and LP
is then eluted by means of a decreasing, linear gradient 2-0.05 M sodium
acetate, pH 7. The eluate is concentrated in a Diaflow XM-50 cell with
slow stirring (see below), dialyzed against 10 mM sodium phosphate,
pH 6, and centrifuged. It is then chromatographed on CM-52 with a
gradient 10-130 mM sodium phosphate, pH 6. After these steps, which
can be accomplished in 3 days, the yield is 7-10 mg/L with $A_{412}/A_{280} \geqslant$
0.90. The final purification and the separation of the subfractions of
LP occur on DEAE-Sephadex. In the authors' opinion the choice of
the buffer for this step remains undecided. Customarily, tris has been
used, but the effect of nitrogenous ligands on LP is still obscure. Bicarbonate elutes one major fraction, but leaves much LP on the column,
even 50 mM at pH 8. Borate (10 mM, pH 9 and 8) resolves LP into a
number of fractions, but the results must be evaluated by means of
EPR and possibly other techniques.

III. ANALYSIS OF THE LACTOPEROXIDASE PROTEIN

Careful analyses failed to disclose significant differences between LP
B1, B2-I, B2-II, and B3 as regards iron content (0.0680-0.0709%) or

carbohydrate content (9.90-10.22%), $E^{1\%}_{1\,cm}$ at 280 nm (14.9-15), or
amino acid composition (Table 1) (6). B4 and B5 accounted together
for less than 10% of the total B group. The A group, on the other
hand, gave $E^{1\%}_{1\,cm}$ = 15.5, a higher iron content (0.0747%) but a lower
carbohydrate content (7.67%). Taken together, these analyses and
the induced transformations related the LP fractions to each other as
below. The horizontal changes within both groups occurred under

$$B1 \to B2_I \to B2_{II} \to B3 \to B4 \to B5$$
$$\downarrow \quad \downarrow \quad \downarrow \quad \downarrow \quad \downarrow \quad \downarrow$$
$$A1 \to A2_I \to A2_{II} \to A3 - \to - \to$$

conditions known to favor deamidization of aspargine or glutamine residues. Thus, ammonium sulfate at 40% saturation and pH 9.4 (4) or 80
mM glycine at pH 10.3 (5) extensively deamidated LP at room temperature within 2 days. Amide nitrogen analyses are not available. The
vertical B → A shift took place during dialysis at 4°C against water or
100 mM phosphate at pH 7, or during the above exposure to glycine.
Analyses revealed that the B to A conversion meant a loss of four glucosamine, six mannose, and one galactosamine residues, also by deamidization.

Table 1 Amino Acid and Carbohydrate Composition of Lactoperoxidase
Fraction B1, Expressed as the Nearest Integral Number per 78,500 g
of Protein

Aspartic acid	71	Cysteine	0
Glutamic acid	61	Cystine	8
Amide nitrogen	62	Tyrosine	15
Threonine	32	Phenylalanine	30
Serine	33	Tryptophan	15
Proline	42	Lysine	34
Glycine	40	Histidine	14
Alanine	37	Arginine	37
Valine	28	Mannose	26
Isoleucine	27	N-acetylglucosamine	14
Leucine	68	N-ac-galactosamine	4
Methionine	8	Sialic acid	0

Source: Ref. 6.

According to this pattern, B1 represents the intact, or least degraded, form of LP. Its amino acid composition gives a molecular weight of 78,431. One atom of iron per molecule should hence give 0.071%, close to the experimental value of 0.0689%. This also means that LP has only one heme group per molecule, in agreement with the magnitude of $\varepsilon_{mM} = 112.3$ cm^{-1} at the Soret maximum.

Sedimentation analysis of fraction B1 gave $S_{20,w}o = 5.19$ S at infinite dilution in 50 mM sodium phosphate, 1% sodium chloride at 20°C (6). The diffusion coefficient $D_{20,w}o = 5.91$ F was independent of the concentration within the range 4.3-10.6 mg $\times$ mL^{-1}. The directly determined partial specific volume at 20°C in the above medium was $\overline{V} = 0.721$ ml $\times$ g^{-1}. The value, calculated from the amino acid and carbohydrate composition, the heme group disregarded, was $\overline{V} = 0.725$ ml $\times$ g^{-1}. The molecular weight of LP B1 as calculated directly from the above values comes out as 76,400, whereas the technique of approach to sedimentation equilibrium gave 78,000. Ferguson (12) plots of the migration rates in gels of different acrylamide concentrations gave a molecular weight of 77,500 (40).

The frictional ratio $f/f_0 = 1.29$ corresponds to axial ratios of 5.6 and 6.3 for prolate and oblate ellipsoids, respectively (6). When LP was adsorbed in a monolayer onto glass ballotini a molecule occupied an average area of 970 (Å)^2. A prolate ellipsoid of the same molecular weight with the axial ratio of 5.6 and with 20% (w/w) of hydration water would require 980 (Å)^2 and a sphere 3100 (Å)^2 at closest packing (15).

The primary structure of LP is unknown. ORD studies in the far ultraviolet region indicated about 17% α-helical structure (19). A recent and detailed study with evaluation of optical and CD spectra revealed 65% β-structure, 23% α-helix, and 12% unordered structure (39). Some information is available about the tertiary structure. SDS-PAGE gel electrophoresis, after pretreatment of LP with 1% SDS, 1% mercaptoethanol, showed a single component, indicating only one peptide chain. Dansylation revealed only one N-terminal amino acid, leucin (39). The previous observation of 0.5 leucine and one blocked N-terminal group (36) was attributed to steric effects from intact disulfide bonds. LP contains 8 disulfide bonds (6) that contribute to the rigidity of the molecule (39).

IV. THE PROSTHETIC GROUP

The inability of acid acetone to separate the heme and protein moieties (11,43) was long taken as evidence for covalent heme-protein bonds. The optical spectrum with four bands within the range 450-650 nm pointed at strong chromophores in the porphyrin ring, as did the initial position, 565 nm, of the α-band of the pyridine hemochromogen spectrum of LP. The silver salt procedure, used to hydrolyze the thioether

bonds in cytochrome C (30), had no effect on the heme-protein bonds
in LP (21,31). Treatment of LP with hydrogen bromide, hydrogen
iodide, or hydrazine in acetic acid, with dry hydrazine, with hydrogen
chloride in methanol, or with strong sodium hydroxide permitted the
subsequent extraction of some ether-soluble heme (16,23). The various structures assigned to such heme might to some extent have been
generated by the reactive chemicals employed. The presumed covalent bonds were tentatively identified as ester or amide bonds (16,
23).

In a milder approach, LP was digested with pronase (7,38). The
major part of the heme could then be extracted by 2-butanone after
acidification. This heme was identified as protoheme by comparison with
pure protohemin or with myoglobin-bound protoheme in the following
tests: Spectra of the pyridine hemochrome and of the heme solution in
butanone, the acid and neutral spectra of the porphyrins, and the
R_f values of the porphyrins in TLC (38). No heme was extracted by
acid butanone from LP in which either hydrogen bonds had been ruptured
by guanidine or disulfide bonds by dithiotreitol. Only if both reagents
were combined could the hemeprotein be split by means of acid butanone (K. G. Paul, P. I. Ohlsson, J. Vanderkooi, unpublished data).
Thus, in summary, it seems well proven that protoheme is the prosthetic group of LP and that no covalent heme-protein bonds exist.

V. STABILITY OF LACTOPEROXIDASE

A. Heat

During pasueurization (i.e., heating to 70°C cor 15 s, whole milk lost
three-quarters of its LP activity (48), whereas partially purified LP
was stable for 15 min at this temperature (46). At 78°C, no time given,
inactivation was complete (2).

B. pH

No systematic study of the time-dependent effect of extreme pH values
on LP seems to be available. Kinetic studies of the rate of formation
of compound I indicated that LP was stable when stored at pH 7 but
was deactivated by storage at pH 3 (20). Some denaturation of LP was
observed at pH < 4 (17). The deamidization of LP by glycine at pH
10.3 for 48 hr at room temperature seemed not to inactivate LP very
much (5).

C. Proteolytic Enzymes

No heme was released by acid butanone after digestion of LP with pepsin
followed by trypsin (21) or chymotrypsin (38). In fact, trypsin and
thermolysin did not inactivate native LP, and chymotrypsin did so only

very slowly (14). Commercial pronase rapidly digested native LP
to fragments from which heme could be extracted (7,38). LP was not
inactivated by the gastric juice from an infant (pH 5) (13), whereas
pepsin at pH 2.5 inactivated LP (14).

D. The "Stickiness" of Lactoperoxidase

Several early reports state that LP is labile, and solutions will easily
become turbid. Sedimentation analyses of LP solutions, concentrated
by ultrafiltration in 50 mM sodium phosphate, pH 7, revealed extensive
polydispersity, although the pattern in disk electrophoresis remained
unchanged. In 10 mM tris at pH 9 no aggregation occurred (6).

Anaerobic conditions are obtained when an inert gas passes over
or through a solution, if necessary with mechanical stirring. Under
such conditions a solution of LP in 50 mM phosphate, pH 7, became
turbid at a rate proportional to the mechanical perturbation. More
surprising, the rate of aggregation also depended upon the material
covering the magnetic bar. Teflon was worst and in decreasing order
siliconized glass, ordinary borosilicate glass, and alkali-boiled glass
(28) (i.e., the more hydrophobic the cover was the more turbidity it
produced). Aggregation also took place with gas bubbling for stirring.
Argon was most harmful, followed by xenon, nitrogen, krypton, helium,
and hydrogen at the same flow rates in terms of milliliters gas per minute. A solution of LP in the above buffer remained clear with unchanged
absorbance when slowly stirred overnight with a magnet, sealed in
alkali-boiled glass, and flushed with helium (28).

LP has a high tendency to adhere to surfaces. This causes a
marked decrease in activity of dilute LP solutions in glass vessels, and
rinsing with only water will not free the vessel from LP. The enzyme
is also firmly adsorbed by tooth enamel. In a study of salivary LP,
Pruitt and Adamson (35) demonstrated that the liquid-phase LP was reduced in direct proportion to the weight of enamel powder added.
Bound LP was enzymatically active and able to inactivate the glycolytic
enzyme hexokinase. The adsorption was irreversible under the conditions of the test and resulted in an elevated LP activity at the morpho-
logical structure to be protected against bacteria.

The structural prerequisites for the aggregation and adsorption
phenomena are largely unknown. However, at close packing on a glass
surface the ellipsoid LP molecules are held in a position, perpendicular
to the surface, by essentially ionic bonds (15). LP is retained by octyl-
Sepharose by what must be hydrophobic bonds (33). The LP molecule
thus seems to be equipped for both ionic and hydrophobic interactions.

VI. OPTICAL SPECTRUM: LIGANDS

Two recent studies of the spectrum of LP Fe(III) at neutral reaction are
available (7,39). The positions of the maxima in the two studies differ

unidirectionally by 0-3.5 nm (a calibration effect?). A third spectrum
(46) is still occasionally quoted, but had been obtained by means of
another type of spectrophotometer on a different type of preparation
and deviates markedly from the other two. The position and absorptivity of the Soret band of LP Fe(III) has been confirmed as 112.3 $\pm$
0.9 (n = 5) mM^{-1} cm^{-1} at 412 nm on a dry weight basis (52). This
value is in full agreement with that of Carlström (6,7). Table 2 therefore gives his absorptivity values of the other maxima with some redetermined positions.

The optical spectrum changes slightly and reversibly upon acidification of the solution. A pK_a value of 3.85 at low ionic strength was
reported long ago (44). More recently a somewhat lower value, 3.46 $\pm$
0.30, in 2 and 20 mM sodium sulfate was obtained (17). The Soret band
of the acid form has migrated to 415 nm with an isosbestic point between
this position and that of the neutral LP, 412 nm. The four-banded
spectrum of the neutral form in visible light persists in the acid form
with slight bidirectional band shifts (17). The conversion of many
Fe(III) hemeproteins from the brown, high-spin to the reddish, low-
spin form within the range pH 8-11 does not occur in LP.

When LP is reduced at neutral reaction with $Pt-H_2$ and a mediator,
a primary product LP Fe(II)-1, is obtained. It rearranges spontaneously into the stable LP Fe(II)-2 (52). The spectra of the two forms are
collected in Table 3. The cycle LPFe(III) $\rightarrow$ LPFe(II)-1 $\rightarrow$ LPFe(II)-2 $\rightarrow$
LPFe(III) with reoxidation by means of air can be repeated several times
The ratio $\Delta A_{565}/\Delta A_{630}$ is always >2.6 during reversible reactions. A

Table 2 Spectra of the Neutral Form of Fe(III) Lactoperoxidase in 200 mM
Sodium Phosphate, pH 6

Species	Absorption maxima Position (nm)/Absorptivity (mM^{-1} cm^{-1})					
Fe(III)[a]	412/112.3	501/9.4[b]	542/7.8		585/5.5	630/5.6
Fe(III)F[c]	411.5/112.2	488.5/9.1	533.5/6.4	560/6.7	590/6.9	615/8
Fe(III)CN[d]	430/100.1	555.5/10.1	595/6.1			
Fe(III)N$_3$[e]	422.5/103.1	595.5/8.9	587/7.2		630/3.7	

[a]Positions redetermined from $dA/d\lambda = 0$ (holmium oxide-calibrated Beckman
DU-7).
[b]$\varepsilon = 8.6$ mM^{-1} cm^{-1} (P. I. Ohlsson and K. G. Paul, unpublished data).
[c]0.5 M NaF. $\varepsilon = 127$ mM^{-1} cm^{-1} at 410 nm (37).
[d]77 mM KCN. $\varepsilon = 89$ mM^{-1} cm^{-1} at 432 nm (10).
[e]0.5 M NaN_3.
Source: Refs. 7 and 52.

Table 3 Spectra of Fe(II) Lactoperoxidase in 100 mM Sodium Phosphate pH 7 [Fe(II)-1,2] or 200 mM Phosphate, pH 6 [Fe(II) CO,CN]

Species	Absorption maxima Position (nm)/Absorptivity (mM^{-1} cm^{-1})				
Fe(II)-1	446/77.8		562/13.6		595
Fe(II)-2	434/94.6		565/14.2		595
Isosbestic points [Fe(II)-1,2]	408	440	502	552	573
Fe(II)CO	424.5/154.5		543/14		577.5/13.7
Fe(II)CN	435/175		537.5/16.2		571.5/21.5

Source: Refs. 7 and 52 and P. I. Ohlsson and K. G. Paul, unpublished data.

lower ratio involves some change that prevents reversibility. Addition of $S_2O_4^{2-}$ to LP causes spectral changes succeeding those due to the reduction. Four spectrally different forms can be discerned. The primary form, LPFe(II)-1, is spontaneously transformed to LPFe(II)-2. The transformation is first-order and highly increasing in rate at lower pH. At pH $\leq$ 4 LPFe(II)-2 changes to a third form, LPFe(II)-3, which probably is a complex between LPFe(II)-2 and $SO_2^{\cdot-}$, the monomer of $S_2O_4^{2-}$. LPFe(II)-3 forms an active ternary complex with $S_2O_4^{2-}$ when LP acts as a dismutase on $S_2O_4^{2-}$ (53). After exhaustion of $S_2O_4^{2-}$ a fourth form with a spectrum similar to LP-H_2O_2 compound III appears. The cycle can be repeated after reoxidation with air.

Reduction of LP in CO-saturated buffers with $S_2O_4^{2-}$ gives two consecutive reduced forms. Transformation rate and pH dependence are the same as without CO (54). Reduction with $S_2O_4^{2-}$ in the presence of CN^- gives only one reduced form with spectrum similar to the spectrum of [LPFe(II)-2] $\cdot$ CO. The spectrum of [LPFe(II)-2] $\cdot$ $SO_2^{\cdot-}$ resembles the spectra of [LPFe(II)-2] $\cdot$ CO and LPFe(II)cyanide (53). The spectrum appearing after addition of NO to electrochemically reduced LP (55) is very close to the spectrum of [LPFe(II)-2] $\cdot$ CO in the visible region.

LP, unlike plant peroxidases, can act as a dismutase in some situations. Thus, in the presence of I^- (56), Br^- (57), or SCN^- (58) it decomposes H_2O_2 to water and O_2. Dithionite at low pH is decomposed catalytically, two molecules of $S_2O_4^{2-}$ being converted to $S_2O_3^{2-}$ + 2 HSO_3^- (53).

Chloride ions do not by themselves alter the optical spectrum of LP Fe(III). However, above an effective chloride ion concentration of ca 1 mM a 10-fold increases in [Cl^-] will increase pK_a by about 0.75.

The 1:1 equilibrium between acid LP and Cl^- gives a $pK_{d,Cl}$ of 2.7
(17). Chloride ions also inhibit the formation of compound I from LP
Fe(III) and H_2O_2 to the effect that the rate constant decreases from
10^7 M^{-1} s^{-1} by an order of magnitude in physiological saline (18).

Cyanide gives a 1:1 complex with LP Fe(III) at neutral reaction
with K_d = 4.2 × 10^{-5} M from kinetic data (10) and 4.6 × 10^{-5} M (10)
or 2.5 × 10^{-5} M (17) from spectrophotometric titrations. The rate of
formation of the cyanide complex is highly pH dependent with a maximum at pH 7.2 (k_{app} ≈ 10^6 M^{-1} s^{-1}) (10). The sigmoid decrease in
reaction rate on both sides was attributed to dissociations of two groups
in the protein with pK_a 6.3 and 7.6. Their possible identities with not
heme-linked imidazole and α-amino groups was discussed. The kinetic
approach did not discriminate between HCN and CN^- as reacting species
(10). The formation of LP compound I is pH independent (20).

The binding of cyanide is not affected by chloride ions at neutral
reaction, but with increasing acidity the two species compete to give
$\Delta pK_{dCN}/\Delta \log[Cl^-]$ about 0.5 (17). It seems possible also that acetic
acid can compete with cyanide for LP Fe(III) (Table 1 in Ref. 10).
Clearly formate and acetate will inhibit the formation of compound I
with H_2O_2 (20). The effect of pH > 9.5 or alternatively nitrogenous
ligands on the formation of the LP Fe(III) cyanide complex may not have
been fully explored.

Fluoride and LP Fe(III) form a 1:1 complex with K_d = (3 ± 2) ×
10^{-4} M, optially titratable within the range pH 3.8-5.4 with no observ-
able trend (37). At higher pH less complex was formed; none above
pH 7. The results were consistent with a mechanism in which HF was
the reacting species with a rate constant of (9.7 ± 0.4) × 10^2 M^{-1} s^{-1}
for its binding to LP.

VII. REDOX POTENTIAL

Two circumstances required a determination of the redox potential
Fe(III)/(II) of LP. It has been concluded from optical and CD data
that the enzyme possesses an unusually narrow heme-accommodating
cleft (39). This might imply a limited exposure of the heme group to
the solvent and consequently a high redox potential (41). Second, the
optical spectrum of LP Fe(III) has some similarity to that of a horseradish peroxidase (HRP) with its 2,4-vinyl groups replaced by acetyl
groups. This substitution raises the redox potential of HRP from −246
mV to −109 mV at pH 7, 25°C (27,50).

We have recently determined the redox potential, E_m, of LP. The
pronounced tendency of LP to aggregate was avoided by using helium
for deaeration and alkali-boiled glass to cover the magnetic stirring bar.
The ability of LP to bind hydrophobically various structures (33) neces-
sitated the use of an excess of mediators. Dithionite is a substrate to
LP (32), and the enzyme was therefore reduced by means of a black

platinum sheet and H_2. With these precautions the direct potentiometric determination yielded the value E_m = -191 ± 2 mV, whereas optical measurements of LP-mediator equilibria gave -188 ± 1 mV, both in triplicate and in 100 mM sodium phosphate, pH 7, 25°C. The value refers to the system Fe(III)/Fe(II)-2, possibly modified by a few millivolts because of complex formation with a mediator. Thus, the redox potential of LP does not differ markedly from that of several other peroxidases.

VIII. THE HEME–ACCOMMODATING POCKET

Remarkably little is known about the nearest surroundings of the protoheme group in LP. Since the primary structure of LP is unknown, no conclusions can be drawn from homologies. Crystals available so far are poor. The heme group can be removed only with serious and irreversible damage to the protein moiety. That excludes the use of such informative techniques as photooxidation, difference titrations, and heme substitutions. Most, but not all, aromatic donor substrates bring about some change in the optical spectrum of LP. However, the changes do not follow the hyperbolic course of a reversible 1:1 equilibrium. This may be related to a possible and simultaneous change in the spin state; the naked LP Fe(III) shows a considerable low-spin component, as is to be expected from its spectrum (54).

A protonization with pK_a 6.3 (or close), found in studies of cyanide binding to LP (10), appears also in turnip peroxidase 1 and 7 and in horseradish peroxidase C, whereas the ionization pK_a 7.6 (51) seems to be unique to LP. The identification of the dissociating groups suffers, as always, from the uncertainty about environmental effects.

The treatment of LP with reagents, specific for various amino acid side chains, has been informative. Reagents directed against arginine (59), tryptophan (59), or histidine (60) had no effect on the activity, nor had SH reagents (61), which is consistent with the absence of cysteine residues in LP (Table 1). Diazotized sulfanilate at pH 9 and 40°C-inactivated LP and analyses revealed two azotyrosine and about one azohistidine residues. The conclusion (60) that two tyrosine residues are essential for LP activity is, however, incorrect. On the contrary the results show that one tyrosine residue is essential for the activity, and that another and nonessential tyrosine residue is equally exposed to the reagent. Possibly a second thought has led to the correct interpretation (61). Obviously the tyrosine residue essential to activity does not have to be located at some "active site."

The carbonyl reagent 1-(ethoxycarbonyl)-2-ethoxy-1,2-dihydroquinoline (EEDQ) irreversibly inhibits LP in a manner suggesting that one carboxyl group is essential to activity (61). Also this group may, or may not, be somewhat remote from the active site. The rate of reaction between LP and H_2O_2 to form compound I was independent of pH down to at least pH 3.1 in steady-state experiments (20), whereas stopped flow gave a decrease in rate with pK_a 3.94 (18). The conversion of the LP form appearing immediately upon reduction LPFe(II)-1 to LPFe(II)-2 is stimulated by protons in a manner suggestive of a pK 3-3.5 (53). EEDQ treatment accelerates this conversion and reduces the H_2O_2 and $S_2O_4^{2-}$ dismutase activities in parallel (53). Thus, various wet chemical procedures point to the existence of at least one acidic, probably carboxylic, group essential to activity.

A detailed study of intact LP by means of MCD and EPR spectroscopy, and comparisons between LP and hemeproteins with known axial ligands, indicated histidine as the proximal and a carboxyl group as the distal ligand at room temperature (62). At 4.2 K, however, LPFe(III) changes to a reddish low-spin form in which a histidine imidazole, as imidazolate, acts as the distal ligand. Resonance Raman (RR) spectroscopy (63) revealed a hexacoordinate high-spin structure in native LP, in agreement with the MCD results (62). LP and the pentacoordinate horseradish peroxidase respond differently to guaiacol and benzhydroxamic acid. Raman spectroscopy gave a dissociation constant of 52 mM for guaiacol with LP compared with 7 mM with HRP C by optical methods (64). The authors (63) concluded that the heme-ligand interactions are of different types in the two peroxidases. Whereas the optically operable binding to HRP is not mediated by the heme group (64), the substrate seems to donate electrons to the lowest unoccupied molecular orbitals in the LP porphyrin and hence interact directly with the heme (63).

MCD and EPR revealed the presence of at least two low-spin species in LPFe(III) (62). Even the presence of high concentrations of cyanide or fluoride failed to convert LP to pure low- or high-spin forms. Considering the lability of LP discussed above, a question about heterogeneities of various LP preparations and their significance may be raised.

One structural feature of the heme-accommodating pocket seems to be established beyond doubt, its ability to shield the heme from the bulk medium. The initial hemochrome spectrum with its α-band at 564 nm is gradually succeeded, at pH 13, by a normal protohemochrome spectrum (23). The 564-nm band is split (7). The stepwise addition of pyridine to a solution of myoglobin Fe(II) disclosed an intermediary hemochrome with its α-band at 563 nm. It was interpreted as a mixed, monohistidine monopyridine hemochrome (38). In the case of the initial LP hemochrome, the restricted access of pyridine to heme would generate the same structure and spectrum.

CD spectra of LP Fe(III) and its cyanide and fluoride derivatives, as well as of LP Fe(II) and its CO and cyanide derivatives, showed split ellipticity bands. This suggests such a narrow pocket that linear iron-ligand bonds could not be formed (39).

Recent results on the rate of formation of compound I with H_2O_2 and $(CH_3)_2CH \cdot OOH$ seem to confirm more of steric hindrance in LP than in HRP (Table 4) (65).

Table 4 Rate Constants (k_1) for the Formation of Compound I Between Lactoperoxidase, Horseradish Peroxidase A or C, and Dihydrogen or Isopropyl Hydrogen Peroxide. 100 mM Sodium Phosphate, pH 7, 25°C

	$k_1(M^{-1} \times s^{-1})$	
Species	H_2O_2	$(CH_3)_2CH \cdot OOH$
HRP A	2×10^6	3.1×10^2
HRP C	15×10^6	800×10^2
LP	18×10^6	2.5×10^2

Source: Ref. 65.

Liquid hydrogen fluoride at dry-ice temperature promptly removes iron from lyophilized cytochrome C, hemoglobin, myoglobin, and horseradish peroxidase A and C but not from catalase or LP (K. G. Paul, P. I. Ohlsson, and J. Vanderkooi, unpublished data). In catalase the heme group is connected to the external medium via a narrow funnel, according to x ray crystallography (26). Another similarity between catalase and LP is found in the spectral response to nitrogenous ligands at low temperatures (54). Thus, in spite of the rapid reaction rate of LP with small hydroperoxides (9) and the enzyme's rather negative redox potential (52), there seems to be ample support from various sources for a conclusion that the protoheme of LP is well hidden.

REFERENCES

1. Agner, K., *Acta Physiol. Scand. 2*, Suppl. 8 (1941).
2. Benard, H., *Hémoglobine et Pigments Apparentes*, Masson & Cie, Paris (1949).
3. Carlström, A., *Acta Chem. Scand. 18*: 2387 (1965).
4. Carlström, A., *Acta Chem. Scand. 20*: 1426 (1966).
5. Carlström, A., *Acta Chem. Scand. 23*: 171 (1969).
6. Carlström, A., *Acta Chem. Scand. 23*: 185 (1969).
7. Carlström, A., *Acta Chem. Scand. 23*: 203 (1969).
8. Carlström, A., and Vesterberg, O., *Acta Chem. Scand. 21*: 271 (1967).
9. Chance, B., *J. Am. Chem. Soc. 72*: 1577 (1950).
10. Dolman, D., Dunford, H. B., Chowdhury, D. M., and Morrison, M., *Biochemistry 7*: 3991 (1968).
11. Elliott, K. A. C., *Biochem. J. 26*: 10 (1932).
12. Ferguson, K. A., *Metabolism 13*: 985 (1964).

13. Gothefors, L., and Marklund, S., *Infec. Immun. 11*: 1210 (1975).

14. Henriksson, A., Ohlsson, P. I., and Paul, K. G., Manuscript in preparation.

15. Honka, E., Ohlsson, P. I., and Paul, K. G., *Acta Chem. Scand. B36*: 273 (1982).

16. Hulquist, D. E., and Morrison, M., *J. Biol. Chem. 238*: 2843 (1963).

17. Kimura, S., and Yamazaki, I., *Arch. Biochem. Biophys. 189*: 14 (1978).

18. Kimura, S., and Tamazaki, I., *Arch. Biochem. Biophys. 198*: 580 (1979).

19. Maguire, R. J., and Dunford, H. B., *Can. J. Biochem. 49*: 666 (1971).

20. Maguire, R. J., Dunford, H. B., and Morrison, M., *Can. J. Biochem. 49*: 1165 (1971).

21. Morell, D. B., *Aust. J. Expt. Biol. Med. Sci. 31*: 567 (1953).

22. Morell, D. B., *Biochem. J. 56*: 683 (1954).

23. Morell, D. B., and Clezy, P. S., *Biochim. Biophys. Acta 71*: 157 (1963).

24. Morrison, M., Hamilton, H. B., and Stotz, E., *J. Biol. Chem. 228*: 767 1957).

25. Morrison, M., and Hultquist, D. E., *J. Biol. Chem. 238*: 2847 (1963).

26. Murthy, M. R. N., Reid, T. J., Sicignano, A., Tanaka, N., and Rossman, M. G., *J. Mol. Biol. 152*: 465 (1981).

27. Ohlsson, P. I., and Paul, K. G., *Biochim. Biophys. Acta 315*: 293 (1973).

28. Ohlsson, P. I., and Paul, K. G., in *Biochemistry, Biophysics, and Environmental Implications of Cytochrome P-450*, Hietanen, E. (Ed.), Elsevier, Amsterdam, p. 805 (1982).

29. Paleus, S., and Neilands, J. B., *Acta Chem. Scand. 4*: 1024 (1950).

30. Paul, K. G., *Acta Chem. Scand. 4*: 239 (1950).

31. Paul, K. G., quoted in Ref. 43 (1950).

32. Paul, K. G., and Ohlsson, P. I., in *Biochemistry, Biophysics, and Regulation of Cytochrome P-450*, Gustafsson, J. A. (Ed.), Elsevier, Amsterdam, p. 331 (1980).

33. Paul, K. G., Ohlsson, P. I., and Henriksson, A., *FEBS Lett. 110*: 200 (1980).

34. Polis, B. D., and Shmukler, H. W., *J. Biol. Chem. 201*: 475 (1953).

35. Pruitt, K. M., and Adamson, M., *Infect. Immun. 17*: 112 (1977).

36. Rombauts, W. A., Schroeder, W., and Morrison, M., *Biochemistry 6*: 2965 (1967).

37. Segal, R., Dunford, H. B., and Morrison, M., *Can. J. Biochem. 46*: 1471 (1968).

38. Sievers, G., *Biochim. Biophys. Acta 579*: 181 (1979).
39. Sievers, G., *Biochem. Biophys. Acta 624*: 249 (1980).
40. Sievers, G., *FEBS Lett. 127*: 253 (1981).
41. Stellwagen, E., *Nature 275*: 73 (1978).
42. Theorell, H., *Adv. Enzymol. 7*: 265 (1947).
43. Theorell, H., in *The Enzymes*, *Vol. 1: 1*, Sumner, J. B., and Myrback, K. (Eds.), Academic Press, New York, N.Y., p. 412 (1951).
44. Theorell, H., and Paul, K. G., *Arkiv Kemi. Geol. Mineral 18A*: 12 (1944).
45. Theorell, H., and Pedersen, K. O., in *The Scedberg*, Almqvist & Wiksell, Uppsala and Stockholm, p. 523 (1944).
46. Theorell, H., and Åkeson, Å., *Arkiv Kemi. Mineral., Geol. 17B*: 7 (1943).
47. Thurlow, S., *Biochem. J. 19*: 175 (1925).
48. Wutrich, S., Richterich, R., and Hostettler, H., *Zeitschrift Lebensmittel-Untersuch. Forsch. 124*: 345 (1964).
49. Yakushiji, E., *Acta Phytochim. 11*: 186 (1939).
50. Yamada, H., Makino, R., and Tamazaki, I., *Arch. Biochem. Biophys. 169*: 344 (1975).
51. Yamazaki, I., Araiso, T., Mayashi, Y., Tamada, H., and Makino, R., *Adv. Biophys. 11*: 249 (1978).
52. Ohlsson, P. I., and Paul, K. G., *Acta Chem. Scand. B37*: 917 (1983).
53. Ohlsson, P. I., *Eur. J. Biochem. 142*: 233 (1984).
54. Smith, M. L., Ohlsson, P. I., Ehrenberg, A., and Paul, K. G., to be submitted for publication.
55. Sievers, G., Peterson, J., Gadsby, P. M. A., and Thomson, A. J., *Biochim. Biophys. Acta 785*: 7 (1984).
56. Magnusson, R. P., aand Taurog, A., *Biochem. Biophys. Res. Commun. 112*: 475 (1983).
57. Piatt, J., and O-Brien, P. J., *Eur. J. Biochem. 93*: 323 (1979).
58. Carlsson, J., *Biochem. Biophys. Res. Commun. 116*: 568 (1983).
59. Mäkinen, K. K., and Mäkinen, P.-L., *Eur. J. Biochem. 123*: 171 (1982).
60. Mäkinen, K. K., and Mäkinen, P.-L., *Biochem. Biophys. Res. Commun. 105*: 1402 (1982).
61. Mäkinen, K. K., *Biochem. Int. 5*: 375 (1982).
62. Sievers, G., Gadsby, P. M. A., Peterson, J., and Thomson, A. J., *Biochim. Biophys. Acta 742*: 659 (1983).
63. Kitagawa, T., Hashimoto, S., Teraoka, J., Nakamura, S., Yajima, H., and Hosoya, T., *Biochemistry 22*: 2788 (1983).
64. Paul, K. G., and Ohlsson, P. I., *Acta Chem. Scand. B32*: 395 (1978).
65. Ohlsson, P. I. and Paul, K. S., *Acta Chem. Scand.* in press (1984).

3

Products of Lactoperoxidase-Catalyzed Oxidation of Thiocyanate and Halides

EDWIN L. THOMAS / *St. Jude Children's Research Hospital, Memphis, Tennessee*

I. INTRODUCTION

Antimicrobial activity (see Chap. 8) of hemoprotein peroxidase enzymes is due to their ability to catalyze H_2O_2-dependent oxidation of halide ions or SCN^- to yield halogens or other oxidizing agents related to the halogens. The halides and SCN^- differ in their ease of oxidation, and peroxidases differ in their ability to catalyze oxidation of these ions. The oxidizing agents formed in these reactions differ in oxidation potential, stability, and solubility.

The oxidizing agents make an electrophilic attack on microbial components, resulting in chemical modification of essential enzymes, transport systems, and other functional components. Sulfhydryl groups are especially susceptible to electrophilic attack, and are usually present in higher amounts than other easily oxidized groups. Aromatic amino acid residues are also susceptible to attack. Most aspects of antimicrobial action can be correlated with chemical modification of these nucleophilic components. Antimicrobial activity is favored by influences that increase the stability of the oxidizing agent, provided that these influences do not interfere with their electrophilic character, or their ability to penetrate microbial membranes.

Although H_2O_2 itself is a powerful oxidizing agent, the H_2O_2 molecule is stabilized and reacts slowly with biological materials. Also, most cells have enzymes that rapidly eliminate H_2O_2. Peroxidase-catalyzed oxidation of halides or SCN^- conserves the oxidizing power of H_2O_2 in forms that react more rapidly, and for which the target cells may have no defense.

II. ENZYMATIC MECHANISM OF HALIDE AND PSEUDO-HALIDE OXIDATION

A. Halide and Pseudohalide Specificity

The thiocyanate ion (SCN^-) is a pseudohalide because of its similarity to the halides. These ions form a series in which the oxidation potential of SCN^- occupies an intermediate position: $F^- < Cl^- < Br^- < SCN^- < I^-$. A powerful oxidizing agent is required to oxidize F^-, whereas I^- is easily oxidized (22). For each ion, X^-, there is a corresponding oxidized form, X_2, which is the halogen, or in the case of SCN^-, the pseudohalogen $(SCN)_2$. Oxidation potentials are in the order: $F_2 > Cl_2 > Br_2 > (SCN)_2 > I_2$. That is, F_2 will oxidize Cl^- to Cl_2, Cl_2 will oxidize Br^- to Br_2, and so on.

The halide specificity of the peroxidases is related to the halide oxidation potential series (36). For example, myeloperoxidase (MPO) catalyzes the oxidation of Cl^-, Br^-, SCN^-, and I^-, whereas lactoperoxidase (LP) catalyzes the oxidation of Br^-, SCN^-, and I^- and horseradish peroxidase (HRP) catalyzes the oxidation only of I^-. Eosinophil peroxidase and chloroperoxidase may have the same specificity as MPO, and thyroid peroxidase the same as LP. No peroxidase catalyzes oxidation of F^-.

It may appear that all peroxidases should have the same halide specificity. That is, if H_2O_2 provides the oxidizing power for MPO-catalyzed oxidation of Cl^-, then it should provide sufficient oxidizing power for oxidation of any of the more readily oxidized ions by any of the peroxidases. However, H_2O_2 does not act directly as the oxidizing agent in peroxidase-catalyzed reactions. Instead, the oxidizing agent is an oxidized form of the peroxidase.

B. Compound I and II States of Peroxidase

The first step in the enzymatic mechanism of hemoprotein peroxidases is the reaction of the enzyme with H_2O_2, which converts the enzyme from the ground state to the compound I state (36). The chemical structure of compound I remains unclear, but it is not an enzyme-substrate $(E \cdot S)$ complex of the peroxidase and H_2O_2. Compound I conserves the oxidizing power of H_2O_2 in the heme moiety including the iron atom and the ligands and possibly in other portions of the enzyme molecule that form the active site. Compound I resembles an $E \cdot S$ complex in that it retains the 2 oxidizing equivalents of H_2O_2. That is, H_2O_2 or compound I will accept 2 electrons (e^-). The transfer of 2 e^- to H_2O_2 reduces H_2O_2 to water, whereas transfer of 2 e^- to compound I returns the enzyme to the ground state.

The agent that oxidizes halide ions or SCN^- is compound I. Therefore, the halide specificity of the peroxidases implies that the compound I states form a series of decreasing oxidation potential: MPO > LP > HRP. The halide series is also generally consistent with rates of oxidation. For example, both the MPO-catalyzed oxidation of Cl^- and the LP-catalyzed oxidation of Br^- are slow except at high concentrations of these ions. However, both enzymes rapidly catalyze I^- oxidation at I^- concentrations of 1-10 μM. The apparent K_m of MPO for Cl^- decreases at low pH, suggesting that protonation of compound I increases the oxidation potential. However, low pH may also influence the interaction of halide ions with compound I. Also, SCN^- appears to compete effectively with I^- for MPO- or LP-catalyzed oxidation, suggesting that influences other than oxidation potential determine rates of oxidation.

The reaction catalyzed by peroxidases can be written

$$H_2O_2 + AH_2 \longrightarrow 2 H_2O + A$$

where AH_2 and A are reduced and oxidized forms of suitable e^- donors. A wide variety of organic compounds can serve as AH_2. With many of these compounds, oxidation proceeds in 2 distinct 1-e^- transfers. The reaction of compound I with AH_2 can result in the 1-e^- reduction of compound I to compound II and oxidation of AH_2 to $AH \cdot$. The transfer of a second e^- from $AH \cdot$ or AH_2 to compound II returns the enxyme to the ground state, completing the catalytic cycle.

Peroxidases also catalyze oxidation of halide ions (X^-).

$$H_2O_2 + X^- \longrightarrow H_2O + OX^-$$

This equation illustrates only one possible mechanism. The oxidized form of the halide ion that is released from the peroxidase active site has not been identified. If the hypohalite ion (OX^-) is formed, it may equilibrate with halogen (X_2), hypohalous acid (HOX), and possibly with complex ions such as X_3^-. The observed products of halide oxidation depend on pH, X^- concentration, and other conditions, and do not necessarily indicate the enzymatic mechanism.

In contrast to the oxidation of many organic compounds, oxidation of halides proceeds by way of a single 2-e^- transfer. It has not been possible to detect compound II during oxidation of halides, and when compound II is formed, it reacts very slowly with halides or SCN^-. This lack of reactivity sets a lower limit for peroxidase antimicrobial activity. At low halide or SCN^- concentrations, the peroxidase reacts with H_2O_2 and then with any 1-e^- donors that may be present to form compound II. Although compound II is continuously reduced to the ground state, the rate of this step is slower than other steps in the catalytic cycle. Therefore, at any instant most of the enzyme molecules are in the compound II state and unavailable for oxidation of halides or SCN^-. At neutral pH and in the presence of proteins or bacteria, the rate of LP-catalyzed oxidation decreases sharply at I^- concentrations below 10 μM or SCN^- concentrations below 3 μM, and the rates are negligible at $[I^-] < 1$ μM or $[SCN^-] < 0.3$ μM (4,45). LP antimicrobial activity shows the same concentration dependence (46-48).

Under biologically relevant conditions, there are always enough 1-e^- donors available to convert compound I to compound II. The peroxidase molecule itself may serve as the 1-e^- donor, because certain amino acid residues of proteins can be oxidized. Frequently, high peroxidase concentrations (or high protein concentrations) result in an unexpected decrease in the rates of peroxidase-catalyzed reactions, particularly at low concentrations of X^- or AH_2. This phenomenon may be due in part to competition by amino acid residues.

The decreased rate of halide or SCN^- oxidation may occur even when the halide or SCN^- concentration is higher than 10 μM, and the peroxidase concentration is in the physiologic range. Oxidation of SCN^- can result in accumulation of unreacted $OSCN^-$, and oxidation of I^- can result in substantial incorporation of I atoms into covalently bound forms, such as iodinated tyrosine residues of proteins. These phenomena deplete the system of SCN^- or I^-, so that SCN^- or I^- fall to the low levels at which oxidation becomes very slow (46-48). This decrease in rates of oxidation can influence LP antimicrobial action, particularly when the target microorganisms consume H_2O_2 at high rates. If oxidation is slow, all of the H_2O_2 may be rapidly lost to H_2O_2-consuming enzymes such as catalase or NADH peroxidase.

C. Turnover of I^- and SCN^-

Although antimicrobial activity is handicapped at low I^- or SCN^-, there is a compensating phenomenon. Each I^- or SCN^- ion can be used more than once. General features of the turnover of I^- and SCN^- are indicated in the equations below, in which X^- is oxidized to X_2, which then oxidizes the reduced microbial components MH_2, with the reduction of X_2 back to X^-.

$$H_2O_2 + 2\ H^+ + 2\ X^- \longrightarrow 2\ H_2O + X_2$$

$$X_2 + MH_2 \longrightarrow 2\ X^- + M + 2\ H^+$$

net

$$H_2O_2 + MH_2 \longrightarrow 2\ H_2O + M$$

The net reaction is peroxidase-catalyzed, X_2-mediated oxidation of microbial components. The X^- acts as a cofactor. That is, both the enzyme and X^- undergo cyclic oxidation and reduction and are not consumed. For this reason, oxidation of microbial components can be proportional to H_2O_2 and independent of I^- or SCN^- over a wide range of I^- or SCN^- concentrations (46-48).

As described above, turnover of X^- is limited by (a) accumulation of unreacted X_2, (b) loss of X^- in reactions that do not reduce X_2 to X^-, and (c) the resulting conversion of the peroxidase to compound II, which slows the rate of X^- oxidation. Nevertheless, turnover of I^- or SCN^- is significant. For example, it is possible to completely inhibit respiration of an *Escherichia coli* suspension with LP, H_2O_2, and 10 μM I^-. Under the same conditions, as much as 100 μM I_2 may be required for complete inhibition (46,47). Therefore, each I^- turns over at least 10 times. Similar results are obtained with SCN^-.

Turnover has caused confusion in studies of peroxidase antimicrobial activity. It was proposed that the peroxidase-H_2O_2-I^- system produces an agent that is more toxic than I_2, because bactericidal action is obtained at low I^- concentrations, whereas higher amounts of added I_2 are required (28). Turnover of I^- accounts for these observations, and indicates that the valid comparison is not between I^- and I_2 but between the amounts of H_2O_2 and I_2.

III. PRODUCTS OF I^- OXIDATION

Peroxidase-catalyzed oxidation of I^- yields I_2 (33). Solutions of I_2 also contain small amounts of HOI and OI^- depending on pH and I^- concentration. At high I^- concentrations, I_3^- is the predominant form:

$$I_2 + I^- \rightleftharpoons I_3^-$$

$$I_2 + H_2O \rightleftharpoons HOI + I^- + H^+$$

$$HOI \rightleftharpoons H^+ + OI^-$$

The I_2, I_3^-, HOI, and OI^- are equivalent in their oxidation state. Interconversion does not require oxidation or reduction. Each contains one I atom of valence +1, or I(+1).

At low I^- concentrations, LP catalyzes direct iodination of suitable e^- donors, such as exposed tyrosine residues of proteins (32,36). This direct iodination is not mediated by a diffusible agent such as I_2. Instead, iodination occurs at the active site of LP and requires that the phenolic portion of the tyrosine residue enter the active site. Although HRP catalyzes oxidation of I^-, it does not catalyze direct iodination.

Direct iodination is the major form of LP-catalyzed iodination at I^- concentrations below 1 μM, and has proved useful in studies on the structure of biological membranes and protein complexes and as a gentle technique for labeling proteins (34-36). The amount of iodination is small, but the high specific radioactivity of I isotopes makes it possible to detect incorporated I. Direct incorporation of SCN^- may occur (3), but the specific radioactivity of $S^{14}CN^-$ or $^{35}SCN^-$ is not sufficient to detect incorporation at low concentrations.

It is doubtful that direct iodination of microbial components contributes to antimicrobial activity, because the amount of iodination is small, SCN^- interferes, exposed tyrosine residues are rarely essential to enzymatic activity, microorganisms have few exposed tyrosine residues on their surface, and exposed microbial surface components are usually not essential to metabolism or growth. Instead, formation of I_2 appears to be the mechanism of antimicrobial action.

IV. PRODUCTS OF SCN⁻ OXIDATION

A proposed scheme (3) for peroxidase-catalyzed oxidqation of SCN^- is as follows:

$$H_2O_2 + 2\ SCN^- + 2\ H^+ \longrightarrow 2\ H_2O + (SCN)_2$$

$$(SCN)_2 + H_2O \longrightarrow HOSCN + H^+ + SCN^-$$

$$HOSCN \rightleftharpoons H^+ + OSCN^-$$

These equations illustrate the relationships of $(SCN)_2$ (thiocyanogen), HOSCN (hypothiocyanous acid), and $OSCN^-$ (hypothiocyanite ion). Each of these agents contains one SCN moiety with an effective oxidation state of +1, or SCN(+1). This proposal does not exclude the possibility that SCN^- is oxidized to HOSCN or $OSCN^-$ without formation of $(SCN)_2$. It is not known whether any of the substances is the oxidized form of SCN^- that is released from the LP-active site.

These equations illustrate the similarity of oxidized forms of SCN^- and those of halides. Despite these similarities, there are significant differences in reactivity. The Cl^- and SCN^- ions or the Cl(+1) and SCN(+1) moieties represent opposite extremes of reactivity, which can be predicted on the basis of the hard-soft acid-base theory (18). Hard

species are those with small-size, high-charge density and low polarizability, whereas Cl^- and $Cl(+1)$ are hard and SCN^- and $SCN(+1)$ are
soft. For example, SCN^- has a larger size with 3 atoms versus 1 for
Cl^-, a lower charge density with one negative charge distributed over
3 atoms, and higher polarizability in that the charge can be considered
to be localized on the S, C, or N atom or distributed over the 3. The
$X(+1)$ moieties in decreasing hardness are $Cl(+1) > Br(+1) > I(+1) >$
$SCN(+1)$.

Hard-hard or soft-soft combinations form stable compounds, whereas hard-soft combinations are unlikely to form or are unstable. For
example, HOCl reacts with amines (RNH_2) to form mono-N-chloramines
(RNHCl), which contain the hard-hard combination of the N-Cl bond
(49,50).

$$HOCl + RNH_2 \longrightarrow RNHCl + H_2O$$

Most RNHCl derivatives hydrolyze slowly if at all. They retain the oxidized character of $Cl(+1)$ and readily oxidize sulfhydryl compounds
(R'SH) to disulfides (R'SSR'):

$$RNHCl + 2\ R'SH \longrightarrow RNH_2 + R'SSR' + H^+ + Cl^-$$

In contrast, HOSCN does not react with RNH_2 to yield N-SCN derivatives in aqueous solutions (52). An illustration of the soft character
of $SCN(+1)$ is the reaction of HOSCN with certain protected protein
sulfhydryl groups to yield sulfenyl thiocyanate derivatives (R'-S-SCN):

$$R'SH + HOSCN \longrightarrow R'-S-SCN + H_2O$$

Although this reaction appears similar to the reaction of HOCl with
RNH_2, the SCN moiety of R-S-SCN does not retain the oxidized character of $SCN(+1)$. Instead, the sulfhydryl sulfur is oxidized. Hydrolysis of R-S-SCN yields SCN^- rather than HOSCN, and the sulfenyl
sulfur remains at the same oxidation state in a sulfenic acid derivative
(R'-S-OH):

$$R'-S-SCN + H_2O \longrightarrow R'-SOH + SCN^- + H^+$$

The oxidized character of the RSOH derivative is illustrated by the
reaction with RSH, in which the sulfenyl sulfur is reduced and RSH is
oxidized:

$$R'-SOH + RSH \longrightarrow R'SSR + H_2O$$

The loss of oxidized character of the SCN moiety of R'SSCN is also
illustrated by exchange with I^-, which yields sulfenyl iodide (R-S-I)
derivatives:

$$R-S-SCN + I^- \rightleftharpoons R-S-I + SCN^-$$

The RSSCN derivative is the predominant form at equal concentrations of I^- and SCN^- (4,15), consistent with the softer nature of the SCN moiety. The hard Cl^- ion does not displace SCN^- from R-SSCN (4).

There are also differences in oxidation potential, solubility, and stability of the X_2, HOX, and OX^- forms of halides or SCN^-. Despite differences in oxidation potential, all are sufficiently powerful oxidizing agents to oxidize microbial components. However, the attack of these agents is electrophilic, so that negatively charged forms such as OX^- or X_3^- may be slow to react. Similarly, negatively charged forms may be slow to diffuse through the hydrophobic barrier of microbial cell membranes. Microbicidal action probably requires chemical modification of intracellular components, so that negatively charged forms may be less effective than X_2 or HOX, which have significant solubility in nonpolar media and can diffuse through biological membranes. Differences in stability may also influence antimicrobial action. If decomposition of the antimicrobial agent is rapid compared with the reaction with microbial components, then less of the agent is available for antimicrobial action. With oxidized forms of the halides, HOX is the least stable form. With oxidized forms of SCN^-, the $(SCN)_2$ form hydrolyzes rapidly and does not achieve a significant concentration in aqueous media (6,58). Indirect evidence was cited for formation of $(SCN)_3^-$ upon addition of SCN^- to solutions of $(SCN)_2$ in organic solvents (22); but other interpretations are possible, and it is unlikely that $(SCN)_3^-$ is found in aqueous solutions.

A. HOSCN/OSCN$^-$

1. *Enzymatic and Chemical Synthesis*

The major product of MPO- or LP-catalyzed oxidation of SCN^- at neutral pH is $OSCN^-$ (2,21). Production of $OSCN^-$ is consistent with the net reaction:

$$H_2O_2 + SCN^- \longrightarrow H_2O + OSCN^-$$

At H_2O_2/SCN^- ratios of 0.5 or less and H_2O_2 concentrations of 0.3 mM or less, about 1 mol of $OSCN^-$ is obtained per mole of H_2O_2. The $OSCN^-$ is stable at neutral to alkaline pH, but high temperature, high SCN^-, low pH, and weak-acid buffers favor decomposition (52).

Alkaline hydrolysis of $(SCN)_2$ also yields $OSCN^-$ (2,21). Dropwise addition of $(SCN)_2$ in CCl_4 to dilute NaOH, followed by careful neutralization with dilute HCl, is the preferred procedure. Provided that the calculated concentration of $(SCN)_2$ in base is less than 0.5 mM, about 1 mole of $OSCN^-$ is obtained per mole of $(SCN)_2$. In contrast, adding $(SCN)_2$ to aqueous media at neutral or acid pH results in rapid decomposition and a poor yield of HOSCN or $OSCN^-$ (2). Efforts to obtain HOSCN or $OSCN^-$ by oxidation of SCN^- with Br_2 in aqueous media or by electrolytic oxidation were unsuccesful (2).

2. Physical and Chemical Characterization

a. Sulfhydryl Oxidation: Identification of $OSCN^-$ (or HOSCN) is based on oxidation of 2 mole of a sulfhydryl compound to the disulfide with recovery of 1 mole of SCN^- (2,21):

$$OSCN^- + 2\ RSH \longrightarrow SCN^- + RSSR + H_2O ,$$

$$HOSCN + 2\ RSH \longrightarrow SCN^- + RSSR + H_2O + H^+$$

Oxidation of 5-thio-2-nitrobenzoic acid (Nbs), which absorbs at 412 nm, to the colorless disulfide provides a convenient and sensitive assay (2). As shown above, the same stoichiometry is obtained with $OSCN^-$, HOSCN, or a mixture of the two. The stoichiometry does rule out $(SCN)_2$, in that reduction of $(SCN)_2$ by 2 RSH would yield 2 SCN^-.

Identification of $OSCN^-$ rather than HOSCN as the predominant form is based on the greater stability of the agent at alkaline pH (2, 21), and the inability to extract the agent into organic solvents from aqueous solutions at neutral pH (2).

Both HOSCN and $OSCN^-$ react with certain protein sulfhydryls to yield R-S-SCN derivatives (3,4). Formation of R-S-SCN or other stable sulfenyl derivatives is due to steric factors that prevent approach of another protein sulfhydryl group (1,24). However, sulfhydryl compounds that can approach the buried R-S-SCN residue will displace SCN^-:

$$R\text{-}S\text{-}SCN + R'SH \longrightarrow RSSR' + SCN^- + H^+$$

The net result is oxidation of 2 sulfhydryls to a disulfide, as observed in the reaction with other sulfhydryl compounds. Neither HOSCN nor $OSCN^-$ reacts rapidly with other biological materials. Reactions with histidine are observed only at high (10 mM) histidine concentrations (5,52). Also, neither HOSCN nor $OSCN^-$ oxidizes 1 of the 2 sulfhydryls of the milk protein β-lactoglobulin (4).

Another assay for HOSCN or $OSCN^-$ is based on the difference between SCN^- concentrations measured in the presence and absence of a sulfhydryl compound (20). The assay for SCN^- is performed in strong acid, and it is assumed that $OSCN^-$ is converted to HOSCN, which decomposes to yield products other than SCN^-. Because the assay measures differences in SCN^- concentration, it is not possible to detect small amounts of $OSCN^-$ in solutions containing large amounts of SCN^-. Also, decomposition of HOSCN may yield SCN^- as one of the products, which would result in underestimation of $OSCN^-$. Finally, strong acid catalyzes nonenzymatic oxidation of SCN^- by H_2O_2 (56, 57). Therefore, the assay does not distinguish between $OSCN^-$ and a mixture of SCN^- and H_2O_2.

Regardless of the assay method, it is important to remove H_2O_2 prior to measuring $OSCN^-$. Catalase can be added to eliminate H_2O_2.

Because H_2O_2 interferes in assays for OSCN$^-$, they cannot be used as continuous assays for OSCN$^-$ production. For example, incubating Nbs with LP, H_2O_2, and SCN$^-$ results in oxidation of Nbs, but oxidation may be due to peroxidase-catalyzed oxidation of Nbs rather than the reaction of OSCN$^-$ with Nbs. Therefore, these assays are limited to measuring the amount of OSCN$^-$ that accumulates, rather than the total amount formed.

b. Absorption Spectrum: Production of OSCN$^-$ can be measured continuously by a nondestructive method based on the weak absorbance at 220−240 nm (19,40). The millimolar extinction coefficient (ε mM) at 235 nm was estimated as 1.29 at pH 6.5 (40), whereas ε mM for H_2O_2 is only 0.07 at 230 nm (16) and 0.04 at 240 nm (7). It is important to correct for absorbance of LP, SCN$^-$, and other components of the reaction mixture (12,40). It is doubtful that this method can be used to measure SCN$^-$ oxidation in biological fluids, because proteins and other materials absorb strongly at these wavelengths. Also, products of decomposition of HOSCN or OSCN$^-$ absorb at these wavelengths (19,40). When OSCN$^-$ decomposes, loss of absorbance does not parallel the loss of OSCN$^-$ (40,54). However, this method may prove useful for studies on rates of SCN$^-$ oxidation under conditions such that there is little decomposition.

In an early-study on oxidation of SCN$^-$, absorbance at 235 nm was shown to decrease at low pH (19). A pK$_a$ of 5.1 was calculated for the agent, from this effect of pH. At that time, methods had not been developed for identifying HOSCN or OSCN$^-$. The authors considered HOSCN, HO$_2$SCN, and HO$_3$SCN as possible structures. Either of the latter 2 structures was considered more likely, in that the yield of substances absorbing at 235 nm was highest when the H_2O_2/SCN$^-$ ratio was high. However, it appears that the agent characterized in that study was HOSCN (41,52). By other methods, a pK$_a$ of 5.3 was calculated for HOSCN (52). Assuming this pK$_a$, and the apparent ε mM of 1.29 at pH 6.5 (40), together with the two-fold decrease in absorbance upon lowering pH from 7 to 4.5 (19), the true ε mM values for HOSCN and OSCN$^-$ would be 0.55 and 1.34, respectively.

c. Partitioning into Organic Solvents: Recently OSCN$^-$ or HOSCN was identified by acidifying and extracting HOSCN into relatively polar organic solvents such as ethyl acetate or octanol (52). The amount of extracted HOSCN is measured from the oxidation of Nbs and from the yield of SCN$^-$ obtained by reduction. The stoichiometry confirms that the extracted form is HOSCN rather than (SCN)$_2$. Oxidation of Nbs and extraction of HOSCN were used to measure and identify OSCN$^-$ in human saliva (51). The characteristic pH profile for extraction provides a method to distinguish between HOSCN or OSCN$^-$ and other oxidizing agents.

Because HOSCN and OSCN$^-$ are in equilibrium, whereas only HOSCN is extracted, measuring the distribution of HOSCN in the organic phase and of HOSCN and OSCN$^-$ in the aqueous phase provide a method for calculating the equilibrium constant for the reaction

$$HOSCN \rightleftharpoons H^+ + OSCN^-$$

A pK_a of 5.3 was calculated for HOSCN, indicating that at pH 5.3 the substance is half in the form of HOSCN and half in the form of OSCN$^-$. The percentage that would be in the form of HOSCN at pH 5, 6, 7, and 8 is 67, 17, 2, and 0.2% (52). Therefore, solutions that contain OSCN$^-$ always contain HOSCN and vice versa, so that the substance may best be described as HOSCN/OSCN$^-$.

   d. Polarographic Techniques: Polarographic analysis has been used to measure oxidation potentials of oxidizing agents produced by the LP-H$_2$O$_2$-SCN$^-$ system (18,41). The half-wave potential (E 1/2) varies with pH, and a pK_a of 5.2 was calculated from this effect (19). At pH 6.5, the E 1/2 for OSCN$^-$ is -0.44 to -0.39 (41). In addition, a short-lived species with an E 1/2 less negative than OSCN$^-$ at -0.2 to -0.25 is formed during decomposition of OSCN$^-$ in the presence of excess H$_2$O$_2$ (41). Although the identity of this species is unknown, these observations indicate that polarographic analysis may be helpful in characterizing the antimicrobial agent(s) produced by the LP system.

   e. Kinetics of Decomposition: Rates of decomposition of HOSCN/ OSCN$^-$ at low concentrations (0.1 mM or less) have been used to characterize HOSCN (52). Decomposition is faster at low pH, and it was assumed that the rate of decomposition depends on HOSCN concentration and that OSCN$^-$ does not participate in the rate-limiting step. A pK_a of 5.3 was calculated for HOSCN, from the effect of pH on the rate constant.

The rate-limiting step appears to be the reaction of HOSCN with SCN$^-$, and high SCN$^-$ concentrations accelerate decomposition. About one-third mol of sulfate (SO$_4^{2-}$) is obtained per mole of the HOSCN/ OSCN$^-$ that is lost to decomposition. At least part of the remaining atoms of HOSCN/OSCN$^-$ is recovered as SCN$^-$ (21,52). Decomposition does not appear to be due to reaction of HOSCN with SCN$^-$ to yield (SCN)$_2$. There is no exchange of the C atoms of HOSCN and SCN$^-$, which would be predicted from the equations below (52):

$$HOSCN + S^{14}CN^- + H^+ \longrightarrow (S^{14}CN)_2 + H_2O,$$

$$(S^{14}CN)_2 + H_2O \longrightarrow HOS^{14}CN + SCN^- + H^+$$

When S^{14}CN is added to HOSCN/OSCN$^-$, no label appears in HOS^{14}CN. When HOS^{14}CN/OS^{14}CN$^-$ is added to SCN$^-$, the amount of label in HOS^{14}CN is not diluted. Therefore, HOSCN/OSCN$^-$ does not appear to be in equilibrium with $(SCN)_2$. This is in contrast to the equilibria between hypohalous acids and halogens.

It was also found that when HOSCN reacts with $^{35}SCN^-$, the SO_4^{2-} obtained in decomposition does not contain the ^{35}S label. This observation indicates that $(SCN)_2$ and $(SCN)_3^-$ are not intermediates in decomposition. However, this observation does not exclude a number of other possible intermediates including NC-SCN, HO_2SCN, and HO_3SCN.

There may be at least 2 other ways in which $HOSCN/OSCN^-$ can be lost. It was proposed that the rate-limiting step in decomposition is the dismutation of 2 HOSCN molecules to yield HO_2SCN (58). This proposal was based on the second-order kinetics of decomposition. However, when the $HOSCN/OSCN^-$ concentration is low (less than 0.5 mM) and the SCN^- concentration is comparable with that of $HOSCN/OSCN^-$, it is likely that the apparent second-order kinetics result from the reaction of HOSCN with SCN^- (52). When SCN^- concentration is increased, decomposition appears first order with respect to $HOSCN/OSCN^-$ concentration (40,52). Nevertheless, dismutation of HOSCN might occur at higher $HOSCN/OSCN^-$ concentrations. At neutral pH, the rate of decomposition of $HOSCN/OSCN^-$ increases sharply at concentrations approaching 0.5 mM. Similar results are obtained with $HOSCN/OSCN^-$ solutions obtained by alkaline hydrolysis of $(SCN)_2$, or by LP-catalyzed oxidation (2). The dramatic increase in the rate of decomposition suggests that a second-order reaction may be involved, in that the rate of such reactions increases as the square of the concentration.

The proposed pathway of decomposition is as follows (55,58):

$$2\ HOSCN \longrightarrow HO_2SCN + SCN^- + H^+,$$

$$HOSCN + HO_2SCN \longrightarrow HO_3SCN + SCN^- + H^+,$$

$$HO_3SCN + H_2O \longrightarrow H_2SO_4 + HCN$$

Only small amounts of cyanide (HCN,CN^-) are observed following decomposition (2), probably because HCN reacts rapidly with HOSCN. This reaction was proposed to yield NC-SCN, which hydrolyzes rapidly to yield cyanate (CNO^-) and SCN^- (57). The proposed stoichiometry under these conditions is as follows (2):

$$4\ HOSCN + H_2O \longrightarrow 3\ SCN^- + CNO^- + SO_4^{2-} + 6\ H^+$$

Because CNO^- decomposes to yield CO_2 and NH_3, the yield of CNO^- may be low. The stoichiometry has not been experimentally evaluated.

Another way in which $HOSCN/OSCN^-$ can be lost is in the reaction with excess H_2O_2. Nonenzymatic oxidation of SCN^- by H_2O_2 was studied at pH 4-12 and pH 2 (56,57). Also, the effect of excess H_2O_2 on the

LP-catalyzed reaction was studied (12). Oxidation of HOSCN, HO_2SCN, and H_2SO_3 by H_2O_2 was proposed to account for oxidation of SCN^- to $SO_4{}^{2-}$, CO_2, and NH_3 (56,57):

$$HOSCN + H_2O_2 \longrightarrow HO_2SCN + H_2O,$$

$$HO_2SCN + H_2O_2 \longrightarrow H_2SO_3 + HOCN,$$

$$H_2SO_3 + H_2O_2 \longrightarrow H_2SO_4 + H_2O,$$

$$HOCN + 2\,H_2O \longrightarrow H_2CO_3 + NH_3$$

The proposed stoichiometry was as follows:

$$4\,H_2O_2 + SCN^- \longrightarrow 2\,H_2O + SO_4{}^{2-} + CO_2 + NH_4{}^+$$

This sequence of reactions does not include HCN, NC-SCN, or HO_3SCN, but the same products and stoichiometry can be obtained in alternative proposals that include these intermediates. At pH 2, NC-SCN and HCN are also obtained as products. The LP-catalyzed reaction was thought to resemble the acid-catalyzed reaction (12), but this apparent similarity may be due to the conditions of the assay for HCN (2). Similarly, LP was reported to catalyze the oxidation of NC-SCN to HCN (12), but this result is probably due to decomposition of $HOSCN/OSCN^-$, which can yield HCN under acid conditions (2).

It would be difficult to obtain conditions under which loss of $HOSCN/OSCN^-$ occurs by only one pathway. For example, when H_2O_2 exceeds 0.5 mM with the $LP-H_2O_2-SCN^-$ system, the reaction of HOSCN with SCN^-, the reaction of 2 molecules of HOSCN with each other, and the reaction of HOSCN with H_2O_2 may contribute to loss of $HOSCN/OSCN^-$. It has also been proposed that LP catalyzes oxidation of $OSCN^-$ (40,41), although alternative mechanisms might be proposed. Because these pathways yield much the same products in somewhat different amounts, it would be a formidable task to determine the relative importance of each pathway, particularly in that SCN^- concentration, pH, and buffer composition influence the results.

Nevertheless, the loss of $HOSCN/OSCN^-$ is of interest in studies of LP antimicrobial action. Loss of $HOSCN/OSCN^-$ may decrease the amount of antimicrobial action. For this reason, it may be best to avoid high concentrations of SCN^-, H_2O_2, or weak acid buffers. On the other hand, a number of possibly toxic substances may be formed as $HOSCN/OSCN^-$ is lost, and these substances may contribute to anti-microbial action.

The observation that SCN^- increases the rate of decomposition of $HOSCN/OSCN^-$ may also have implications for efforts to increase LP antimicrobial action in biological fluids. The SCN^- concentration in bovine milk is low, and adding SCN^- along with H_2O_2 may be required

for antimicrobial action (10). It appears that SCN^- is present in
adequate amounts for antimicrobial action in human saliva (44,53), but
it may be necessary to add SCN^- to obtain the highest possible yield
of $HOSCN/OSCN^-$ when saliva is supplemented with a high concentration (0.7 mM) of H_2O_2 (44). Feeding SCN^- in substantial amounts to
experimental animals is toxic to the thyroid gland, and may result in an
increased rather than decreased incidence of dental caries (37). These
effects may be related in that proper thyroid function is required for
normal saliva flow (30,37). However, it is possible that accelerated
decomposition of $HOSCN/OSCN^-$ contributes to these results.

  f. Formation of N-SCN Derivatives: One approach to increasing
the stability of $HOSCN/OSCN^-$ is to add compounds that yield stable
N-SCN derivatives. For example, $HOSCN/OSCN^-$ reacts with sulfon-
amide compounds ($R-SO_2-NH_2$) to yield thiocyanatosulfonamides ($R-SO_2-NH-SCN$). This reaction increases the stability of oxidizing activity because the HOSCN concentration is decreased, and the N-SCN
derivatives retain the oxidized character of the SCN(+1) moiety (52).
The N-SCN derivatives may oxidize sulfhydryls directly, or may
hydrolyze to yield $HOSCN/OSCN^-$, which acts as the oxidizing agent:

$$HOSCN + RSO_2NH_2 \longrightarrow RSO_2NHSCN + H_2O),$$

$$RSO_2NHSCN + 2\ R'SH \longrightarrow RSO_2NH_2 + R'SSR' + SCN^- + H^+$$

  Certain N-SCN derivatives have greater solubility in organic solvents than does HOSCN. Therefore, formation of these nonpolar N-
SCN derivatives favors stability and partitioning into the organic
phase during extraction of oxidizing agents from saliva or milk (54),
which may be useful for measuring $HOSCN/OSCN^-$ in these fluids.
The lipid solubility of these N-SCN derivatives suggests that they could
facilitate attack of the LP system on intracellular components of microorganisms. However, N-SCN derivatives hydrolyze readily, so that
high concentrations of RSO_2NH_2 are required to favor formation of the
N-SCN derivative.

  The N-SCN derivatives of amines can be obtained when water is
excluded, as in the reaction of $(SCN)_2$ with amines in organic solvents
(6,22,58).

$$(SCN)_2 + RNH_2 \longrightarrow RNHSCN + RNH_3^+ + SCN^-$$

The RNH_3^+ and SCN^- precipitate together as the amine salt, leaving
a pure solution of the RNHSCN derivative. Such a solution might be
useful as a nonenzymatic source of $HOSCN/OSCN^-$, in that these derivatives hydrolyze instantly in water:

$$RNHSCN + H_2O \longrightarrow RNH_2 + HOSCN$$

B. $(SCN)_2$

1. Synthesis and Characterization

Synthesis of $(SCN)_2$ is performed by reacting Br_2 with an excess
of a suspension of $Pb(SCN)_2$ in CCl_4 (58). Fading of the $(Br)_2$ color
provides a way to monitor the reaction. Provided that the concentration
of $(SCN)_2$ is low (<50 mM), the solvent and $Pb(SCN)_2$ are free of water,
and the solvent is not permitted to evaporate, the $(SCN)_2$ is quite
stable and convenient to use. Formation of a yellow precipitate indicates decomposition.

The εM of $(SCN)_2$ in CCl_4 is 140 at 295 nm (5). Alternatively,
$(SCN)_2$ is measured by adding the solution in CCl_4 directly into 0.1
M NaI with rapid mixing, to obtain oxidation of I^- to I_2, which can
then be titrated with thiosulfate (58). In contrast, if $(SCN)_2$ is allowed
to hydrolyze to yield $HOSCN/OSCN^-$ and then I^- is added, little or no
I_2 is formed, and the oxidizing activity disappears rapidly (2). Decomposition may be due to formation of an unstable $(SCN)_2 I^-$ complex
ion (13). An assay for $HOSCN/OSCN^-$ was developed based on formation of a short-lived species (20), possibly $(SCN)_2 I^-$. The ε mM attributed to $(SCN)_2 I^-$ was 41.1 at 302 nm (13). The $I_2(SCN)^-$ complex
ion was also proposed, and the ε mM was 42.9 at 303 nm (29). The
interhalogen compound ISCN has also been proposed (13,29).

2. Reactivity and Decomposition

In organic solvents, $(SCN)_2$ reacts with a wide variety of functional groups to yield alkyl or aryl thiocyanate derivatives (6,58).
The reaction of $(SCN)_2$ with unsaturated lipids has been used to measure double bonds (58).

Evidence for peroxidase-catalyzed formation of $(SCN)_2$ is that incubation of the $LP-H_2O_2-SCN^-$ system with tyrosine, tryptophan, or
histidine results in chemical modification of these aromatic amino acids
(3). Similar modification is obtained when the amino acids are amide-
linked as residues of proteins. Bacterial components are chemically
modified in the same way (48). The same derivatives are obtained by
adding $(SCN)_2$ in CCl_4 to aqueous solutions of amino acids or proteins
(3) or to bacterial suspensions (54).

In contrast, when LP, H_2O_2, and SCN^- are incubated together
and then the amino acids are added, or when $(SCN)_2$ in CCl_4 is added
to water and then the amino acids are added, little or no chemical
modification is obtained. These results suggest that LP catalyzes the
oxidation of SCN^- to $(SCN)_2$. If the amino acids are present when
$(SCN)_2$ is formed, $(SCN)_2$ reacts with the amino acids. If the amino
acids are not added until after the hydrolysis of $(SCN)_2$ is complete,
then no reaction occurs.

Although this interpretation may be logically derived from the
observations, there are other observations that suggest a different

interpretation (3,4). First, a number of derivatives of the amino
acids are obtained. Only one of these derivatives contains the S and
C portions of the SCN moiety in a 1:1 ratio. The other derivatives
contain only the C portion. Second, the amount of C incorporated into
these derivatives is much less than 1 mol/mol of H_2O_2. Third, incorporation of C reaches a maximum value at high ratios of H_2O_2 to SCN^-,
rather than at the 1:2 ratio that would favor $(SCN)_2$ formation. These
observations suggest that another highly reactive, short-lived, oxidized form of SCN^- may be formed in small amounts during peroxidase-
catalyzed oxidation of SCN^-, and during hydrolysis and decomposition
of $(SCN)_2$ at neutral pH.

C. NC-SCN

Another agent that may be formed is the pseudohalogen NC-SCN. The
structure and reactivity of this compound is thought to more closely
resemble that implied by the structure NC-SCN and the name cyanogen
thiocyanate, rather than $S(CN)_2$ and the trivial name, sulfur dicyanide
(25). NC-SCN may be considered to contain a CN(+1) moiety or
SCN(+1) moiety. Therefore, NC-SCN is closely related to interhalogens such as ICl.

The reactivity of interhalogens is dominated by the more readily
oxidized portion. For example, ICl is closer to I_2 in its reactivity than
to Cl_2. Therefore, NC-SCN should resemble cyanogen, $(CN)_2$, rather
than $(SCN)_2$, and the reaction of NC-SCN with biological materials may
result in incorporation of the CN moiety. As described above, incubation of bacteria, proteins, or aromatic amino acids with $LP-H_2O_2-SCN^-$
results in incorporation of the C atom of SCN^- to a greater extent than
the S atom. Therefore, the results suggest that small amounts of NC-
SCN may be formed when the ratio of H_2O_2 to SCN^- is high, when
$HOSCN/OSCN^-$ concentration exceeds 0.5 mM, or when conditions
favor decomposition of $HOSCN/OSCN^-$ (22).

Interestingly, NC-SCN is one of the many agents that were proposed to be responsible for antimicrobial activity of the LP system (38),
prior to the time at which oxidation of SCN^- to $HOSCN/OSCN^-$ was
recognized. Chemically synthesized NC-SCN was shown to have antibacterial activity. Synthesis of NC-SCN is performed by reacting
cyanogen iodide (ICN) with AgSCN in organic solvents (25,55). Hydrolysis of NC-SCN yields CNO^- and SCN^-, so that measurements of
CNO^- may provide an indirect method for detecting $NC-SCN^-$. However, CNO^- may also arise from reactions involving HO_2SCN (22).

Oxidation of SCN^- in the presence of CN^- yields CNO^-, due to
formation and hydrolysis of NC-SCN (12). It was shown that CN^-
reacts rapidly and stoichiometrically with $HOSCN/OSCN^-$, resulting in
loss of oxidizing activity (2). This reaction can be used as a test for
$HOSCN/OSCN^-$, although CN^- also reacts with halogens. Adding [14]CN^-

to bacteria in the presence of HOSCN/OSCN$^-$ results in incorporation of ^{14}C into bacterial components (54), but it has not been established whether this reaction is due to N^{14}C-SCN formation, or to the reaction of ^{14}CN$^-$ with R-SSCN derivatives (4), which yields alkyl thiocyanate or isothiocyanate derivatives:

$$\text{R-S-SCN} + {}^{14}\text{CN}^- \longrightarrow \text{RS}{}^{14}\text{CN} + \text{SCN}^-$$

$$\text{RS}{}^{14}\text{CN} \longrightarrow \text{RN}{}^{14}\text{CS}$$

Although the reactivity of NC-SCN is best understood in terms of the unsymmetrical structure, the 2 C atoms may be equivalent in the sense that label introduced from S^{14}CN$^-$ or ^{14}CN$^-$ may be equivalent:

$$\text{N}{}^{14}\text{C-SCN} \rightleftharpoons \text{NC-S}{}^{14}\text{CN}$$

D. HO$_2$SCN and HO$_3$SCN

Cyanosulfurous acid (HO$_2$SCN) and cyanosulfuric acid (HO$_3$SCN) have been proposed as intermediates in decomposition of (SCN)$_2$ or HOSCN/ OSCN$^-$ and during oxidation of SCN$^-$ by excess H$_2$O$_2$. Their properties and reactivity are almost completely unknown, but they have been proposed to contribute to antimicrobial activity (19,40,41). Chemically synthesized HO$_3$SCN was short-lived in water (23). Antimicrobial activity has not been studied. By analogy to oxidized forms of halides, HO$_2$SCN and HO$_3$SCN would be expected to act as oxidizing agents, although not necessarily to be more effective than HOSCN/ OSCN$^-$. Short-lived compounds or compounds with a broad reactivity may be less effective as antimicrobial agents than compounds that are stable and that react with a single class of essential biological materials.

E. Other Agents

The possibility that SCN$^-$ might undergo 1-e$^-$ oxidation by compound II raises the possibility that short-lived radicals such as $\cdot$ SCN might be produced. However, the 2-e$^-$ oxidation of SCN$^-$ by compound I is favored. Radical mechanisms involving $\cdot$ (SCN)$_2$ or OSCN^{2-} have been proposed for nonenzymatic oxidation of SCN$^-$ under special conditions (8,9). No evidence was obtained for a radical mechanism of nonenzymatic oxidation of SCN$^-$ by H$_2$O$_2$ (56,57).

Production of HCN was proposed to account for toxicity of SCN$^-$ (59) and the antimicrobial activity of the LP-H$_2$O$_2$-SCN$^-$ system (12). However, the amounts of HCN that are formed are small (2), and far below the level required to inhibit *E. coli*. Also, bacteria which do not contain cytochrome oxidase, such as the streptococci and lactobacilli, are almost entirely unaffected by HCN. Results that implied that substantial amounts of HCN were formed during LP-catalyzed oxidation of

SCN$^-$ (12) were apparently due to the conditions of the assay for HCN (2).

It was proposed (39) that peroxidase-catalyzed oxidation of halides yields an activated form of O_2 known as singlet oxygen, $^1O_2$. This proposal is based on the analogy to the reaction of HOCl with H_2O_2, which yields $^1O_2$. Under strongly alkaline conditions, the deprotonated forms (OCl$^-$ and HO$_2^-$) react to yield $^1O_2$, which rearranges with the emission of light to yield O_2 (11,17). Chemiluminescence (emission of light) is detected during peroxidase-catalyzed reactions, but does not necessarily indicate formation of $^1O_2$. A wide variety of chemical reactions are chemiluminescent (31).

Rearrangement of $^1O_2$ to O_2 is faster than reactions of $^1O_2$ with other substances, because the latter reactions cannot exceed the rate of diffusion-limited reaction. Therefore, if $^1O_2$ is produced, O_2 will be the major product. The LP-H_2O_2-SCN$^-$ system does not yield O_2, as measured with the O_2 electrode in deaerated solutions (54). Therefore, $^1O_2$ does not contribute to antimicrobial activity.

V. INTERACTION OF I$^-$ AND SCN$^-$

Antimicrobial activity of LP in biological fluids is complicated by the presence of both I$^-$ and SCN$^-$. The SCN$^-$/I$^-$ ratio is usually 10:100, and SCN$^-$ competes effectively with I$^-$ for peroxidase-catalyzed oxidation (14,42,43), suggesting that the influence of I$^-$ would be negligible. However, (SCN)$_2$ oxidizes I$^-$ to I$_2$, so that oxidation of SCN$^-$ in the presence of I$^-$ might yield I$_2$ indirectly. Oxidation of even small amounts of I$^-$ might be significant, in that the LP-H_2O_2-SCN$^-$ system is primarily bacteriostatic, whereas the LP-H_2O_2-I$^-$ system is bactericidal. In addition, there are many other possible interactions of I$^-$ and SCN$^-$, including formation of ISCN, (SCN)$_2$I$^-$, or I$_2$SCN$^-$, and exchange reactions of I$^-$ and SCN$^-$ with sulfenyl derivatives.

To determine whether these interactions may be of biological significance, studies on LP antimicrobial activity were carried out in the presence of both SCN$^-$ and I$^-$, at varying SCN$^-$/I$^-$ ratios. Methods were as described previously (46-48) with gram-negative bacteria (*E. coli* ML 308-225). The results are relevant only to these bacteria, and more complex results are obtained with gram-positive organisms, such as streptococci. Therefore, the results do not rule out the possibility that supplementing biological fluids with I$^-$ might be useful. The results suggest that supplementing with HRP or HRP and I$^-$ might result in increased bactericidal action.

In Fig. 1, bactericidal action is expressed as the logarithm of the ratio of the number of bacteria in an untreated control (6×10^8 cells/ml) to the number of viable bacteria remaining after exposing the sample to the LP system. A value of zero indicates no killing, a value of 4 in-

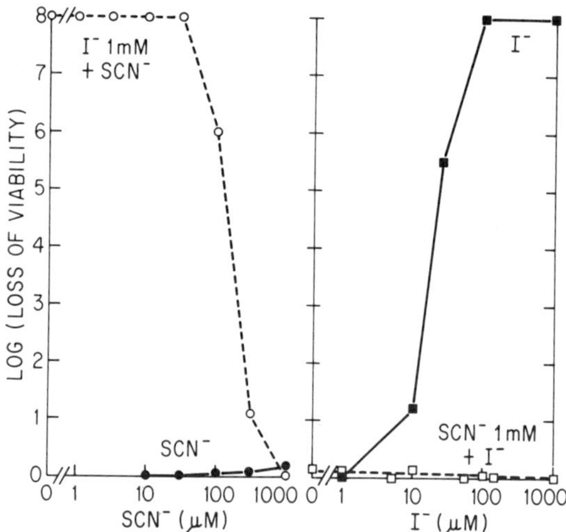

Figure 1 Bactericidal action.

dicates that 1 cell in 10,000 remained viable, and values of 8 indicate that within the limits of measurement, the sample was sterilized.

Figure 1 (left, lower curve) shows results with constant H_2O_2 (0.3 mM) and varying SCN⁻. Little or no killing was observed. The bacteria were diluted and plated within 15 min after exposure to the LP system, to prevent the slow bactericidal action of HOSCN/OSCN⁻. These results do not indicate that the LP system had no effect. As described below, bacterial metabolism was inhibited. However, bacteria exposed to the LP-H_2O_2-SCN⁻ system under these conditions recover and grow to yield colonies.

Figure 1 (left, upper curve) shows killing with 0.3 mM H_2O_2, 1 mM I⁻, and varying SCN⁻. In the absence of SCN⁻, complete killing was obtained, but SCN⁻ interfered at SCN⁻/I⁻ ratios as low as 0.1, and SCN⁻ completely blocked killing at a ratio of 1. In Fig. 1 (right) the relation of SCN⁻ and I⁻ is reversed. With I⁻ alone (upper curve), complete killing was obtained with 0.1 mM I⁻. When SCN⁻ was 1 mM and I⁻ was varied (lower curve), killing was blocked by SCN⁻. Other studies have shown that SCN⁻ interferes with bactericidal activity (26,27).

The experiment in Fig. 1 was also performed replacing LP with HRP, which catalyzes I⁻ oxidation but not SCN⁻ oxidation. Provided that the H_2O_2 concentration was relatively high (0.3 mM), SCN⁻ did not interfere with killing by the HRP-H_2O_2-I⁻ system. These results indicated that the effect of SCN⁻ in Fig. 1 was due to competition of SCN⁻ and I⁻ for LP-catalyzed oxidation.

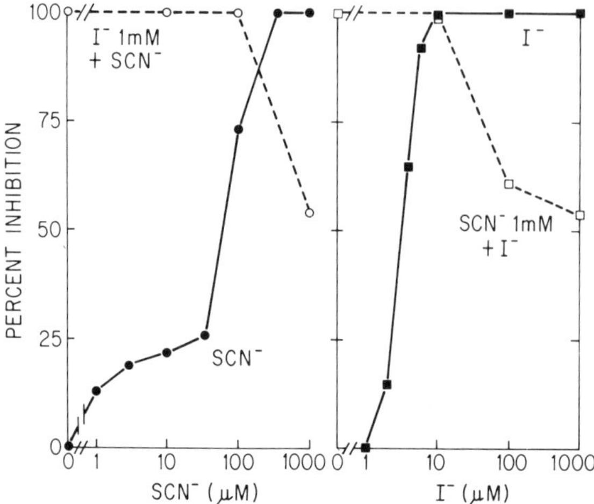

Figure 2 Inhibition of respiration.

Figure 2 shows results of an experiment identical to that in Fig. 1, but in which inhibition of respiration rather than bactericidal action was measured. Figure 2 (left, lower curve) shows that the LP-H_2O_2-SCN^- system inhibited respiration, though it did not kill the bacteria under these conditions. Figure 2 (left, upper curve) shows that with 1 mM I^- and no SCN^-, 100% inhibition was obtained. When SCN^- was added at concentrations greater than 0.1 mM, SCN^- interfered. At I^-/ SCN^- = 1, antagonism was observed. That is, the LP system was more effective with I^- alone or SCN^- alone than when both I^- and SCN^- were present. In Fig. 2 (right), 100% inhibition was obtained with I^- as low as 10 μM. When both I^- and SCN^- were present, antagonism was observed.

In other experiments, I^- caused rapid decomposition of HOSCN/ $OSCN^-$, accounting for the antagonism observed when both I^- and SCN^- were present. This rapid decomposition also interfered with the slow bactericidal action of HOSCN/$OSCN^-$, which requires several hours of exposure for significant killing.

In summary, of the many possible interactions of SCN^- and I^- in LP antibacterial activity, two interactions appeared significant. First, SCN^- and I^- competed for oxidation. Second, I^- increased the rate of decomposition of HOSCN/$OSCN^-$. Both of these interactions diminished bactericidal activity against gram-negative bacteria, although bacterio-static activity was less affected. In contrast, SCN^- had only a small effect on bactericidal activity of the HRP-H_2O_2-I^- system, and this ef-fect was overcome by adding more H_2O_2.

ACKNOWLEDGMENTS

This research was supported by research grant DE 04325 from the National Institute of Dental Research, by Cancer Center Support grants CA 08480 and CA 21765 from the National Cancer Institute, and by ALSAC. I thank my collaborators Drs. T. Aune and M. Morrison, and also Dr. G. Schonbaum for helpful discussions, K. A. Pera and M. M. Jefferson for technical assistance, and P. Nicholas for manuscript preparation.

REFERENCES

1. Allison, W. S., *Acc. Chem. Res. 9*: 293 (1976).
2. Aune, T. M., and Thomas, E. L., *Eur. J. Biochem. 80*: 209 (1977).
3. Aune, T. M., Thomas, E. L., and Morrison, M., *Biochemistry 16*: 4611 (1977).
4. Aune, T. M., and Thomas, E. L., *Biochemistry 17*: 1005 (1978).
5. Bacon, R. G. R., and Irwin, R. S., *J. Chem. Soc.*: 778 (1958).
6. Bacon, R. G. R., in *Organic Sulfur Compounds*, Kharasch, N. (Ed.), Pergamon Press, New York, p. 306 (1961).
7. Beers, R. F., Jr., and Sizer, I. W., *J. Biol. Chem. 195*: 133 (1959).
8. Behar, D., Bevan, P. L. T., and Scholes, G., *J. Phys. Chem. 76*: 1537 (1972).
9. Betts, R. H., and Dainton, F. S., *J. Am. Chem. Soc. 75*: 5721 (1953).
10. Björck, L., Claesson, O., and Schuthess, W., *Milchwissenschaft 34*: 726 (1979).
11. Brown, R. J., and Ogryzlo, E. A., *Proc. Chem. Soc.*: 117 (1964).
12. Chung, J., and Wood, J. L., *Arch. Biochem. Biophys. 141*: 73 (1970).
13. Clark, B. R., and Skoog, D. A., *Anal. Chem. 47*:2458 (1975).
14. Coval, M. L., and Taurog, A., *J. Biol. Chem. 242*: 5510 (1967).
15. Cunningham, L. W., *Biochemistry 3*: 1629 (1964).
16. George, P., *Biochem. J. 54*: 267 (1953).
17. Held, A. M., and Hurst, J. K., *Biochem. Biophys. Res. Commun. 81*: 878 (1978).
18. Ho, T.-L., *Chem. Rev. 75*: 1 (1975).
19. Hogg, D. M., and Jago, G. R., *Biochem. J. 117*: 779 (1970).
20. Hoogendoorn, H., in *Proceedings, Microbial Aspects of Dental Caries*, Sp. Suppl. Microbiology Abstracts, Stiles, H. M., Loesche, W. J., and O'Brien, T. C. (Eds.), p. 353 (1976).
21. Hoogendoorn, H., Piessens, J. P., Scholtes, W., and Stoddard, L. A., *Caries Res. 11*: 77 (1977).

22. Hughes, M. N., in *Chemistry and Biochemistry of Thiocyanic Acid and its Derivatives*, Newman, A. A. (Ed.), Academic Press, New York, p. 8 (1975).

23. Jander, G., Grattner, B., and Scholz, G., *Chem. Ber. 80*: 279 (1947).

24. Kharasch, N., in *Organic Sulfur Compounds*, Kharasch, N. (Ed.), Pergamon Press, New York, p. 375 (1961).

25. Kitching, W., Smith, R. H., and Wilson, I. R., *Aust. J. Chem. 15*: 211 (1962).

26. Klebanoff, S. J., *J. Exp. Med. 126*: 1063 (1967).

27. Klebanoff, S. J., *J. Bacteriol. 95*: 2131 (1968).

28. Klebanoff, S. J., *Semin. Hematol. 12*: 117 (1975).

29. Lewis, C. L., and Skoog, D. A., *J. Am. Chem. Soc. 84*: 1101 (1962).

30. Madson, K. O., in *Dietary Chemicals vs. Dental Caries*, Gould, R. F. (Ed.), American Chemical Society, Washington, D.C. (1970).

31. Mendenhall, G. D., *Angnew. Chem. Int. Ed. Engl. 16*: 225 (1977).

32. Morrison, M., Gayse, G., and Danner, D. J., in *Biochemistry of the Phagocytic Process*, Schultz, J. (Ed.), North-Holland, Amsterdam, p. 51 (1970).

33. Morrison, M., Bayse, G. S., and Michaels, A. W., *Anal. Biochem. 42*: 195 (1971).

34. Morrison, M., Bayse, G. S., and Webster, R. G., *Immunochemistry 8*: 289 (1971).

35. Morrison, M., Gates, R. E., and Huber, C. T., in *Membrane Transformations in Neoplasia*, Schultz, J., and Block, R. E. (Eds.), Academic Press, New York, p. 33 (1974).

36. Morrison, M., and Schonbaum, G. R., *Ann. Rev. Biochem. 46*: 861 (1976).

37. Muhlemann, H. R., Meyer, R. W., Konig, K. G., and Marthaler, T. M., *Helv. Odontol. Acta 5*: 18 (1961).

38. Oram, J. D., and Reiter, B., *Biochem. J. 100*: 382 (1966).

39. Piatt, J. F., Cheema, A. S., and O'Brien, P. J., *FEBS Lett. 74*: 251 (1977).

40. Pruitt, K. M., and Tenovuo, J., *Biochim. Biophys. Acta 704*: 204 (1982).

41. Pruitt, K. M., Tenovuo, J., Andrews, R. W., and McKane, T., *Biochemistry 21*: 562 (1982).

42. Sörbo, B., and Ljunggren, J. G., *Acta Chem. Scand. 12*: 479 (1958).

43. Tenovuo, J., *Archs oral Biol. 23*: 899 (1978).

44. Tenovuo, J., Månsson-Rahemtulla, B., Pruitt, K. M., and Arnold, R., *Infect. Immun. 34*: 208 (1981).

45. Thomas, E. L., and Aune, T. M., *Biochemistry 16*: 3581 (1977).

46. Thomas, E. L., and Aune, T. M., *Antimicrob. Agents Chemother.* *13*: 1000 (1978).
47. Thomas, E. L., and Aune, T. M., *Antimicrob. Agents Chemother.* *13*: 1006 (1978).
48. Thomas, E. L., and Aune, T. M., *Infect. Immun. 20*: 456 (1978).
49. Thomas, E. L., *Infect. Immun. 23*: 522 (1979).
50. Thomas, E. L., *Infect. Immun. 25*: 110 (1979).
51. Thomas, E. L., Bates, K. P., and Jefferson, M. M., *J. Dent. Res. 59*: 1466 (1980).
52. Thomas, E. L., *Biochemistry 20*: 3273 (1981).
53. Thomas, E. L., Bates, K. P., and Jefferson, M. M., *J. Dent. Res. 60*: 785 (1981).
54. Thomas, E. L., unpublished results.
55. Walden, P., and Audrieth, L. F., *Chem. Rev. 5*: 339 (1928).
56. Wilson, I. R., and Harris, G. M., *J. Am. Chem. Soc. 82*: 4515 (1960).
57. Wilson, I. R., and Harris, G. M., *J. Am. Chem. Soc. 83*: 286 (1961).
58. Wood, J. L., *Org. React. (N.Y.) 3*: 240 (1946).
59. Wood, J. L., in *Chemistry and Biochemistry of Thiocyanic Acid and its Derivatives*, Newman, A. A. (Ed.), Academic Press, New York, p. 156 (1975).

4

Steady-State Kinetics of Lactoperoxidase-Catalyzed Reactions

WILLIAM G. BARDSLEY / *The University of Manchester and St. Mary's Hospital, Manchester, England*

I. INTRODUCTION

Lactoperoxidase (LP), like other peroxidases such as horseradish peroxidase (HRP) and myeloperoxidase (MPO), catalyzes the reactions

$$H_2O_2 + AH_2 = 2H_2O + A$$

or

$$H_2O_2 + 2AH = 2H_2O + 2A$$

where AH_2 is a two-electron equivalent and AH a one-electron equivalent reducing agent. The enzyme forms intermediate species called
compounds I and II, as in the sequence

$$LP + H_2O_2 \longrightarrow \text{compound I} + H_2O$$

$$\text{Compound I} + AH_2 \longrightarrow \text{compound II} + AH\cdot$$

$$\text{Compound II} + AH_2 \longrightarrow LP + AH\cdot$$

where the species $AH\cdot$ is a free radical. This species undergoes further reactions, such as

$$2AH\cdot \longrightarrow A + AH_2$$

as well as other reactions. A number of excellent reviews describing
the definitive experiments that suggested this scheme are available
(30,50,56,72).

Caution must be exercised in the interpretation of the steady-
state kinetics of peroxidases. One complication is that the free radical
products formed during the reaction can react with enzyme species
leading to loss of enzyme activity. Another difficulty is that steady-
state kinetics can never reveal details about complicated sequences
such as those leading up to compound I. It is principally the number
of species reacting with substrate or releasing product and the sequence in which these events occur that are amenable to investigation
by steady-state methods. Another source of artifacts is the interaction
among the various enzyme species that are possible. For instance, a
good example of the complexities that can occur is provided by the fact
that, in open systems, peroxidase-catalyzed reactions can show sus-
tained oscillations (24,48,71,73).

In this chapter, I shall employ the nomenclature introduced by
Cleland (13-15) to describe kinetic schemes. (It is unfortunate that
in this system of nomenclature "A" has been used to represent the substrate and in the peroxidase system "A" will therefore represent H_2O_2.
However, "A" has also been used traditionally in the peroxidase literature to represent electron or hydrogen donors. This ambiguity in
usage should cause no difficulty in the present chapter, since the
meaning of "A" will be clear in the context.) Let A be H_2O_2, B be a
hydrogen donor, and P the free radical product. Then, since H_2O is
not counted as a reactant, we can summarize the classic peroxidase
mechanism as in scheme 1 of Fig. 1. EA is compound I, F is compound
II, and the scheme is a ping-pong mechanism. It is probable that, at
low substrate concentrations, this is the main reaction pathway, but
the fact is that this scheme does not fit the initial rate data over a
wider range of substrate concentrations. It is, of course, possible to
add the reaction of another A species giving a dead-end complex FA
(i.e., compound III as in scheme 2 of Fig. 1). This scheme now permits

substrate inhibition by excess of A (H_2O_2) but is still not sufficiently comprehensive to account for the kinetics over an extended range of substrate concentration.

II. THE STEADY-STATE KINETICS OF LACTOPEROXIDASE

A. Published Work Relevant to the Steady-State Kinetics of Lactoperoxidase

Concerning the kinetic behavior of lactoperoxidase, all subsequent work can be seen to stem from the pioneering studies of Chance (6,7). By rapid-flow and more leisurely techniques, he demonstrated that LP formed the same sequence of intermediates as HRP. Rate constants were estimated, and it was shown that, although reaction between LP and H_2O_2 was usually more rapid than that between compound II and electron donor, this was not a general rule. The concept of a sharp pH optimum was challenged as it was established that the rate of reaction between compound II and electron donors showed no systematic variation in the range pH 3.6-6.7. The anomalous kinetics that occur due to irreversible destruction by H_2O_2 were emphasized, and it was pointed out that when this is taken into account the estimates for rate constants with LP were higher than corresponding values for HRP. leading to the conclusion that LP is a more active enzyme than HRP. A scholarly compilation by Maehly and Chance (39) is a useful source for alternative assay methods for catalases and peroxidases. Further details of the kinetics of LP were then unraveled in an important series of papers by Dunford and coworkers (17,40,41,57). Changes in the Soret region of the LP spectrum were exploited to study the binding of Fluoride. This process followed pseudo-first-order kinetics with a rate constant of $(9.7 \pm 0.4) \times 10^2$ M^{-1} s^{-1} that was pH independent in the range pH 3.8-5.4 (57). The binding of cyanide was studied by temperature-jump experiments in the range pH 4.55-10.60, and this was found to depend upon two ionizable groups with pK_a values similar to a histidine-imidazole and a free α-amino group of an amino acid residue (17). It was concluded that these ionizable groups were not ligands of the heme. Maguire et al. investigated the pH dependence of k_1, the second-order rate constant for compound I formation, using steady-state kinetics in the presence of saturating concentrations of hydroquinone and guaiacol (40). They found a value of $k_1 = (9.2 \pm 0.9) \times 10^6$ M^{-1} s^{-1}, in good agreement with Chance's value of 2×10^7 M^{-1} s^{-1} (7), and this was pH independent in the range pH 3-10.8. However, attention was drawn to the fact that k_1 decreased with time at pH 3, a process that was slower at pH 7. The reaction of LP compound II with iodide was found to be rather complex (41). The apparent rate constant was resolved according to

$$k_{obsd} = k_1[I^-] + k_2[I^-]^2$$

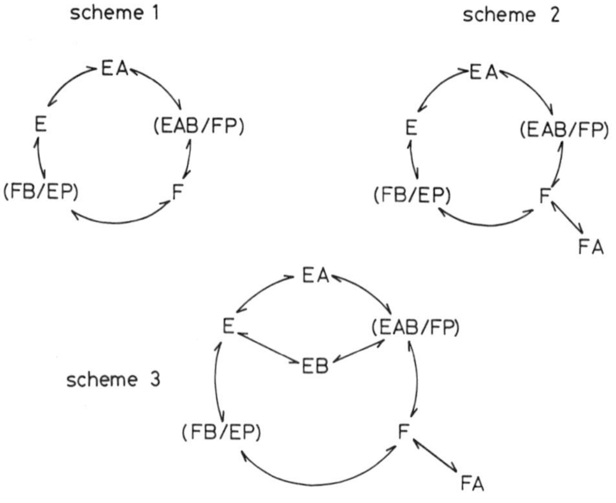

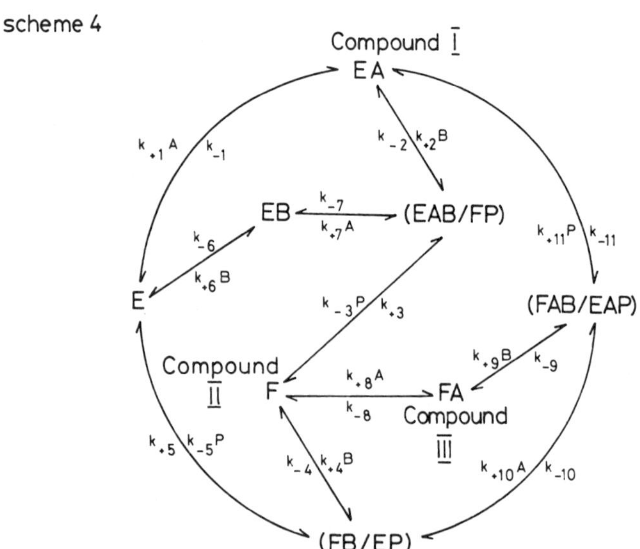

Figure 1 Possible reaction mechanisms for LP-catalyzed reactions. The symbol A represents H_2O_2, B is ABTS, and P is the radical cation. The stoichiometry is actually

$$H_2O_2 + 2ABTS = 2P^+ + 2OH^-,$$

but this is abbreviated to

$$A + 2B = 2P$$

and the pH dependence of k_1 and k_2 in the range pH 2.0-10.1 was interpreted in terms of an acid dissociation outside this pH range. Kimura and Tamasaki recently reported a heme-linked ionization of pK_a = 3.5 and, from the chloride dependence of the absorbance, suggested that chloride formed a complex with the acid form of the enzyme with a dissociation constant of pK = 2.7 (33). Subsequently (34), they reinvestigated the spectra of compounds I, II, and III, confirmed Chance's value of 0.2s for the half-time for spontaneous conversion of compound I into compound II, but disputed the earlier claim (40) concerning the pH independent of k_1. Lamas (36) has performed a number of experiments that show that LP catalyzes both iodination and the coupling reaction in thyroglobulin more efficiently than chloramine T and has suggested that the enzyme is involved in both reactions beyond simply providing the active form of iodine. The precise mechanisms are still obscure, and this is also true for the iodination of lipids, although progress is now being made in determining the reaction products as, for instance, the identification by Boeynaems et al. (5) of an iodo-δ-lactone as the product of LP-catalyzed iodination of arachidonic acid. The iodination reaction catalyzed by LP is of considerable significance in contemporary biochemistry, but detailed steady-state work is not available. Bayse et al. (4) recorded that HRP did not catalyze the reaction, but at neutral pH LP readily brought about the iodination of peptides containing tyrosine. The rate was proportional to enzyme concentration, a ping-pong mechanism was claimed, K_m values were measured, and they emphasized the confusion that can arise in attempting to measure iodination spectrophotometrically due to the complications arising from the coupling reactions. Threatte et al. (64) have supported the value of iodide-specific electrodes for measuring LP-catalyzed iodination of tyrosine and details of the experimental conditions required for vectorial labeling of membranes, namely LP = 10^{-7} M, $[I^-]$ < 10^{-6} M, $[H_2O_2]$ < 10^{-4} M, are provided by Morrison (44). It has been suggested that LP compound I catalyzes the iodination of thyroglobulin and compound II catalyzes thyroid hormone synthesis (65,78). Also, a more detailed understanding of the LP-catalyzed oxidation of thiocyanate to hypothiocyanite is now possible due to polarographic (91) and kinetic studies (92,97).

Turning now to a number of recent publications on miscellaneous topics that impinge on the subject of LP kinetics, attention is first

---

Figure 1 (Continued) Scheme 1: the classical peroxidase scheme where EA is compound I and F is compound II; scheme 2: the classic peroxidase scheme enlarged to allow dead-end substrate inhibition brought about by the formation of FA (i.e., compound III); scheme 3: further enlargement of the classic scheme by allowing random addition of A or B; scheme 4: the greater cyclic mechanisms combining all of the previous features and also allowing additional pathways permitting product release via compound III (11,60,95).

drawn to the purification of LP using affinity chromatography described by Pommier and Cahnmann (53). This exploits the knowledge
that glutathione and cysteine bind to LP, producing a red shift in the
Soret band. The binding is promoted by diiodotyrosine but reversed
by iodide or guaiacol. Goitrogens are oxidized by LP, but this leads
to inactivation. Not surprisingly, since it is probably at the basis of
the biological activity, this aspect of LP chemistry has attracted a good
measure of attention. Edelhoch et al. (19), for instance, undertook a
serious kinetic study of the interactions of LP, iodide, and thiourey-
lene drugs. They found that iodide binds to LP with a dissociation
constant of 2×10^{-5} M, and it was not consumed at pH 8.8 during the
oxidation of N-acetyltyrosylamide or various goitrogens. Differential
equations were set up to account of the inactivation of LP by a combination of autoinactivation in dilute solutions, and the effect of antithyroid
drugs and appropriate rate and binding constants were estimated. At
an earlier date Chang and Schroeder (9) suggested that tyrosine residues in LP could be oxidized by H_2O_2, leading to inactivation, but they
also undertook an investigation of the inactivation of LP that occurs
when the enzyme is allowed to react with 3-amino-1:2:4-triazole and
H_2O_2 at pH 7. Four to five tyrosine residues and two residues of histidine were lost during this process. When LP was incubated with
phenylhydrazine, isopropylphenylhydrazine, or phenyldiimide, inactivation occurred, and Allison and coworkers (1) showed that 1 mol
of phenylhydrazine was bound per 40,000 g of LP. They suggested
that it was possible for the phenyldiimide to interact with the heme
moiety but likely that the hydrazine reacted elsewhere. Mäkinen and
Mäkinen have studied the destruction of LP by butadienone-sensitized
photochemical inactivation (84,85). Numerous amino acid residues were
involved, and they cautioned against interpretation of results in terms
of specific effects on arginyl residues. However, time-dependent irreversible inactivation by diazotized sulfanilate led to labeling of two
tyrosine and two histidine residues (86). Attempted labeling of histidine residues by diethylpyrocarbonate, methyl-4-nitrobenzene sulfonate,
and rose bengal revealed no essential histidines, and hence it was
concluded that LP has two essential tyrosyl residues.

Løvstad (38) followed up the earlier observation that chlorproma-
zine is oxidized to stable red-colored free radicals by HRP with a
study of several important phenothiazine derivatives as substrates for
LP. An attempt was made to assess the effect of substituents in the
2- and 10-positions of the phenothiazine ring, and a table of K_m values
and V_{max} values was given. The production of free radicals during
LP-catalyzed reactions is evidently an important area, and evidence of
what can be achieved is provided by the sort of studies carried out by
Yamazaki and Piette (70). They used an electron paramagnetic resonance spectrometer adapted with a flow apparatus to study the radicals
produced by HRP and also ascorbic acid oxidase and gave equations to
describe the steady-state concentration and dismutation of these species.

On the subject of the effect of excess H_2O_2 on peroxidases, the paper
by Erman and Yonetani deserves mention (20). With cytochrome C peroxidase, a 10-fold excess of H_2O_2 gave a complex reaction involving
release of molecular oxygen from compound I, but also oxidation of the
heme group and various amino acid residues in the proteins occurred.
The thermal instability of LP has been mentioned several times, and
attention is drawn to the work of Tamura and Morita (63). They resolved the heat denaturation of Japanese radish peroxidase into three
processes: dissociation of protohemin from the holoperoxidase, a
conformational change in the apoperoxidase, and modification or degradation of protochemin. Recovery of activity occurred at neutral
pH but not at pH 5 or pH 9. Binding of LP to glass can lead to apparent time-dependent losses of activity, and a study of this phenomenon
has confirmed the elongated form of the LP molecule with a positively
charged end (80).

It has been the custom in peroxidase studies to ignore deviations
from Michaelis-Menten kinetics, and a welcome exception to this prac-
tice is the recent paper on the selenium-glutathione peroxidase of rat
liver by Splittgerber and Tappel (61). The enzyme showed complex
kinetics, including hysteretic effects, and these authors made a determined attempt to interpret the behavior in terms of a model involving
several oxidation-reduction forms of the catalytic site complicated by
slow transition between enzyme forms. Finally, no review of the LP
literature would be complete without again referring to the fact that,
although LP compound III does not decompose into LP as easily as
HRP compound III decomposes into HRP, Nakamura et al. (45) were
able to select appropriate experimental conditions for substained oscillations.

The relationship of LP to other peroxidases such as chloroperoxidase (CPO), thyroid peroxidase (TPO), myeloperoxidase (MPO),
eosinophilic peroxidase (EPO), intestinal peroxidase (IPO), and
salivary peroxidase is of interest. It may be that there are special
kinetic properties that suit each enzyme for its specific biological
function, but as yet the literature dealing with such possibilities is
sparse. CPO catalyzes the halogenation reaction

$$AH + X^- + H_2O_2 = AX + H_2O + OH^-$$

but chlorite can act as both oxidant and chlorine donor. In fact,
chlorite reacts rapidly with HRP to give compound X, which may be
the halogenating intermediate in the chlorite reaction (10). However,
in the absence of a halogen acceptor, compound X decays to give
chloride and compound I, the reactions being strongly pH dependent.

The alkaline transitions of CPO have been examined in the near-
ultraviolet and visible region over a pH range of 6-12 (82), and a
study of the dismutation of chlorite to form chlorine dioxide, chlorate,
and oxygen has established that inactivation of the enzyme by chlorine

dioxide causes loss of the Soret absorption band of the native enzyme
(94). It is clear that CPO catalyzes the peroxidation of chloride and
bromide to molecular chlorine and bromine when there is no organic
substrate present to act as halogen receptor. What is not yet completely settled is the role of free halogen or other intermediates in
halogenation. Libby et al. (83) present strong evidence that chlorination does not involve free chlorine but the evidence is less clear
regarding bromine, and free iodine is held to be mandatory for iodination reactions. A study of the steroselectivity of the halogenation
reaction by Ramakrishnam et al. (93) led them to conclude that active-
site chlorination proceeds without appreciable stereoselectivity, but
bromination involved prior formation of free bromine and its release
into solution.

TPO differs from the other peroxidases by being membrane
bound, and so proteolysis and detergent treatment are required to
prepare the enzyme. There is evidence for formation of intermediates
similar to those of the classic scheme (47), but of course the coupling
reaction is especially significant because of the importance of this process in thyroid hormone synthesis. Virion et al. (65) have studied the
kinetics of iodination and coupling with TPO and LP, as well as the
absorbance at 430 nm due to compound III, and concluded that different enzyme-H_2O_2 species are involved. They reported that the
coupling reaction began after a lag period that was independent of the
concentration of iodide, thyroglobulin, or enzyme and from the kinetic
data tentatively suggested that the iodination reaction involved compound I but the coupling reaction required compounds II or III.

Further experiments in support of this scheme have been published
(78), and evidence for the function of free iodide as a regulator of
the simultaneous iodination of thyroglobulin and synthesis of iodothy-
ronines is accumulating (98). Yamazaki and coworkers have recently
turned attention to the kinetics of TPO. An important comparison of
LP and TPO (89) was published, and it was established that TPO reacted with methylmercaptoimidazole similarly to but more rapidly than
LP. Subseqently, the catalytic intermediates during iodination were
explored (90), leading to the determination of rate constant values by
stopped-flow methods. Steady-state kinetics were also employed to
study the regulation of the iodination reaction (88). A study of TPO
kinetics with guaiacol over extended ranges of substrate concentration
was analyzed using the F test to support a rate equation of degree 3:3
in guaiacol and 4:4 in peroxide (60). A Monte Carlo simulation study of
the statistical power of the F test reinforced the conclusion that fourth-
order and third-order terms were difficult to detect but second-order
ones were quite easy to identify (77). This is exactly what was found
experimentally (60). Whereas all peroxidases oxidize iodide, only CPO
and MPO catalyze chlorination reactions effectively. Chloride binds
to MPO, altering the absorption spectrum (62) in the Soret region.
Amino acids give chloramines that rapidly degrade spontaneously,

an exception being formation of the stable taurine chloramine. Naskalski (46) has made a study of the kinetics of chlorination of taurine,
paying particular attention to the inactivation of MPO that occurs
during catalysis and has suggested that the H_2O_2- and pH-dependent
inactivation could be involved in natural regulatory mechanisms to limit
the effect of MPO inside the phagocytic vesicle.

Thomas et al. (96) have performed an interesting study of the incorporation of amines into proteins that occur during MPO-catalyzed
oxidation of chloride to chlorite. Chloroamines were produced as intermediates, but it was concluded that the phenomenon was not likely to
be involved in the antimicrobial activity. Recent steady-state kinetic
studies with CPO have revealed substrate inhibition by high peroxide
concentration and confirmed that the actual kinetic scheme must be
quite complicated (94).

MPO also differs from LP in having a molecular weight of 140,000
and containing two hemes. Whereas acetone precipitation serves to remove the heme from HRP, the prosthetic group is linked covalently in
LP and is especially stable in the case of MPO. Because of this stability, Wu and Schultz (69) suggested the possibility of an amide linkage.
It is evident that, like HRP and catalase, MPO forms a compound I type
of species that decays to compound II with a half-time of the order of
100 msec (29). Like LP, MPO is not homogeneous (21), and reductive
cleavage of MPO produces two enzymatically active hemimyeloperoxi-
dases (2). Work on the subunit structure is well advanced (26), in-
equivalence of heme binding has been confirmed (27), and affinity
chromatography has been developed (42). The possible involvement
of superoxide anion (35) or singlet oxygen in MPO oxidations has re-
ceived attention (28,31), and MPO does interfere with the determination
of superoxide dismutase activity (49,55).

Recent evidence from 1270 nm chemiluminescence in the LP, H_2O_2,
Br^- system has also been interpreted as favoring the production of
singlet oxygen to account for cytotoxicity and chemiluminescence (79).

Like LP, solid-state MPO has been used for catalytic iodination of
protein (18). A comparison of the properties of EPO and MPO (43)
shows that there are only minor differences in the kinetic properties
of these two enzymes. Similar pH optima were found, inactivation by
excess H_2O_2 was reported, and both enzymes were inhibited by cyanide
and azide. The only distinct difference was found with p-phenylenediamine, which was much better as a hydrogen donor for EPO than for
MPO. Protoporphyrin IX may be the cofactor of EPO, and the optical
and EPR spectra of EPO, IPO, and HRP are similar and somewhat different to those of MPO (68).

B. ABTS as Hydrogen Donor

The reagent 2,2'-azino-di-(3-ethylbenzthiazoline-6-sulfonic acid)
(ABTS) was originally used for cerium studies (32,37) but was intro-

duced into peroxidase studies as an ideal reagent. It is relatively
nontoxic when compared with some other hydrogen donors, is available
in purified form, forms a well-defined reaction product with high absorbance, and is more sensitive than other known chromogens (23,67).
The manufacturer's claims have been endorsed by several groups (11,
16,25,54), and ABTS is now established as an excellent reagent for
peroxidase studies. The reagent produces a metastable radical cation
with a strong absorbance around 412 nm where the reagent itself has
low background absorbance. The radical species disproportionates
slowly into an azodication and starting material. Although this reaction
does not interfere with kinetic studies, it is a minor nuisance in that
product-inhibition studies cannot be performed in the straightforward
way possible with other enzymes where the reaction products are available in quantity as pure, stable reagents.

It is possible to titrate HPR with ABTS and H_2O_2 and calculate an
equilibrium constant for the reaction. Also, using extended ranges of
ABTS and H_2O_2 concentrations, it has been claimed that kinetic evidence requires a rate equation of degree 3:3 in ABTS and 4:4 in
H_2O_2 (11). Scheme 4 of Fig. 1 shows the greater cyclic mechanism that
was suggested to account for these findings in the case of HRP and
cervical mucus peroxidases (95). This mechanism was arrived at by considering how the classic peroxidase mechanism of schemes 1 and 2 could
be extended to account for higher-degree terms in the rate equation.
There is always a problem when using synthetic substrates since pecu-
liar reaction pathways can operate that are normally "silent" with the
biologically relevant substrates. Another possible criticism is that,
in the analyses of horseradish and cervical mucus peroxidases, no statistical procedures were used. However, the F test has been used to
establish a high-degree rate equation for thyroid peroxidase with
guaiacol, and again the greater cyclic mechanism was proposed (60).
Some recent evidence covering these questions is now presented.

C. Computer Studies with the Greater Cyclic Mechanism

At present there is no generally accepted method for characterizing rate
equations. With fairly simple rate equations, it is possible to regress
directly to the rate equation expressed as a function of the individual
rate constant. However, if scheme 4 of Fig. 1 is the peroxidase scheme,
then the rate equation is too complicated for this until such time as
several of the rate constants can be determined independently. However, we might ask whether such a kinetic scheme can give certain
types of curves like the ones observed experimentally and, although
this type of analysis has been attempted for simple mechanisms (22),
there seems no hope of performing the necessary algebra with rate
equations of the sort we are now considering.

To find out whether the possible $v(S)$ and double reciprocal plots
for this mechanism, with ABTS varied and H_2O_2 fixed, are as exten-

sive as those that are available to arbitrary rational functions of degree 3:3 with positive coefficients, we decided not to ask whether certain curves occur but rather how probable such curves are. This method has been used previously to characterize 2:2 mechanisms (59). For the 3:3 mechanisms, we wrote a program that used the known facts concerning the algebra and geometry of such rate equations (3). For rate constants chosen from a chemically reasonable range, it was concluded that the greater cyclic mechanism can give most of the possible 3:3 curves (66). In particular, pronounced substrate-inhibition curves, such as the ones given by peroxidases, are highly probable with rate constant values suggested by kinetic studies with peroxidases (60). The probability that the correct degree of the rate equation can be estimated for the greater cyclic mechanism has been computed (77), and the tendency to give sigmoid (75) or substrate-inhibited curves (76) when there is no specific restraint on the relative magnitude of rate constant values has also been obtained.

D. The Reactions Between Lactoperoxidase, ABTS, and H_2O_2

The titration of ABTS by H_2O_2 in the presence of LP is shown in Fig. 2. At pH 5.6 the ABTS peak is stronger than in more acid solution having $\varepsilon = 3.8 \times 10^4$ at 340 nm. The radical cation, P, has $\varepsilon = 3.8 \times 10^4$ at 413 nm, but also has an absorbance of 15% of this value at 340 nm. When this is taken into account, the data from Fig. 2 give an equilibrium constant of

$$K_{eq} = \frac{[P^2]}{[ABTS]^2[H_2O_2]}$$

$$= (3.7 \pm 2.4) \times 10^5 M^{-1}$$

When equilibration has been reached, the peak at 413 nm decays as the radical disproportionates to give the azodication that then contributes to the absorbance at 340 nm. The stoichiometry is

$$2P \xrightarrow{k_1} \text{azodication} + \text{ABTS}$$

but in the presence of H_2O_2 a further reaction occurs according to

$$2P + H_2O_2 \xrightarrow{k_2} 2 \text{ azodication}$$

For H_2O_2 concentration below 10 mM we have

$$\frac{dP}{dt} = -(2k_1 + 2k_2[H_2O_2])P^2$$

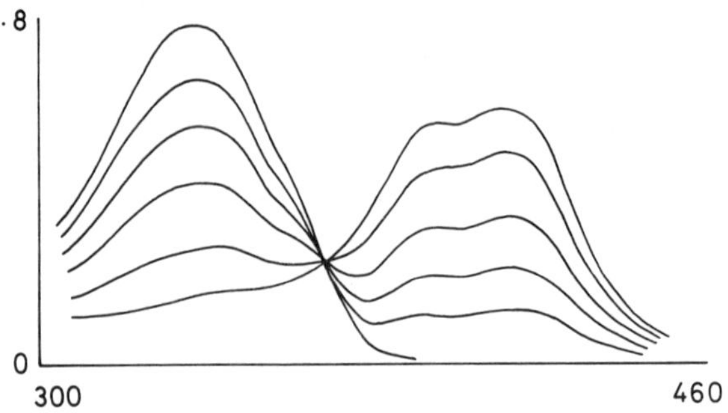

wavelength (nm)

Figure 2 The absorbtion spectra of ABTS and the radical cation. The curve with the highest absorbance at 340 nm is 0.02 mM ABTS in 0.2 M acetate buffer, pH 5.6. The next five curves result from successive additions of 2.5 µl of a solution containing H_2O_2 (1 mM) and lactoperoxidase (10^{-7} M). The spectral changes occurred very rapidly and allowed the calculation of an equilibrium constant but, on standing for several hours, the spectra could be seen to change as the radical disproportionated. This was accelerated by adding excess H_2O_2.

or

$$\frac{1}{P} - \frac{1}{P_0} = k_0 t$$

where

$$k_0 = 2k_1 + 2k_2[H_2O_2] \text{ and } P_0 = P(0)$$

The values of k_1 and k_2 were calculated to be

$$k_1 = 0.5 \text{ M}^{-1} \text{ s}^{-1}$$

$$k_2 = 2 \times 10^3 \text{ M}^{-2} \text{ s}^{-1}$$

but higher-order kinetics were found for $[H_2O_2] > 10$ mM, and in the range 10 mM $< [H_2O_2] < 100$ mM it is best to take $k_0 = 45$ s^{-1} to avoid overestimating the disappearance of the radical cation. So it is clear that any experiments designed to study the rates of LP-catalyzed oxidation of ABTS by H_2O_2 over long time periods should take this decay into account. For instance, if the radical cation solution had an absorbance of 0.1, then over a 1-hr period this would decrease to 0.09 in the presence of 1 mM H_2O_2 but to 0.07 in the presence of 100 mM H_2O_2.

There is a much more serious problem concerning the steady-state measurement of LP-catalyzed reactions, and this is illustrated in Fig. 3(a). When 10^{-10} M LP solutions are incubated with ABTS fixed at 1 mM and H_2O_2 much less than 0.1 mM, the rate of product formation with time is approximately linear over at least 15 min. Slight curvature can be seen over longer time periods, but this can be shown to be due to substrate depletion since, when H_2O_2 is added continuously to maintain the solutions at 0.01 mM, the rate is linear for over half an hour. In the range $H_2O_2 = 0.1$ mM to $H_2O_2 = 1$ mM, the reaction rate increases dramatically but the P(t) profiles are clearly curves. This is due to destruction of the enzyme since, if reaction is conducted in 1 mM H_2O_2 until product formation ceases, addition of fresh enzyme causes the cycle to be repeated. As the H_2O_2 concentration increases up to 100 mM, the reaction rate decreases but the P(t) profiles become less curved. We have studied this phenomenon over a wide range of substrate concentrations, and the result is reproducible and may be summarized thus: the rate of inactivation of LP during the reaction increases as the reaction rate increases.

A number of experiments designed to illuminate this phenomenon are now described. When a concentrated solution of LP is diluted to concentrations more appropriate for an assay, say from 10^{-7} to 10^{-10} using large volumes to minimize losses due to adsorption onto the glass surfaces (81), it is possible to measure a very slow decay at 23°C with a first-order rate constant of $(1.57 \pm .37) \times 10^{-5}$ s^{-1}. This is increased slightly by ABTS but is quite insufficient to account for the inactivation. In the presence of H_2O_2, LP undergoes irreversible destruction by a complex process. Using data in the range 1 mM < $[H_2O_2]$ < 100 mM, the behavior can be accommodated by the time-dependent inhibition model of Childs and Bardsley (12) according to the scheme

$$E + I \underset{k_{-1}}{\overset{k_1}{\rightleftharpoons}} EI \underset{k_{-2}}{\overset{k_2}{\rightleftharpoons}} EI^*$$

where

$$I = H_2O_2$$

The rate constants were estimated to be

$$k_1 = (1.67 \pm 0.56) \times 10^2$$

$$k_{-1} = 0.73 \pm 0.24$$

$$k_2 = (8.5 \pm 0.09) \times 10^{-4}$$

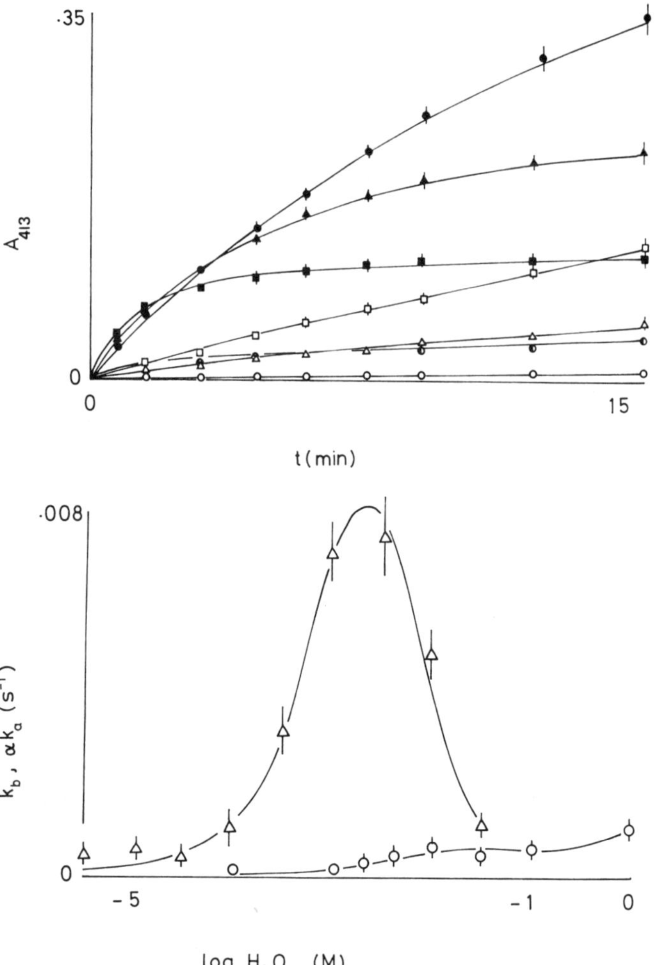

Figure 3 The initial rate of LP-catalyzed reaction between ABTS and H_2O_2. (a): The absorbance change at 413 nm when LP (10^{-10} M) is incubated in ABTS (1 mM) with H_2O_2 at these concentrations: $\circ$, 0.00316 mM; $\triangle$, 0.01 mM; $\square$, 0.0316 mM; $\bullet$, 0.1 mM; $\blacktriangle$, 0.316 mM; $\blacksquare$, 1 mM; $\circ$, 3.16 mM. As the H_2O_2 increases still further, up to 100 mM, the curvature decreases and the rates become very low. The curves are best fit curves obtained by regression to the equation for suicide inhibition derived in the text, and the points are means of five determinations. (b): The parameters involved in suicide inhibition as functions of the log (base 10) of molar H_2O_2 concentration. $\circ$, k_b values obtained for fitting first-order decay to the data for inactivation by H_2O_2. $\triangle$, k_a α parameters obtained by regression to the data of Fig. 3(a). It is clear that inactivation is mainly due to this effect except at 100 mM H_2O_2 when k_b and k_a α are more comparable. k_a is the rate constant for suicide inactivation and α is the proportion of enzyme in the form of EP complexes leading to suicide inhibition.

$$k_{-2} = (2.56 \pm 0.19) \times 10^{-6}$$

using regression of v/v_0 as a function of H_2O_2 and time to the equation

$$\frac{E + EI}{E_0} = \frac{k_{-2}(k_1 I + k_{-1})}{\lambda_1 \lambda_2} + \frac{k_1 I k_2}{\lambda_1(\lambda_2 - \lambda_1)} \exp\lambda_1 t - \frac{k_1 I k_2}{\lambda_2(\lambda_2 - \lambda_1)} \exp\lambda_2 t$$

where λ_1 and λ_2 satisfy the characteristic equation

$$\lambda^2 + (k_1 I + k_{-1} + k_2 + k_{-2})\lambda + k_{-1}k_{-2} + k_1 I(k_2 + k_{-2}) = 0$$

Over shorter time periods, covering the range down to 80% loss of activity, these data can also be approximately modeled by a first-order process, with pseudo-first-order rate constants varying from $(1.21 \pm 0.24) \times 10^{-4}$ s^{-1} to $(1.07 \pm 0.02) \times 10^{-3}$ as H_2O_2 varies from 0.1 mM to 1 M [Fig. 3(b)]. Only at the higher concentrations of H_2O_2, say $[H_2O_2] > 10$ mM, could this provide an important contribution to the decay and, as we have seen, the P(t) profiles become less curved at higher H_2O_2 concentrations. So we must conclude that the radical cation produced by the reactions inactivates the enzyme. To test this hypothesis, LP was incubated at 23°C, pH 5.6 with P (synthesized from ABTS and ceric ammonium sulfate) at a concentration of 0.04 mM. This concentration is much higher than that produced during the steady-state kinetics and yet, over a 20-min period, there was only a modest loss in enzyme activity. We must conclude that when P is produced at the enzyme-active site there are two alternatives: either P is released or P never leaves the enzyme but takes part in a chemical reaction leading to loss of enzyme activity.

To model ABTS as a suicide substrate for LP, consider, at fixed substrate concentration, a steady state in which a proportion of the total enzyme, α say, is in the form of the EP species. Then we would have

$$E = \underset{(1 - \alpha)}{\overline{E}} + \underset{\alpha E}{EP}$$

where

E = total active enzyme

$\overline{E}$ = Σ all active species not reacting with P

EP = Σ all species reacting with or releasing P

Now, suppose EP releases product with a rate constant k_c, or reacts with product to give EP* with a rate constant k_a. To this we must add denaturation with rate constant k_b due to the effect of H_2O_2 leading to the scheme:

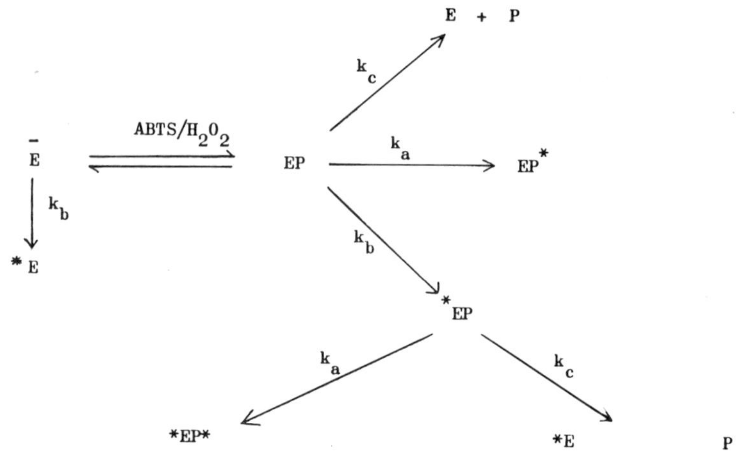

The governing equations when $k_a \gg k_b$ and $k_c \gg k_b$ are

$$\frac{dP}{dt} = k_c \alpha E \frac{k_a + k_b + k_c}{k_a + k_c}$$

and

$$\frac{dE}{dt} = -(k_a \alpha + k_b)E$$

leading to

$$\frac{d^2P}{dt^2} = -(k_a \alpha + k_b)\frac{dP}{dt}$$

and finally, the approximation

$$P = \frac{v_0}{k_a \alpha + k_b}\{1 - \exp[-(k_a \alpha + k_b)t]\}$$

where

$$v_0 = dP/dt \text{ at } t = 0$$

Figure 3(a) shows the best fit curves obtained by regression to this equation and the estimates for k_b and $k_a\alpha$ shown in Fig. 3(b) suggest a value of $k_a \sim 10^{-2}\ s^{-1}$ since, at maximum rates of inactivation, it is not unreasonable to assume that $\alpha \to 1$.

In order to assess the extent to which these various causes contribute to the curvature of the P(t) plot, we need an expression for P(t) allowing for decay due to the disproportionation of the radical and also its oxidation by H_2O_2. An argument to obtain such an expression first assumes that $P_0(t)$ would be the amount if no further chemistry occurred, that is,

$$P_0 = v_0 t$$

However, due to the disproportionation of P and reaction between P and H_2O_2 we actually have,

$$\frac{dP}{dt} = v_0 - k_0 P^2$$

where $k_0 = 2k_1 + 2k_2[H_2O_2]$ as discussed previously.

Since $dP/dt > 0$, we have the formula

$$\frac{P(t)}{P_0(t)} = \frac{\tanh(\sqrt{v_0 k_0}\, t)}{\sqrt{v_0 k_0}\, t}$$

From the calculations shown in Table 1, it is quite clear that the major contribution to curvature of the P(t) plot is suicide inhibition. However, if steady-state measurements are conducted at 100 mM H_2O_2 concentrations, there will be a progressively more important contribution to nonlinearity of the P(t) plot due to inactivation of LP by H_2O_2. Also, it should be noted that the ε_{413} value of the radical cation is decreased by some 5% in 10 mM H_2O_2 and about 25% in 100 mM H_2O_2.

E. The Optimum pH

The steady-state rate of reaction was determined as a function of pH with several different combinations of substrate concentrations, and the pH profiles were fitted by Michaelis pH functions for 2 and 3 ionizing species. A third-order equation gave a satisfactory fit to data as seen in Fig. 4. The pH optimum was different at each set of substrate concentrations and so the pH dependence cannot simply be due to the ionization of two or three major species. It seems that any pH value between 5 and 6 could be chosen for kinetic studies, and we performed all of our experiments in 0.2 M acetate buffer pH 5.6.

F. Thermal Stability

LP is stable indefinitely as an ammonium sulfate suspension at 4°C, but when this suspension is diluted to give 10^{-7}-10^{-10} M solutions, multiphase decay in activity is observed. The cause of this decay is not known at present, but it can be even more complicated if small volumes are used due to appreciable adsorption of LP onto glass sur-

Table 1 Inactivation of LP During Catalysis[a]

| | (i) | (ii) | | (iii) | | (iv) | |
| | Spontaneous decay | Denaturation due to H_2O_2 | | Production of azodication | | Suicide inhibition | |
	23°C	1 mM H_2O_2	100 mM H_2O_2	1 mM H_2O_2	100 mM H_2O_2	1 mM H_2O_2	31.7 mM H_2O_2
1 min	1	0.99	0.97	1	1	0.65	0.93
2 min	1	0.98	0.94	1	1	0.42	0.86
5 min	1	0.96	0.85	1	0.97	0.11	0.68
15 min	0.99	0.88	0.63	0.99	0.80	0.001	0.31

[a]The change in rate of product formation, $v = dP/dt$, with time is due to several causes, namely: (i) spontaneous decay due to loss of enzyme activity on dilution; (ii) denaturation due to the chemical reaction between H_2O_2 and LP; (iii) decay of the radical cation, P, due to inactivation by disproportionation and reaction with H_2O_2; and (iv) inactivation by suicide inhibition. The rate, $v = dP/dt$, as a proportion of $v_0 = dP/dt$ at $t = 0$ is calculated according to equations given in the text.

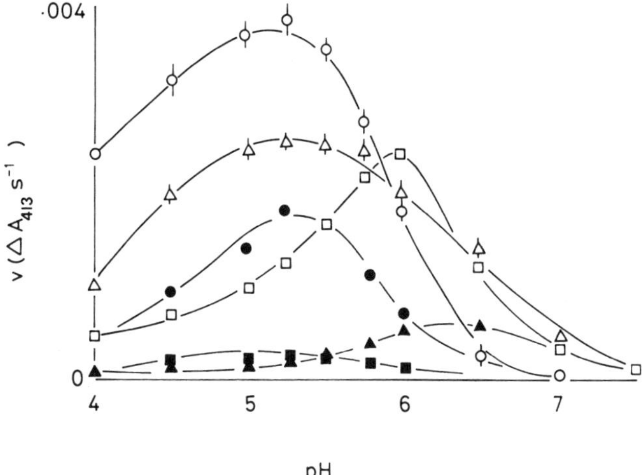

Figure 4 pH profiles for the LP-catalyzed reaction between ABTS and H_2O_2. Initial rates were determined with a variety of substrate concentrations using 0.2 M acetate buffers in the range pH 4-6 but using phosphate up to pH 7.5. Points are means of five determinations, and the curves are the best fit curves for third-order Michaelis pH functions at the following substrate concentrations: ○, ABTS (1 mM) and H_2O_2 (1 mM); △, ABTS (10 mM) and H_2O_2 (1 mM); □, ABTS (0.1 mM) and H_2O_2 (0.1 mM); ●, ABTS (0.1 mM) and H_2O_2 (0.1 mM); ▲, ABTS (1 mM) and H_2O_2 (0.01 mM); ■', ABTS (0.01 mM) and H_2O_2 (0.01 mM).

faces (81). This complication was avoided by the use of large volumes in the experiments described in this chapter.

There is a rapid initial decay lasting an hour or so followed by a steady decline lasting for several weeks at temperatures around 6-8°C. Figure 5 shows the dependence of this process on temperature, and the fitted curves are for regression to the scheme

$$E_1 \underset{k_{-1}}{\overset{k_1}{\rightleftharpoons}} E_2 \xrightarrow{k_2} E_3{}^*$$

where E_2 and $E_3{}^*$ are assumed to be inactive. The equation describing this decay is

$$\frac{E_1}{E_0} = \frac{k_1}{\lambda_2 - \lambda_1}\left(\frac{\lambda_1 + k_2}{\lambda_1}\exp\lambda_1 t - \frac{\lambda_2 + k_2}{\lambda_2}\exp\lambda_2 t\right)$$

where

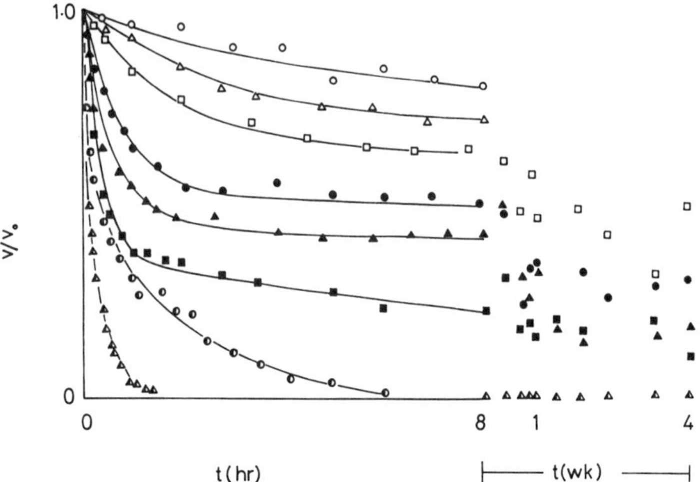

Figure 5 Thermal denaturation of LP. A suspension of LP (5 mg ml^{-1}) in ammonium sulfate (3.2 M) phosphate buffer (0.1 M) pH 7 was diluted 1:100 with 0.2 M acetate buffer, pH 5.6, and stored for 1 hr to equilibrate. At time t = 0, 0.5 ml of this solution was added to 9.5 ml of 0.2 M acetate buffer, pH 5.6, at the required temperature, that is: ○, 2°C; △, 23°C: □, 30°C; ●, 40°C; ▲, 50°C; ■, 60°C; ◌, 62.5°C; △, 65° and 70°C. At appropriate intervals of time, enzyme activity remaining was estimated in triplicate giving the points shown. After 8 hr the solutions at 30°, 40°, 50°, 60°, and 65°C were cooled, placed in a refrigerator at 6 ± 2°C and assayed as convenient for another month. The curves are fitted by regression to a two-stage denaturation model as discussed in the text.

$$\lambda_{1,2} = \frac{1}{2}\left[-(k_1 + k_{-1} + k_2) \pm \sqrt{(k_1 + k_{-1} - k_2)^2 + 4k_{-1}k_2}\right]$$

as described by Childs and Bardsley (12). The decay constant k_2 was too small compared with k_1 and k_{-1} to be estimated by regression analysis at temperatures below 50°C. At the end of some 8 hr of heat inactivation, the solutions were maintained in a refrigerator at 6 ± 2°C. No recovery of activity occurred. Instead, the activity continued to decline steadily, and from the combined results obtained for decay down to about 40% residual activity over 1 month, k_2 was estimated to be $(3.60 \pm 0.41) \times 10^{-7}$ s^{-1} at 6 ± 2°C.

G. The Plot of v([E₀])

It is very important in kinetic studies to be sure that the initial rate is proportional to enzyme concentration over a wide range. For instance, in the decay of activity due to heat or H_2O_2, rates can be measured down to 1% of the starting values. Nonlinearity of the $v([E_0])$ plot can be caused by a variety of artifacts but also, if an enzyme is present in several states of aggregation which are significantly different kinetically and if the rate of polymerization is fairly rapid and is affected by changes in substrate concentration, then the $v([E_0])$ plot will be curved. Shindler and Bardsley (58) previously reported such curvature for LP, and a reinvestigation was undertaken using five determinations at each $[E_0]$ concentration over three orders of magnitude. The experiment was repeated at several substrate concentrations, and the results can be seen in Fig. 6. The data were fitted with a hierarchy of polynomial models. At low substrate concentrations the F test showed no significant improvement on adding quadratic terms and, although upward curvature was seen at higher substrate concentrations, it was concluded that this was not significant. Hence, there is no evidence for deviations from linearity in the $v([E_0])$ plot and no evidence for kinetically significant enzyme polymerization with LP at pH 5.6. As mentioned, at higher substrate concentrations there was some evidence of upward curvature, and this is best seen by the fact that the weighted regression lines in Fig. 6(a) underestimated the highest point. In view of the fact that suicide inhibition is less important at higher enzyme concentrations, it is probable that initial rates were somewhat underestimated with higher substrate concentrations and low enzyme concentrations, giving the appearance of upward curvature in the $v([E_0])$ plot. The double log plot of Fig. 6(b) shows all of the data points, and in this space there seems no convincing evidence for systematic upward curvature.

H. The Plot of $v([H_2O_2])$ at Fixed ABTS Concentrations

The data of Fig. 7 show that with H_2O_2 varied pronounced substrate inhibition occurs, but the turning point moves to higher H_2O_2 concentrations with increasing ABTS concentrations. The F test showed a significant improvement for 3:3 as opposed to 2:2 but no significant improvement with a 4:4 function. The highest-degree numerator terms were very small and so we conclude that high H_2O_2 concentrations lead to pileup of the LP in compound III, and this has the character of a dead-end complex. The rate equation is 2:2 or possibly 3:3 in H_2O_2, and we draw attention to the shape of the curves in Fig. 7 and that of Fig. 3(b). This suggests that at H_2O_2 concentrations around 1 mM a reaction pathway is preferred that is very efficient but passes through one enzyme intermediate species which undergoes the suicide inhibition. It is unlikely that this species is compound III since when this species predominates reaction rate and inactivation rate are both low.

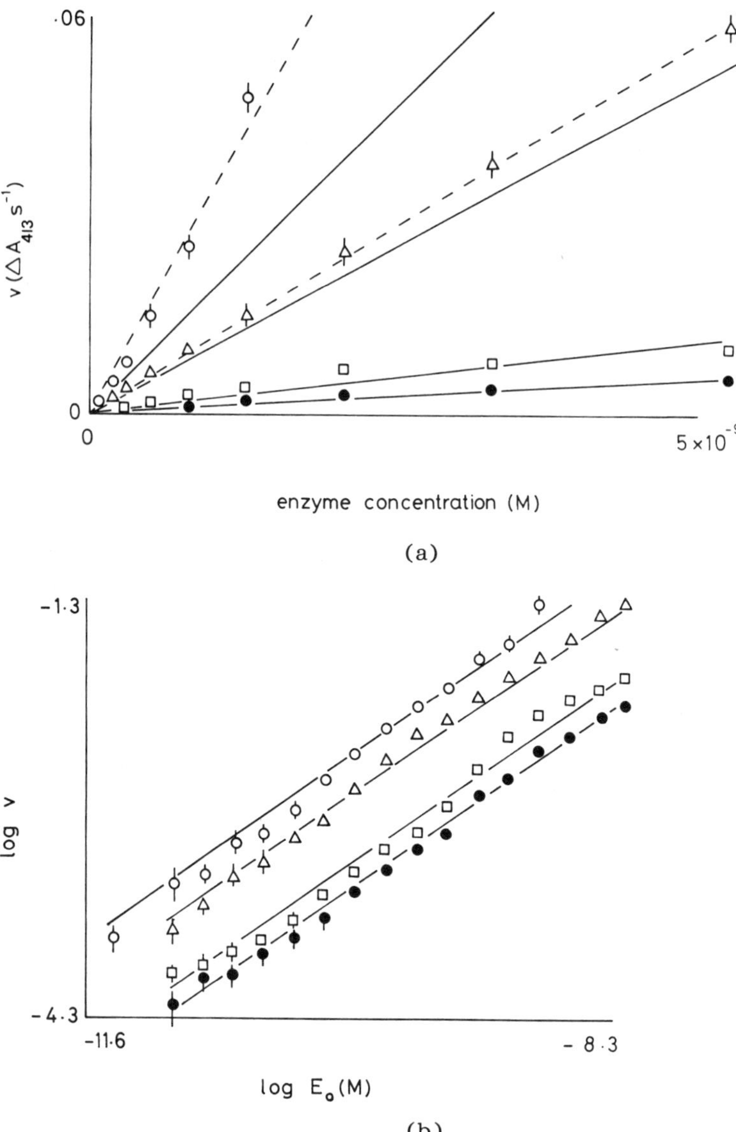

Figure 6 The dependence of initial rate on enzyme concentration. LP solutions of concentrations 5×10^{-10} M, 5×10^{-9} M, and 5×10^{-8} M were made up, and by suitable dilutions the initial rate of reaction was measured for 2.5×10^{-12} M $\leqslant$ LP $\leqslant 6.3 \times 10^{-9}$ M using substrate concentrations as follows: $\circ$, ABTS = 1 mM, H_2O_2 = 1 mM; $\triangle$, ABTS = 1 mM, H_2O_2 = 0.1 mM; $\square$, ABTS = 1 mM, H_2O_2 = 0.0316 mM; $\bullet$, ABTS = 1 mM, H_2O_2 = 0.01 mM. The lowest concentration of enzyme was fixed by the difficulty in measuring initial rates, and the highest concen-

I. The Profile of $v([ABTS])$ at fixed H_2O_2 Concentrations

Like Fig. 7, the kinetic profiles shown in Fig. 8 have turning points that move to higher concentrations of ABTS as the H_2O_2 concentration increases. The F test gave a significant improvement for degree 3:3 as opposed to 2:2, but no improvement for 4:4. The highest-degree numerator terms were significant, and so we conclude that the LP rate equation is degree 2:2 or 3:3 in ABTS.

III. CONCLUSIONS

We have seen that LP is a very difficult enzyme to study by steady-state methods. Yet, this is the standard technique used to estimate the enzyme during purification procedures, and so an attempt must be made to identify the various sources of error, to assign a catalytic mechanism, and to derive a plausible rate equation. Using ABTS as hydrogen donor, the radical cation product is sufficiently stable for kinetic studies lasting up to 15 min. For times much in excess of this, especially in strong solutions, the decay due to disproportionation and oxidation by H_2O_2 should be taken into account. The spontaneous denaturation of LP should also be considered during lengthy measurements, for example of enzyme eluted from columns or gels. To estimate LP, it is permissible to use any pH value between 4.5 and 6.5, and it is also reasonable to assume that the amount of enzyme present is proportional to the initial rate. The assay is relatively insensitive to ABTS concentration in the range 0.5 mM < [ABTS] < 15 mM, but the choice of H_2O_2 concentration is more problematical. If H_2O_2 concentrations less than 0.01 mM are used, the reaction rate is reasonably constant but rather low so that time periods of about 15 min are required for accurate measurements. If values of H_2O_2 concentration around 0.1-1 mM are used, the reaction rate is much more rapid, but suicide inhibition becomes pronounced. If pressed to specify the best condi-

---

Figure 6 (Continued)   tration was determined by substrate depletion and the physical impossibility of measuring such rapid reaction rates with conventional apparatus. Points displayed are means $\pm$ SD from five determinations. (a): Over a linear scale it is not possible to show the fit to all of the points. The solid lines are the best fit lines for unweighted regression, and the dashed line is for weighted regression. From this it is possible to see the upward curvature when the assays are performed using higher substrate concentrations. (b): The complete $v([E_0])$ data in double logarithmic space (base 10). The lines are the unweighted best fit lines to the equation $v = k\,[E_0]$ in this space (i.e., $\log v = \log K + \log [E_0]$. The fit to a family of parallel lines is not very good, but when all the difficulties inherent in the assay are considered, there is no convincing evidence of systematic deviation from linearity.

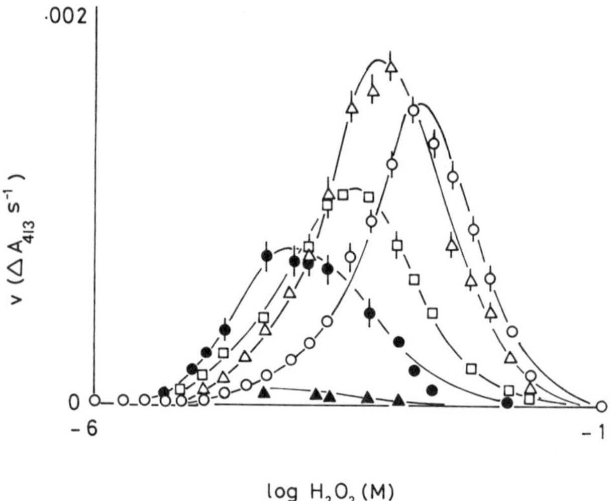

log H_2O_2 (M)

Figure 7 The dependence of initial velocity on log (base 10) of molar H_2O_2 concentration with ABTS fixed. The initial rate was determined at 23°C with LP (10^{-10} M), 0.2 M acetate buffer, pH 5.6, H_2O_2 in the range 0.001-100 mM, and ABTS fixed as follows: ○, 2.5 mM; △, 1 mM; □, 0.4 mM; ●, 0.1 mM; and ▲, 0.01 mM. The experimental points are means of five determinations and the curves are the best fits for functions of degree 3:3. The results of the F test on the sum of weighted residuals squared for these curves were: ○, 3:3 better than 2:2 (99% level); △, 2:2 better than 1:1 (99% level); □, 3:3 better than 2:2 (95% level); ●, 3:3 better than 2:2 (99% level); ▲, 2:2 better than 1:1 (99% level). In no case was a 4:4 curve justified, but in all cases a 2:2 curve was a statistically significant improvement over a 1:1 curve.

tions for an assay of LP, then [ABTS] = 1 mM, [H_2O_2] = 0.1 mM, pH 5.6 could be suggested since this gives a high initial rate and the suicide inhibition is not too serious if rates are determined over a 1- to 2-min period. However, Mäkinen and Tenovuo (87) suggest shorter reaction time and lower substrate concentrations to estimate lower LP levels. Any assay of LP that is conducted in a discontinuous manner will clearly underestimate the velocity, and so it is recommended that LP determinations be conducted continuously and as quickly as possible after mixing the reagents together to minimize the artifacts. By conventional techniques, it is possible to mix the reagents and commence recordings at 413 nm within 15 sec.

Now we must see if we can calculate a steady-state rate equation for LP of the form

$$v = f([E_0], A, B, P)$$

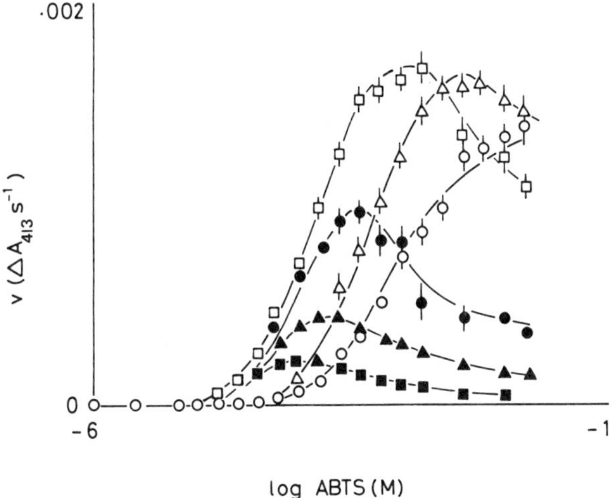

Figure 8 The dependence of initial velocity on log (base 10) of molar
ABTS concentration with H_2O_2 fixed. The initial rate was determined
at 23°C with LP (10^{-10} M), 0.2 M acetate buffer, pH 5.6, ABTS in the
range 0.001–15.85 mM, and H_2O_2 fixed as follows: ○, 3.16 mM; △, 1.0
mM; □, 0.316 mM; ●, 0.1 mM; ▲, 0.0316 mM; and ■, 0.01 mM. The experimental points are means of five determinations and the curves are
the best fit for functions of degree 3:3. The results of the F test
on the sum of weighted residuals squared for these curves were: ○,
2:2 better than 1:1 (99% level); △, 2:2 better than 1:1 (99% level);
□, 3:3 better than 2:2 (99% level); ●, 3:3 better than 2:2 (95% level);
▲, 3:3 better than 2:2 (95% level); ■, 2:2 better than 1:1 (99% level).
In no case was a 4:4 curve justified, but in all cases a 2:2 curve was
a statistically significant improvement over a 1:1 curve.

where v is the initial rate measured as a tangent to the P(t) profile at
t = 0 and where

$[E_0]$ = enzyme concentration

A = H_2O_2 concentration

B = hydrogen donor concentration

P = product concentration

f = an appropriate function

Despite publication of K_m and V_{max} values by numerous workers
in the LP area, the fact remains that LP does not obey Michaelis-Menten

kinetics if data points are spread over a wide concentration range.
This has been acknowledged by Polis and Shmukler (52), who published a nonlinear double reciprocal plot, by Pickering et al. (51) who
gave a bell-shaped semilogarithmic plot with H_2O_2, and by Shindler
and Bardsley (58) who claimed substrate inhibition with both ABTS and
H_2O_2 and suggested grounds for considering the presence of cubic
terms in the rate equation. In order to decide on a suitable rate equation, we shall consider the unpublished data presented in this review.
This refers to the bovine milk enzyme as supplied by Boehringer,
Mannheim (413:280 > 0.6) at 23°C in 0.2 M acetate buffer pH 5.6 using
ABTS as B, the hydrogen donor, and we shall only consider the case
P = 0. To facilitate discussion, we shall consider sequentially the
mechanisms of Fig. 1.

A Rate Equation for the Classic Peroxidase Scheme

The rate equation for the classic Chance mechanism (8) of scheme 1,
Fig. 1 is

$$\frac{v}{[E_0]} = \frac{\alpha_{11}AB}{\beta_{00} + \beta_{01}B + \beta_{10}A + \beta_{11}AB}$$

where

$$\alpha_{11} = 2k_{+1}k_{+2}k_{+3}k_{+4}k_{+5}$$

$$\beta_{00} = k_{-1}k_{+4}k_{+5}(k_{-2} + k_{+3})$$

$$\beta_{01} = k_{+2}k_{+3}k_{+4}k_{+5}$$

$$\beta_{10} = k_{+1}[k_{+2}k_{+3}(k_{-4} + k_{+5}) + k_{+4}k_{+5}(k_{-2} + k_{+3})]$$

$$\beta_{11} = k_{+1}k_{+2}k_{+4}(k_{+3} + k_{+5})$$

This is 1:1 in both A and B, after cancellation of B between numerator
and denominator, and predicts linear double reciprocal plots with both
substrates. It is clearly not able to accommodate the steady-state
kinetics of LP.

A Rate Equation for the Classic Peroxidase Scheme Allowing
Compound III as a Dead-End Complex

The rate equation for the classic scheme allowing compound III formation
as in scheme 2 of Fig. 1 is

$$\frac{v}{[E_0]} = \frac{\alpha_{11}AB}{\beta_{00} + \beta_{01}B + \beta_{10}A + \beta_{11}AB + \beta_{20}A^2}$$

where

$$\alpha_{11} = 2k_{+1}k_{+2}k_{+3}k_{+4}k_{+5}k_{-8}$$

$$\beta_{00} = k_{-1}k_{+4}k_{+5}k_{-8}(k_{-2} + k_{+3})$$

$$\beta_{01} = k_{+2}k_{+3}k_{+4}k_{+5}k_{-8}$$

$$\beta_{10} = k_1k_{-8}[k_{+2}k_{+3}(k_{-4} + k_{+5}) + k_{+4}k_{+5}(k_{-2} + k_{+3})]$$

$$\beta_{11} = k_{+1}k_{+2}k_{+4}k_{-8}(k_{+3} + k_{+5})$$

$$\beta_{20} = k_{+1}k_{+2}k_{+3}k_{-8}(k_{-4} + k_{+5})$$

This equation is a distinct improvement over the previous ones. It is
1:2 in A and 1:1 in B, but must be rejected since it does not allow for
the substrate inhibition given by excess B.

A Rate Equation for the Classic Peroxidase Scheme Allowing Random Additions of A or B Dead-End Inhibition Due to Compound III Formation

The scheme under consideration is that of scheme 3 in Fig. 1, and
this leads to the rate equation

$$\frac{v}{[E_0]} = \frac{\alpha_{11}AB + \alpha_{21}A^2B + \alpha_{12}AB^2}{\beta_{00} + \beta_{10}A + \beta_{01}B + \beta_{20}A^2 + \beta_{11}AB + \beta_{02}B^2 + \beta_{30}A^3 + \beta_{21}A^2B + \beta_{12}AB^2}$$

where

$$\alpha_{11} = 2k_{+3}k_{+4}k_{+5}k_{-8}(k_{-1}k_{+6}k_{+7}k_{+1}k_{+2}k_{-6})$$

$$\alpha_{21} = 2k_{+1}k_{+2}k_{+3}k_{+4}k_{+5}k_{+7}k_{-8}$$

$$\alpha_{12} = 2k_{+2}k_{+3}k_{+4}k_{+5}k_{+6}k_{+7}k_{-8}$$

$$\beta_{00} = k_{-1}k_{+4}k_{+5}k_{-6}k_{-8}(k_{-2} + k_{+3} + k_{-7})$$

$$\beta_{10} = k_{-8}(k_{-1}k_{+3}k_{+4}k_{+5}k_{+7} + k_{+1}k_{+3}k_{-4}k_{-6}$$

$$+ k_{-1}k_{+3}k_{-4}k_{+6}k_{+7} + k_{+1}k_{+2}k_{+3}k_{+5}k_{-6}$$

$$+ k_{-1}k_{+3}k_{+5}k_{+6}k_{+7} + k_{+1}k_{-2}k_{+4}k_{+5}k_{-6}$$

$$+ k_{+1}k_{+3}k_{+4}k_{-6} + k_{-1}k_{-2}k_{+4}k_{+5}k_{+7}$$

$$+ k_{+1}k_{+4}k_{+5}k_{-6}k_{-7})$$

$$\beta_{01} = k_{+4}k_{+5}k_{-8}[(k_{-1}k_{+6} + k_{+2}k_{-6})(k_{+3} + k_{-7}) + k_{-1}k_{-2}k_{+6}]$$

$$\beta_{20} = k_{+1}k_{+2}k_{+3}k_{-4}k_{-6}k_{+8} + k_{-1}k_{+3}k_{-4}k_{+7}k_{+8}$$
$$+ k_{+1}k_{+2}k_{+3}k_{+5}k_{-6}k_{+8} + k_{-1}k_{+3}k_{+5}k_{+6}k_{+7}k_{+8}$$
$$+ k_{+1}k_{+3}k_{+4}k_{+5}k_{+7}k_{-8} + k_{+1}k_{+2}k_{+3}k_{-4}k_{+7}k_{-8}$$
$$+ k_{+1}k_{+2}k_{+3}k_{+5}k_{+7}k_{-8} + k_{+1}k_{-2}k_{+4}k_{+5}k_{+7}k_{-8}$$

$$\beta_{11} = k_{-8}(k_{+1}k_{+2}k_{+3}k_{+4}k_{-6} + k_{-1}k_{+3}k_{+4}k_{+6}k_{+7}$$
$$+ k_{+2}k_{+3}k_{+4}k_{+5}k_{+7} + k_{+2}k_{+3}k_{-4}k_{+6}k_{+7}$$
$$+ k_{+2}k_{+3}k_{+5}k_{+6}k_{+7} + k_{+1}k_{+2}k_{+4}k_{+5}k_{-6}$$
$$+ k_{+4}k_{+5}k_{+6}k_{+7}k_{-1} + k_{-2}k_{+4}k_{+5}k_{+6}k_{+7}$$
$$+ k_{+1}k_{+2}k_{+4}k_{+5}k_{-7})$$

$$\beta_{02} = k_{+2}k_{+4}k_{+5}k_{+6}k_{-8}(\bar{k}_{+3} + k_{-7})$$

$$\beta_{30} = k_{+1}k_{+2}k_{+3}k_{+7}k_{+8}(k_{-4} + k_{+5})$$

$$\beta_{21} = k_{+2}k_{+7}[k_{+3}k_{+6}k_{+8}(k_{-4} + k_{+5}) + k_{+1}k_{+4}k_{-8}(k_{+3} + k_{+5})]$$

$$\beta_{12} = k_{+2}k_{+4}k_{+6}k_{+7}k_{-8}(k_{+3} + k_{+5})$$

This rate equation is 2:3 in A and 2:2 in B and can thus account for the substrate inhibition given by both substrates. The chemistry involved is reasonable, and the only novel assumption involved is the proposition that, whereas LP with A gives compound I, which is detected spectrophotometrically, prior combination of LP with the hydrogen donor is also feasible. This alternative random pathway was not detected in classic work since the LP-B complex does not possess distinct spectral characteristics. However, Kitagawa et al. (80) have recently reported a resonance Raman study of heme-substrate interactions in LP showing differences between plant and animal peroxidases but establishing beyond doubt the binding of electron donors to peroxidases in the absence of H_2O_2. For instance, benzohydroxamic acid caused a spectral shift with HRP but none with LP, whereas guaiacol shifted the spectrum of LP but not HRP. So the possibility of random addition of either ABTS or H_2O_2 in the kientic sequence required by the steady-state data is reinforced by this independent physical evidence. The only feature that this mechanism cannot accommodate is the F test showing that the v versus ABTS data are fitted rather better by degree 3:3 than degree 2:2.

A Rate Equation for the Greater Cyclic Mechanism

The rate equation for scheme 4 of Fig. 1 is 4:4 in A and 3:3 in B and too lengthy to print. Unlike HRP (11), thyroid peroxidase (60), and cervical mucus peroxidase (95), there is no compelling evidence to adopt this scheme for LP. It seems that with LP compound III has more of the character of a dead-end complex and so the pathways involving k_{+9}, k_{-9}, k_{+10}, k_{-10}, k_{+11}, and k_{-11} are relatively silent. Presumably, most of the reaction flux avoids these pathways except at high ABTS concentration. Only under these forcing conditions is reaction flux diverted into these pathways, and this could account for the statistical evidence for improvement in fit on increasing the degree from 2:2 to 3:3. In view of the numerous sources of error with LP, it could be, however, that this statistical evidence is spurious. Accordingly, we propose scheme 3 of Fig. 1 as the simplest mechanism to account for the steady-state kinetics of LP with ABTS and H_2O_2 in acetate buffer pH 5.6, 23°C and conclude that the extra pathways involved in the greater cyclic mechanism are less important with LP than with HRP, TPO, and cervical mucus peroxidase.

ACKNOWLEDGMENTS

I thank J. S. Shindler for our initial experiments with LP; F. Solano Muñoz, J. L. Iborra, and J. A. Lozano for providing unpublished data on thyroid peroxidase; K. J. Indge, J. P. Kavanagh, J. M. Wardell, and A. J. Wright for assistance with computation; R. M. Wood for help with mathematical analysis; and H. B. Dunford for providing me with useful information in advance of publication. The help given to me by P. B. McGinlay in performing the experiments described in this chapter is gratefully acknowledged as is the skilled secretarial assistance of J. S. Crombie. Above all, I thank R. E. Childs who helped me to respond to our experience with the ABTS-HRP system by developing an interest in complex kinetics.

REFERENCES

1. Allison, W. S., Swain, L. C., Tracy, S. M., and Benitez, L. V., *Arch. Biochem. Biophys. 155*: 400 (1973).
2. Andrews, P. C., and Krinsky, N. I., *J. Biol. Chem. 256*: 4211 (1981).
3. Bardsley, W. G., *J. Theor. Biol. 65*: 281 (1977).
4. Bayse, G. S., Michaels, A. W., and Morrison, M., *Biochim. Biophys. Acta 284*: 30 (1972).
5. Boeynaems, J. M., Reagan, D., and Hubbard, W. C., *Lipids 16*: 246 (1981).

6. Chance, B., *Science 109*: 204 (1949).

7. Chance, B., *J. Am. Chem. Soc. 72*: 1577 (1950).

8. Chance, B., *Arch. Biochem. Biophys. 41*: 416 (1952).

9. Chang, J. Y., and Schroeder, W. A., *Arch. Biochem. Biophys. 156*: 475 (1973).

10. Chiang, R., Rand-Meir, T., Makino, R., and Hager, L. P., *J. Biol. Chem. 251*: 6340 (1976).

11. Childs, R. E., and Bardsley, W. G., *Biochem. J. 145*: 93 (1975).

12. Childs, R. E., and Bardsley, W. G., *J. Theor. Biol. 53*: 381 (1975).

13. Cleland, W. W., *Biochim. Biophys. Acta 67*: 104 (1963).

14. Cleland, W. W., *Biochim. Biophys. Acta 67*: 173 (1963).

15. Cleland, W. W., *Biochim. Biophys. Acta 67*: 188 (1963).

16. Cockle, S. M., and Harkness, R. A., *Br. J. Obstet. Gynaecol. 85*: 776 (1978).

17. Dolman, D., Dunford, H. B., Chowdhury, D. M., and Morrison, M., *Biochemistry 7*: 3991 (1968).

18. Dubin, A., and Silberring, J., *Anal. Biochem. 72*: 372 (1976).

19. Edelhoch, H., Irace, G., Johnson, M. L., Michot, J. L., and Nunez, J., *J. Biol. Chem. 254*: 11822 (1979).

20. Erman, J. E., and Yonetani, T., *Biochim. Biophys. Acta 393*: 343 (1975).

21. Gelberg, N. T., and Schultz, J., *Arch. Biochem. Biophys. 148*: 407 (1972).

22. Gerdinand, W. C., *Biochem. J. 98*: 278 (1966).

23. Gawenh, K., Wielinger, H., and Werner, W., *Z. Anal. Chem. 252*: 222 (1970).

24. Goldbeter, A., and Caplan, S. R., *Ann. Rev. Biophys. Bioeng. 5*: 449 (1976).

25. Groome, N. P., *J. Clin. Chem. Clin. Biochem. 18*: 345 (1980).

26. Harrison, J. E., Pabalan, S., and Schultz, J., *Biochim. Biophys. Acta 493247* (1977).

27. Harrison, J. E., and Schultz, J., *Biochim. Biophys. Acta 536*: 341 (1978).

28. Harrison, J. E., Watson, B. D., and Schultz, J., *FEBS Lett. 92*: 327 (1978).

29. Harrison, J. E., Araiso, T., Palcic, M. M., and Dunford, H. B., *Biochem. Biophys. Res. Commun. 94*: 34 (1980).

30. Hayaishi, O., in *Oxygenases*, Academic Press, New York, 1962.

31. Held, A. M., and Hurst, J. K., *Biochem. Biophys. Res. Commun. 81*: 878 (1978).

32. Hünig, S., Balli, H., Conrad, H., and Schott, A., *Ann. Chem. 676*: 36 (1964).

33. Kimura, S., and Yamazaki, I., *Arch. Biochem. Biophys. 189*: 14 (1978).

34. Kimura S., and Yamazaki, I., *Arch. Biochem. Biophys. 198*: 580 (1979).
35. Klebanoff, S. J., *J. Biol. Chem. 249*: 3724 (1974).
36. Lamas, L., *Eur. J. Biochem. 96*: 93 (1979).
37. Lang, H., Hönel, H., and Hahn, H., *Z. Anal. Chem. 201*: 321 (1964).
38. Løvstad, R. A., *Gen. Pharmacol. 11*: 331 (1980).
39. Maehly, A. C., and Chance, B., in *Methods of Biochemical Analysis*, Glick, D. (Ed.), Vol. 1, Interscience, New York, p. 357 (1954).
40. Maguire, R. J., and Dunford, H. B., *Can. J. Biochem. 49*: 1165 (1971).
41. Maguire, R. J., and Dunford, H. B., *Biochemistry 11*: 937 (1972).
42. Merrill, D. P., *Prep. Biochem. 10*: 133 (1980).
43. Migler, R., and DeChatelet, L. R., *Biochem. Med. 19*: 16 (1978).
44. Morrison, M., *Methods Enzymol. 70*: 214 (1980).
45. Nakamura, S., Yokota, K., and Yamazaki, I., *Nature 222*: 794 (1969).
46. Naskalski, J. W., *Biochim. Biophys. Acta 485*: 291 (1977).
47. Ohtaki, S., Nakagawa, H., and Yamazaki, I., *FEBS Lett. 109*: 71 (1980).
48. Olsen, L. F., and Degn, H., *Biochim. Biophys. Acta 523*: 321 (1978).
49. Patriarca, P., Dri, P., and Snidoro, M., *J. Lab. Clin. Med. 90*: 289 (1977).
50. Paul, K. G., in *The Enzymes*, Boyer, P. B. Lardy, H., and Myrback, K. (Eds.), Academic Press, New York, p. 227 (1963).
51. Pickering, A., Oram, J. D., and Reiter, B., *J. Dairy Res. 29*: 151 (1962).
52. Polis, B. D., and Shmukler, H. W., *J. Biol. Chem. 201*: 475 (1953).
53. Pommier, J., and Cahnmann, H. J., *J. Biol. Chem. 254*: 3006 (1979).
54. Porstmann, B., Porstmann, T., and Nugel, E., *J. Clin. Chem. Clin. Biochem. 19*: 435 (1981).
55. Rest, K. F., and Spitznagel, J. K., *Biochem. J. 166*: 145 (1977).
56. Saunders, B. C., Holmes-Siedle, A. G., and Stark, B. P., in *Peroxidase*, Butterworths, London (1964).
57. Segal, R., and Dunford, H. B., *Can. J. Biochem. 46*: 1470 (1968).
58. Shindler, J. S., and Bardsley, W. G., *Biochem. Biophys. Res. Commun. 67*: 1307 (1975).
59. Solano-Muñoz, F., Bardsley, W. G., and Indge, K. J., *Biochem. J. 195*: 589 (1981).

60. Solano-Muñoz, F., Iborra, J. L., Lozano, J. A., and Bardsley, W. G., *Int. J. Biochem. 15:* 1195 (1983).

61. Splittgerber, A. G., and Tappel, A. L., *J. Biol. Chem. 254:* 9807 (1979).

62. Stelmaszynska, T., and Zgliczynski, J. M., *Eur. J. Biochem. 45:* 305 (1974).

63. Tamura, Y., and Morita, Y., *J. Biochem. 78:* 561 (1975).

64. Threatte, R. M., Fregly, M. J., Field, F. P., and Jones, P. K., *J. Pharm. Sci. 68:* 1530 (1979).

65. Virion, A., Pommier, J., Deme, D., and Nunez, J., *Eur. J. Biochem. 117:* 103 (1981).

66. Wardell, J. M., Bardsley, W. G., Kavanagh, J. P., and Wood, R. M., *J. Theor. Biol. 95:* 465 (1982).

67. Werner, W., Ray, H.-G., and Wielinger, H., *Z. Anal. Chem. 252:* 224 (1970).

68. Wever, R., Hamers, M. N., Weening, R. S., and Roos, D., *Eur. J. Biochem. 108:* 491 (1980).

69. Wu, N. C., and Schultz, J., *FEBS Lett. 60:* 141 (1975).

70. Yamazaki, I., and Piette, L. H., *Biochim. Biophys. Acta 50:* 62 (1961).

71. Yamazaki, I., Yokota, K., and Nakajima, R., *Biochem. Biophys. Res. Commun. 21:* 582 (1965).

72. Yamazaki, I., in *Molecular Mechanisims of Oxygen Activation,* Hayaishi, O. (Ed.), Academic Press, New York, p. 535 (1974).

73. Yokota, K., and Yamazaki, I., *Biochemistry 16:* 1913 (1977).

74. Andrews, P. C., and Krinsky, N. I., *J. Biol. Chem. 257:* 13240 (1982).

75. Bardsley, W. G., and Wright, A. J., *J. Mol. Biol. 165:* 163 (1983).

76. Bardsley, W. G., Solano-Muñoz, F., Wright, A. J., and McGinlay, P. B., *J. Mol. Biol. 169:* 597 (1983).

77. Burguillo, F. J., Wright, A. J., and Bardsley, W. G., *Biochem. J. 211:* 23 (1983).

78. Courtin, F., Deme, D., Virion, A., Michot, J. L., Pommier, J., and Nunez, J., *Eur. J. Biochem. 124:* 603 (1982).

79. Kanofsky, J. R., *J. Biol. Chem. 258:* 5991 (1983).

80. Kitagawa, T., Hashimoto, S., Teraoka, J., Nakamura, S., Yajima, H., and Hosova, T., *Biochemistry 22:* 2788 (1983).

81. Honka, E., Ohlsson, P. I., and Paul, K. G., *Acta Chem. Scand. B36:* 273 (1982).

82. Lambeir, A.-M., and Dunford, H. B., *Arch. Biochem. Biophys. 220:* 549 (1983).

83. Libby, R. D., Thomas, J. A., Kaiser, L. W., and Hager, L. P., *J. Biol. Chem. 257:* 5030 (1982).

84. Mäkinen, K. K., and Mäkinen, P.-L., *Eur. J. Biochem. 123:* 171 (1982).

85. Mäkinen, K. K., and Mäkinen, P.-L., *FEBS Lett.* *137*: 276 (1982).
86. Mäkinen, K. K., and Mäkinen, P.-L., *Biochem. Biophys. Res. Commun.* *105*: 1402 (1982).
87. Mäkinen, K. K., and Tenovuo, J., *Anal. Biochem.* *126*: 100 (1982).
88. Nakamura, M., Yamazaki, I., Nakagawa, H., and Ohtaki, S., *J. Biol. Chem.* *258*: 3837 (1983).
89. Ohtaki, S., Nakagawa, H., Nakamura, M., and Yamazaki, I., *J. Biol. Chem.* *257*: 761 (1982).
90. Ohtaki, S., Nakagawa, H., Kimura, S., and Yamazaki, I., *J. Biol. Chem.* *256*: 805 (1981).
91. Pruitt, K., Tenovuo, J. Andrews, R. W., and McKane, T., *Biochemistry* *21*:562 (1982).
92. Pruitt, K., and Tenovuo, J., *Biochim. Biophys. Acta* *704*: 204 (1982).
93. Ramakrishnan, K., Oppenhuizen, M. E., Saunders, S., and Fisher, J., *Biochemistry* *22*: 3271 (1983).
94. Shahangian, S., and Hager, L. P., *J. Biol. Chem.* *256*: 6034 (1981).
95. Shindler, J. S. Childs, R. E., and Bardsley, W. G., *Eur. J. Biochem.* *65*: 325 (1976).
96. Thomas, E. L., Jefferson, M. M., and Grisham, M B., *Biochemistry* *21*: 6299 (1982).
97. Wever, R., Kast, W. M., Kasinoedin, J. H., and Boelens, R., *Biochim. Biophys. Acta* *709*: 212 (1982).
98. Wildberger, E., Von Gruenigen, C., Kohler, J., Kohler, H., and Studer, H., *Eur. J. Biochem.* *130*: 485 (1983).

5

Genetic Variation of Salivary Peroxidase

EDWIN A. AZEN / *University of Wisconsin, Madison, Wisconsin*

I. INTRODUCTION: GENETIC POLYMORPHISMS IN PAROTID SALIVA

Parotid saliva has proven especially useful for genetic studies of protein polymorphisms and, for these studies, has distinct advantages over the whole saliva. Thus, unlike whole saliva, the parotid fluid is relatively uncontaminated with food, bacteria, or cell debris. Since it is a thin watery secretion with lower mucus content, it is easier to handle and process than is whole saliva. Furthermore, many parotid fluid proteins are more stable and less rapidly degraded in parotid fluid than when the same proteins are studied in the whole saliva.

We and other workers previously described genetic polymorphisms
in parotid saliva among a number of proteins, including salivary peroxidase, proline-rich proteins, amylase, vitamin B_{12}-binding proteins,
and histidine-rich basic proteins. Some of these data were recently
reviewed (4). Since this review, several other genetic protein polymorphisms were discovered in parotid saliva (7-10,28,39,48,62). These
salivary polymorphisms may prove especially useful in defining genetic
variability in populations and individuals, in understanding molecular
mechanisms of protein variations, in elucidating evolutionary patterns,
and in studying genetic linkage relationships. The salivary protein
polymorphisms may also be useful in studying the genetic background
of common dental diseases.

I will now discuss in more detail genetic polymorphisms found
among the many proline-rich proteins (PRPs) since, as will be shown
later, there is an important relationship between salivary peroxidase
(SAPX) and one acidic PRP called the parotid acidic (Pa) protein.
The PRPs constitute about 70% of the human salivary proteins (32).
They are unique in their composition of amino acids. Glycine, glutamic
acid, and proline together constitute about 75% of the amino acid residues, with proline alone constituting 25% of a typical protein in this
family. Among the PRPs, there is a great diversity of molecular sizes,
ionic charges, and number of carbohydrates and phosphate groups
(11,12,14,17,22,32,34,35,37,45,46).

Although the members of the PRP family show some differences,
they also show striking common properties including similar amino acid
compositions (11,12,14,15,22,32,34,35,37,49) and amino acid sequences
(29,41,45,46,49,50-53), immunologic relatedness (9,19,33,48), and
close linkage of their genetic determinants on one of the autosomal
human chromosomes (2,8-10,47,48,54,62). We have termed the closely
linked group of genes producing the PRPs the salivary protein gene
complex (SPC) (54). Each of the genes are expressed in saliva as
different polymorphisms, so that different combinations of variations
in these proteins are seen in different individuals in all racial groups
studied (2,4,8-10,27,28,48,54,62). The frequent expression of null
types (that is, the absence of one or more PRPs in saliva) is an unusual and notable characteristic of a number of the recognized polymorphisms of the SPC. Recently, human PRP genes have been isolated,
cloned, and partially characterized by restriction mapping and DNA
sequencing (55).

I will discuss later, more fully, one of the polymorphic PRPs (the
Pa protein) in reference to the SAPX proteins, but, at this point,
would like to mention briefly some of its general features. The Pa
protein has a molecular weight in the range of 50,000-150,000 with an
isoelectric point in the range of 3.9-4.5 (17). It is also phosphoryla-
ted (6) and disulfide bonded (3,4). Thus, it is present in the saliva
as a presumed dimer and can be dissociated by 2-mercaptoethanol into
a thiol monomer (Pa-SH). The Pa protein is absent from some salivas.

As will be discussed later, the presence of the Pa protein correlates perfectly with a modified form of SAPX, and the absence of the Pa protein with an unmodified form of SAPX. We postulate, on the basis of evidence to be presented later, that the Pa protein is a direct modifier of the SAPX protein by protein-protein interaction through disulfide bond formation.

II. ELECTROPHORETIC DESCRIPTION OF THE DIFFERENT GENETICALLY DETERMINED FORMS OF SAPX

We previously found in parotid saliva genetic variants of SAPX with different electrophoretic mobilities in acid slab polyacrylamide gels stained with p-phenylenediamine and hydrogen peroxide (3). The two most common genetic types are shown in Fig. 1, channels 7 and 8. Channel 7 shows the slow type (SAPX 2, major band labeled S), and channel 8 shows the fast type (SAPX 1, major band labeled F). We also found an uncommon variant termed SAPX 3 (not shown in Fig. 1), which migrates slower than SAPX 2. We also studied myeloperoxidase extracted from the leukocytes of 45 randomly collected samples from whites in order to compare its electrophoretic pattern with that of SAPX. A major band migrating faster than the major fast SAPX band was observed. We found no genetic variation of myeloperoxidase in this small sample in contradistinction to the results with the SAPX proteins.

III. INHERITANCE OF SAPX TYPES AND POPULATION DATA

We studied 14 families (3) and found that the expression of the gene determining the slow SAPX 2 type is completely dominant, whereas that of the gene determining the fast SAPX 1 type is recessive. Clearly in this study, SAPX 1 × SAPX 1 matings always give SAPX 1 offspring, whereas SAPX 2 × SAPX 2 matings occasionally give SAPX 1 offspring (Table 1). If we assume autosomal inheritance with expression of the gene determining the SAPX 2 type being completely dominant and that determining the SAPX 1 type being recessive, the numbers of expected offspring closely fit the observed values (Table 1). These family data fit the genetic hypothesis. Expected values for Table 1 were determined using the following gene frequencies of SAPX for whites. Among 101 randomly collected samples from whites, gene frequencies are: SAPX 1 = 0.787, SAPX 2 = .208 and SAPX 3 = 0.005. (SAPX 3 is an uncommon dominantly expressed variant in whites.)

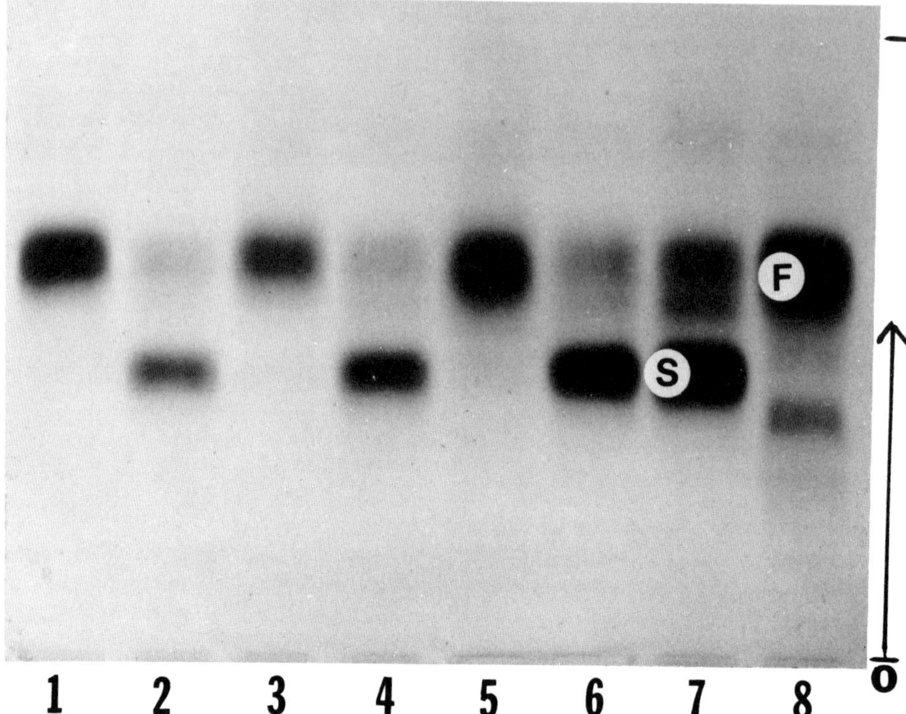

Figure 1 2-Mercaptoethanol dissociates SAPX 2 to give SAPX 1. Parotid saliva was incubated with 2-mercaptoethanol at 37°C. The incubation mixture contained parotid saliva of SAPX 2 type, 2-mercaptoethanol $(5 \times 10^{-4}$ M), and aprotinin (200 U/ml). Samples were electrophoresed. in an acid polyacrylamide slab gel and were stained with p-phenylenediamine. There was no effect of 2-mercaptoethanol on the SAPX 1 type, but the same effect of 2-mercaptoethanol was seen on the SAPX 3 type (not shown). Channels: 1, treated, 15 min; 2, untreated, 15 min; 3, treated, 30 min; 4, untreated, 30 min; 5, treated, 60 min; 6, untreated, 60 min; 7, fresh control, SAPX 2 type; 8, fresh control, SAPX 1 type. (From Ref. 3.)

IV. EVIDENCE FOR MODIFICATION OF SAPX

We found strong evidence (although it is not conclusive) that the electrophoretically slower-migrating forms of SAPX (SAPX 2 and SAPX 3) represent modified forms of the faster-migrating form, SAPX 1 (3).

First, family data indicate completely codominant expression of the SAPX 2 and SAPX 3 types, whereas the SAPX 1 type shows recessive

Table 1 Salivary Peroxidase Types in 14 Families

	Offspring			
	SAPX 1		SAPX 2	
Parental type	Observed	Expected	Observed	Expected
SAPX 1 × SAPX 2 (4)	6	5.7	7	7.3
SAPX 2 × SAPX 2 (4)	2	3.6	10	8.4
SAPX 1 × SAPX 1 (6)	21	21	0	0

Source: Ref. 3.

inheritance. A classic parallel example is the ABO blood group system
(44) where type A and B modifications are expressed as codominant
characteristics, whereas the unmodified type O is recessive. Second,
the presumed modified forms of SAPX (SAPX 2 and SAPX 3) show
larger molecular weights than the presumed unmodified form (SAPX 1).
The molecular weights of SAPX 1 and SAPX 2 were determined in polyacrylamide gels (25). The molecular weight of SAPX 1 is in the range
of 68,000-76,000 and that of SAPX 2 in the range of 93,000-126,000.
Third, the larger molecular weight, slower-migrating forms (SAPX 2
and SAPX 3) can be converted to the smaller and faster-migrating form
(SAPX 1) by splitting disulfide bonds. Thus, as is shown in Fig. 1,
channels 1-6, treatment of parotid saliva with 2-mercaptoethanol converts the SAPX 2 type to the SAPX 1 type. From this experiment, it
appears likely that 2-mercaptoethanol has dissociated a disulfied bonded complex between the SAPX 1 protein and another unidentified molecule. We later present evidence that this unidentified molecule may be
the Pa protein thiol monomer (Pa-SH). We were not successful in detecting by protein staining the material dissociated from the SAPX 2
and SAPX 3 complexes. If the unidentified complexing molecule is a
protein, its concentration may be too low to detect by standard protein staining.

V. CORRELATION IN SALIVA BETWEEN GENETIC
VARIANTS OF Pa AND SAPX PROTEINS

When saliva samples were typed for both the Pa and SAPX protein polymorphisms, we were surprised to find a perfect correspondence between Pa and SAPX genetic types. The presence of the Pa protein
in either its common form (Pa 1) or much less common form (Pa 2)
correlates perfectly with "modified" SAPX types (SAPX 2 and SAPX 3),

respectively. On the other hand, the absence of the Pa proteins
(Pa 0) correlates perfectly with the presence of the "unmodified"
SAPX 1 type. A study of randomly collected saliva samples (3) shows
a perfect correlation between Pa 1 and SAPX 2 types, and between Pa
0 and SAPX 1 types as is demonstrated in Table 2. The perfect correlation of the uncommon Pa 2 type with the uncommon SAPX 3 type was
observed in one family (not shown in Table 2).

Although there is a perfect correspondence of genetic types, the
Pa 1 and SAPX 2 proteins are not the same for the following reasons.
First, they migrate with different electrophoretic mobilities in gels.
Furthermore, neuraminidase modifies SAPX (as assessed by electro-
phoretic changes in mobilities) but does not affect the Pa proteins.
Finally, after autoincubation of saliva, endogenous proteolysis causes
partial degradation of the SAPX 2 protein but does not affect the Pa 1
protein.

VI.   THE Pa PROTEIN THIOL MONOMER (Pa–SH)
MAY MODIFY SAPX

The data presented in the previous sections strongly indicate that
the Pa protein thiol monomer (Pa–SH) may modify SAPX 1 through disulfide bond formation. These data include the following. First, the
occurrence of the Pa 1 and Pa 2 proteins correlates perfectly with that
of the codominantly inherited SAPX 2 and SAPX 3 types, and the Pa 0
types with the recessively inherited SAPX 1 type, respectively.
Second, the Pa 1, SAPX 2, and SAPX 3 proteins are shown to be disul-
fide-bonded molecules. Third, 2-mercaptoethanol, a disulfide-splitting
agent, converts the modified SAPX 2 and SAPX 3 types to the unmodified SAPX 1 type.

On the basis of these data, it is postulated that under suitable
conditions the following reactions might occur:

Table 2   Randomly Collected Saliva
Samples From 101 Whites, 17 Blacks,
and 8 Chinese Typed for SAPX and Pa

	Pa+	Pa−	
SAPX 1	0	80	80
SAPX 2	46	0	46
Total	46	80	126

Reduction of Pa dimer:

Pa dimer + molecule with reactive $-SH \rightarrow$ Pa monomer + mixed disulfide

(Pa 1)-S-S-(Pa 1) + 2R-SH $\rightarrow$ 2(Pa 1)-SH + RSSR

Oxidation of Pa monomer:

Pa monomer + SAPX 1 + oxidizing agent $\rightarrow$ SAPX 2 + water

(Pa 1)-SH + (SAPX 1)-SH + [0] $\rightarrow$ (SAPX 1)-S-S-(Pa 1) + H_2O

A similar reaction might occur between the Pa 2 monomer and SAPX 1 to give SAPX 3. From our studies, the postulated modifier has a molecular weight in the range of 17,000-58,000. This molecular weight roughtly fits the expectation for the postulated Pa 1 monomer. However, it will be necessary to characterize biochemically the different SAPX types in order to either prove or disprove this modification hypothesis.

VII. BIOLOGICAL AND CLINICAL CONSIDERATIONS OF THE SAPX PROTEIN POLYMORPHISM

Does the occurrence of genetic variants of SAPX proteins in the saliva have any biological significance? This question is important, since many studies note the occurrence and significance of an antibacterial system consisting of peroxidase, thiocyanate (SCN^-), and hydrogen peroxide (20,30,31,36,42). As a first step in answering this question, we investigated enzymatic activities of SAPX in individuals with different genetically determined SAPX types (5). SAPX enzyme activities were assessed using a p-phenylenediamine substrate (38). In comparing randomly collected salivas of 47 SAPX 1 and 31 SAPX 2 types, we found no significant differences in any of the parameters studied, including age, sex, smoking history, SAPX enzyme activity, protein concentration, SCN^- concentration, or flow rate. Smokers showed significantly higher levels of SCN^- ($p = < 0.0001$), lower SAPX enzyme activity ($p = 0.005$), and greater age ($p = 0.0003$) compared with nonsmokers. Significant correlations were found between salivary flow rate and SCN^- concentration ($r = -0.34$, $p = 0.05$), SAPX enzyme activity and age ($r = -0.38$, $p = 0.001$), SAPX enzyme activity and protein concentration ($r = 0.26$, $p = 0.02$), and salivary SCN^- concentration and age ($r = 0.23$, $p = 0.05$).

Although we did not find significant quantitative differences in SAPX enzyme activities between the two groups (SAPX 1 and SAPX 2), perhaps future studies, in which other substrates (including oral pathogenic bacteria) are used and a more refined kinetic analysis is done, might reveal differences. However, in the study referred to previously (5), we did find a suggestive difference in the frequency distributions of SAPX enzyme activities in the two populations (SAPX 1 and SAPX 2). The frequency distribution of the SAPX 2 type appeared bimodal with overlap of the two modes. However, the frequency distribution of the SAPX 1 type appeared unimodal. If bimodality of the frequency distribution of the SAPX 2 type can be confirmed, the most likely explanation would be the presence of a subtle molecular (perhaps genetic) heterogeneity in the non-SAPX material (perhaps the Pa protein thiol monomer) complexed to the SAPX protein.

It is possible that different genetic variants of SAPX may vary in function. Thus, the different SAPX proteins may vary in their enzymatic activities or in their binding to different substrates or bacteria, or they may show differences in their stabilities in solution or at tooth surfaces. The effect of SAPX at the tooth surfaces may be important, since SAPX has been shown to be one of the factors controlling bacterial plaque formation (26). It is interesting that SAPX has been shown to bind to a variety of surfaces such as enamel, human salivary sediment, hydroxyapatite powder, and various species of streptococci. Other workers (40) showed that SAPX is concentrated at tooth surfaces by adsorption, and it is believed that bound forms of SAPX may be more stable than the soluble forms (43). Thus, if the various forms of SAPX differ in their binding properties, they may also differ in their stabilities.

If the Pa protein (an acidic Pr protein) is complexed to SAPX, then these complexed forms of SAPX may share some biological properties with the class of acidic Pr proteins. For example, it has been shown that acidic Pr proteins bind avidly to hydroxyapatite and to tooth enamel (1,21) and also bind calcium (13,15). The acidic Pr proteins may also play a role in governing calcium concentration in saliva (23,24,41). The protein-bound phosphate of acidic Pr proteins may be important in binding calcium to the proteins and in attaching the proteins to enamel surfaces (16).

There are conflicting clinical data for the possible role of PRP in oral disease. Studies in caries-free and caries-resistant adults (56, 57) show no relationship of some genetic PRP phenotypes to disease susceptibility. Other studies (58) show no evidence that the caries status and propensity to calculus formation are associated with abnormal levels of acidic PRP. However, two other studies show possible relationships between PRP genetic phenotypes and dental disease (59,60). One of these studies (59) is of particular interest since the Pa+ phenotype (also SAPX 2) is associated with an increased DMFS score compared with the Pa0 phenotype (also SAPX 1). Another study (61) showed no significant differences in components of the lactoperoxidase system in caries-resistant versus caries-susceptible adults. Clearly, more studies are needed to clarify the biochemical, biological, and functional properties of the SAPX protein variants and their possible clinical relationships.

VIII. SUMMARY

Salivary peroxidase (SAPX) exists in several genetically determined
forms that differ in molecular weight, SAPX 2 and SAPX 3 types being
larger than the SAPX 1 type. Two of these forms (SAPX 2 and SAPX
3) are probably complexes of SAPX 1 with the acidic PRPs, Pa 1 and
Pa 2 thiol monomers, respectively, through disulfide bond formation.
The biological significance of these findings has not been determined.

ACKNOWLEDGMENT

This study was supported by a grant from the National Institutes
of Dental Research (DEO 3658-17), and is Paper No. 2550 of the Laboratory of Genetics, University of Wisconsin, Madison, Wisconsin.

REFERENCES

1.   Armstrong, W. G., *Arch. Oral Biol. 15*: 1001 (1970).
2.   Azen, E. A., and Denniston, C. L., *Biochem. Genet. 12*: 109
     (1974).
3.   Azen, E. A., *Biochem. Genet. 15*: 9 (1977).
4.   Azen, E. A., *Biochem. Genet. 16*: 79 (1978).
5.   Azen, E. A., *Arch. Oral Biol. 23*: 801 (1978).
6.   Azen, E. A., *Arch. Oral Biol. 23*: 1173 (1978).
7.   Azen, E. A., and Denniston, C., *Biochem. Genet. 17*: 909
     (1979).
8.   Azen, E. A., Hurley, C. K., and Denniston, C., *Biochem.
     Genet. 17*: 257 (1979).
9.   Azen, E. A., and Denniston, C., *Biochem. Genet. 18*: 483
     (1980).
10. Azen, E. A., and Denniston, C., *Biochem. Genet. 19*: 475
     (1981).
11. Bennick, A., and Connell, G. E., *Biochem. J. 123*: 455 (1971).
12. Bennick, A., *Biochem. J., 145*: 557 (1975).
13. Bennick, A., *Biochem. J. 155*:163 (1976).
14. Bennick, A., *Biochem. J. 163*: 229 (1977).
15. Bennick, A., *Biochem. J. 163*: 241 (1977).
16. Bennick, A., Cannon, M., and Madapallimattam, G., *Biochem.
     J. 183*: 115 (1979).
17. Friedman, R. D., and Merritt, A. D., *Am. J. Hum. Genet. 27*:
     304 (1975).
18. Friedman, R. D., Merritt, A. D., and Rivas, M. L., *Am. J.
     Hum. Genet. 27*: 292 (1975).
19. Friedman, R. D., and Karn, R. C., *Biochem. Genet. 15*: 549
     (1977).

20. Hamon, C. B., and Klebanoff, S. J., *J. Exp. Med.* *137*: 438
     (1973).
21. Hay, D. I., *Arch. Oral Biol.* *18*: 1517 (1973).
22. Hay, D. I., and Oppenheim, F. G., *Arch. Oral Biol.* *19*: 627
     (1974).
23. Hay, D. I., and Grøn, P., in *Proceedings—Microbial Aspects
     of Dental Caries,* Sp. Supp. Microbiol. Abst., Stiles, H. M.,
     Loesch, W. I., and O'Brien, T. C., (Eds.), pp. 143 (1977).
24. Hay, D. I., and Schlessinger, D. H., in *Proceedings of the
     International Symposium on Calcium Binding Proteins and
     Calcium Function in Health and Disease,* Wasserman, R. W.
     (Ed.), North Holland, New York (1977).
25. Hedrick, J. L., and Smith, A. J., *Arch. Biochem. Biophys.*
     126: 155 (1968).
26. Hoogendoorn, H., and Moorer, R., *Odontol. Revy 24*: 355
     (1973).
27. Ikemoto, S., Minaguchi, K., Suzuki, K., and Tomita, K.,
     Science 197: 378 (1977).
28. Ikemoto, S., Minaguchi, K., Tomita, K., and Suzuki, K.,
     Ann. Hum. Genet. (Lond.) 43: 11 (1979).
29. Isemura, S., Saitoh, E., and Sanada, K., *J. Biochem. 87*:
     1071 (1980).
30. Iwamoto, Y., and Matsumura, T., *Arch. Oral Biol. 11*: 667
     (1966).
31. Iwamoto, Y., Nakamura, R., Tsunemitsu, A., and Matsumura,
     T., *Arch. Oral Biol. 13*: 1015 (1968).
32. Kauffman, D. L., and Keller, P. J., *Arch. Oral Biol. 24*: 249
     (1979).
33. Kousvelari, E. E., and Oppenheim, F. G., *Biochim. Biophys.
     Acta 578*: 76 (1979).
34. Levine, M. J., Ellison, S. A., and Bahl, O. P., *Arch. Oral
     Biol. 18*: 827 (1973).
35. Levine, M., and Keller, P. J., *Arch. Oral Biol. 22*: 37 (1977).
36. Morrison, M., and Steele, W. F., in *Biology of the Mouth,*
     Publication No. 89, American Association for the Advancement
     of Science, Washington, D.C., p. 89 (1968).
37. Oppenheim, F. G., Hay, D. I., and Franzblau, C., *Biochem-
     istry 10*: 4233 (1971).
38. Pilz, H., O'Brien, J. S., and Heipertz, R., *Clin. Biochem. 9*:
     85 (1976).
39. Pronk, J. C., and Frants, R. R., *Hum. Hered. 29*: 181 (1979).
40. Pruitt, K. M., and Adamson, M., *Infect. Immun. 17*: 112
     (1977).
41. Schlessinger, D. H., Jacobs, R., and Hay, D. I., in *Peptides,
     Proceedings of the 5th American Peptide Symposium,* Goodman,
     M., and Meinhofer, J. (Eds.), Wiley, New York, p. 56 (1977).

42. Slowey, R. R., Eidelman, S., and Klebanoff, S. J., *J. Bacteriol. 96*: 575 (1968).
43. Tenovuo, J., and Kurkijarvi, K., *Arch. Oral Biol. 26*: 309 (1981).
44. Watkins, W. M., *Science 152*: 172 (1966).
45. Wong, R. S. C., Hoffman, T., and Bennick, A., *J. Biol. Chem. 254*: 4800 (1979).
46. Wong, R. S. C., and Bennick, A., *J. Biol. Chem. 255*: 5943 (1979).
47. Yu, P. L., Karn, R. C., Merritt, A. D., Azen, E. A., and Conneally, P. M., *Am. J. Hum. Genet. 32*: 555 (1980).
48. Azen, E. A., and Yu, P. L., *Biochem, Genet. 22*: 1 (1984).
49. Bennick, A., *Mol. Cell. Biochem. 45*: 83 (1982).
50. Kauffman, D., Wong, R., Bennick, A., and Keller, P., *Biochemistry 21*: 6558 (1982).
51. Saitoh, E., Isemura, S., and Sanada, K., *J. Biochem. 93*: 883 (1983).
52. Shimomura, H., Kanai, Y., and Sanada, K., *J. Biochem. 93*: 857 (1983).
53. Schlessinger, D. H., Jacobs, R., and Hay, D. I., in *Peptides, Proceedings of the Sixth American Peptide Symposium*, Gross, E. and Meienhofer, J. (Eds.), Pierce Chemical Co., Rockford, Ill., p. 133 (1979).
54. Goodman, P. A., Yu, P. L., Azen, E. A., and Karn, R. C., *Am. J. Hum. Genet. 34*: 182A (1982).
55. Azen, E., Lyons, K., McGonigal, T., Barrett, N., Clements, S., Maeda, N., Vanin, E. F., Carlson, D., and Smithies, O. *Proc. Natl. Acad. Sci. 81*: 5562 (1984).
56. Anderson, L. C., Lamberts, B. L., and Bruton, W. F., *J. Dent. Res. 61*: 393 (1982).
57. Anderson, L. C., and Mandel, I. D., *J. Dent. Res. 61*: 1167 (1982).
58. Mandel, I. D., and Bennick, A., *J. Dent. Res. 62*: 943 (1983).
59. Yu, P. L., Bixler, D., Goodman, P. A., Azen, E. A., and Karn, R. C. (submitted for publication).
60. Friedman, R. D., Azen, E. A., Yu, P. L., Green, P. A. Karn, R. C., and Merritt, A. D., *Hum. Hered. 30*: 372 (1980).
61. Mandel, I. D., Behrman, J., Levy, R., and Weinstein, D. J., *J. Dent. Res. 62*: 922 (1983).
62. Azen, E. A., and Yu, P. L., *Biochem. Genet. Supress. 22*: 1065 (1984).

6

The Peroxidase System in Human Secretions

JORMA O. TENOVUO / *Institute of Dentistry, University of Turku, Turku, Finland*

I. INTRODUCTION

After the first report of peroxidase activity in bovine milk (26), almost 20 years elapsed before a significant purification of this enzyme was reported and the name lactoperoxidase (LP) was used (119). Later, several relatively simple procedures for the isolation and purification of cow's milk LP in very high yield were developed (2,62,73).

The basic work of mapping the localization of LP at the tissue level was done by Morrison and coworkers (63-66). With immunochemical and isolation studies they demonstrated LP in the salivary, lacrimal, harderian and mammary glands but not in any other bovine tissues. Subsequent studies of human secretions have shown peroxidase activity in saliva (93), tears (125), cervical mucus (92), milk (25), and nasal glands (128). However, recently it was shown that there is no detectable LP secreted in human milk (60). The peroxidase activity observed in human milk is probably derived from milk leukocytes.

LP is also present in the salivary glands of pig (66), monkeys (54, 55), rats (56), guinea pigs (46), and hamsters (46), and peroxidase activity has been detected in rat lacrimal gland (56), as well as in sow (58) and guinea pig milk (96). In mouse, rat, and guinea pig, peroxidase activity has been found also in the larynx (38), tracheal epithelium (11,129), stomach (6), and colon (126). Peroxidase activity is also present in hog intestine mucosa (95).

Other peroxidases in the human body include neutrophil myeloperoxidase (89), eosinophil peroxidase (130), glutathione peroxidase (22), thyroid peroxidase (1), and uterine peroxidase (92). Human breast cancer tissue also contains peroxidase activity of unknown origin (36). This activity has been suggested to be estrogen dependent (18), but contradictory views have also been presented (39). Various human peroxidases, their sources, and proposed functions in vivo are presented in Table 1.

II. THE PEROXIDASE SYSTEM IN THE HUMAN MOUTH

A. Salivary Peroxidase

1. Origin and Nature of Peroxidase Activity in Saliva

The presence of peroxidase activity in human saliva has been known for many years, but it was not until the early 1950s that the first actual peroxidase assays were made (67,70). Although the source of the enzyme was unknown, it was suggested that the enzyme was probably derived from the salivary gland. Later it was demonstrated that in the human the "salivary" or "iodide" peroxidase (because of possible function in the metabolism of iodide) is present in the acini of the parotid glands (66,93) and that the enzyme has catalytic properties similar to those of bovine LP (86,103,108). Salivary peroxidase has common antigenic determinants with bovine LP (85) and similar heterogeneity and molecular weight distribution (32,115). Indeed, the similarity of the peroxidases from bovine milk, bovine salivary glands, and human saliva has led to the designation of the human salivary gland peroxidase as lactoperoxidase (64).

In contrast to bovine LP, human salivary LP has never been purified in high yield. The only significant purifications of human LP, reported from whole saliva (32) and parotid saliva (93), show that the human enzyme is a weakly basic protein with a molecular weight of

Table 1 Peroxidases in the Human Body

Enzyme	Source	Proposed function
Salivary peroxidase	Saliva	ψ
Lacrimal peroxidase	Lacrimal fluid	Antimicrobial ψ
Myeloperoxidase	Neutrophils	Antimicrobial
	Monocytes	Cytotoxic (tumor cells, platelets, etc.)
	Milk?	
Eosinophil peroxidase	Eosinophils	Antimicrobial
		Tumoricidal
Glutathione peroxidase	Erythrocytes	Integrity of cell membrane
Thyroid peroxidase	Thyroid gland	Iodine metabolism
Uterine peroxidase	Cervical mucus	Antimicrobial?
		Protein crosslinking?
Breast cancer peroxidase	Mammary tumors	?

80,000-100,000. Unfortunately, Slowey et al. (93), who obtained a 1026-fold purification, did not study the chemical characteristics of the enzyme. They showed that the purified product was devoid of amylase, lysozyme, and IgA but was antibacterial against *Lactobacillus acidophilus*. Revis (85) demonstrated in immunodiffusion experiments that antiserum to the purified bovine LP recognized both human parotid saliva and the immunogen. However, in immunoelectrophoresis the parotid saliva peroxidase had a less cathodal migration than bovine LP. This difference in mobility may be due to complexing of the positively charged human enzyme with one of the negatively charged proteins found in high concentration in parotid saliva (85). Indeed, Azen (4) demonstrated complexes between parotid peroxidase and some acidic proteins in saliva. Although all available evidence suggests that human salivary peroxidase is similar to bovine LP, no final conclusions should be drawn until successful purification and characterization of the human enzyme have been achieved. Thus, the name *lactoperoxidase* may not be appropriate for human salivary peroxidase, especially since recent observations suggest that the peroxidase in human milk is not lactoperoxidase (60). Therefore, instead of lactoperoxidase the name *salivary peroxidase* will be used in this article.

2. Heterogeneity of Salivary Peroxidase

Human salivary peroxidase has been shown to exist in multiple forms (33,34,52,115), a property which is also characteristic of bovine milk LP. Carlström (9) showed bovine milk LP to be extensively heterogenous and to consist of 10 electrophoretically different subfractions and, by chromatography on DEAE-Sephadex, Paul et al. (73) separated bovine LP into 5 fractions. Extensive chromatographic studies have indicated that human salivary peroxidase exists both in high (mol. wt. $\geqslant$150,000) and low (mol. wt. ~ 75,000) molecular weight forms that can be found in both whole and parotid saliva (52,115). The high molecular weight form may represent a peroxidase aggregate (91,115), although some complexing with other salivary constituents may also occur (4). The high molecular weight form is more stable than the low molecular weight form (115). Azen has thoroughly reviewed the genetic heterogeneity of salivary peroxidase in Chap. 5.

Human salivary peroxidase is heterogeneous with respect to electrophoretic mobility (4,34,52) as well as molecular weight. Depending on the technique used, the following pI values have been reported for parotid salivary peroxidase: 9.7, 7.1, and 6.4 (34), 8.1 (52,115), and 7-7.8 (52). With whole saliva, the values range from 4.3 (52,76, 115), 6.5 (76), and 8.1 (52,115) to 8.6 (76). Slight activity with pI values of 3.8, 7.3, and 9.5 has also been observed (76).

In conclusion, human parotid saliva peroxidase seems to have properties similar to bovine LP: molecular weight approximately 75,000, basic pI, and tendency to occur in aggregates or bound to acidic proteins. However, in whole saliva the profile of activity is more complex. Part of the activity in whole saliva is probably derived from oral leukocytes (52,53,70) (e.g., crevicular fluid leukocytes can release large quantities of myeloperoxidase) (45). There seems to be a positive correlation between orogranulocyte peroxidase activity and the severity of periodontal disease (43). It is also known that dental plaque is able to release myeloperoxidase from polymorphonuclear (PMN) leukocytes (99). The amount of peroxidase found in various oral samples is given in Table 2.

Peroxidases have been shown to act as marker enzymes in estrogen-responsive tissues, such as uterus and mammary gland (36). Recently, it was observed that the activity of human salivary peroxidase increased significantly during ovulation (13) and, therefore, it was suggested that salivary peroxidase assay may serve as an indicator for ovulation. However, further studies (Fig. 1) revealed that, although there is an increase in salivary peroxidase activity during the preovulatory period

Table 2 Reported Average Concentrations of Peroxidase, Thiocyanate (SCN^-), Hypothiocyanite ($OSCN^-$), and Iodide (I^-) in Various Oral Samples

	Peroxidase[a] ($\mu g/ml$)	SCN^- (μM)	$OSCN^-$ (μM)	I^- (μM)
Parotid saliva	1-13[b]	760-900[b,g]	52[b]	1-2[g]
Whole saliva				
Stimulated	2-13[b,c]	840-1400[b,h,i,m]	10-34[b,c,k]	10[i,m]
Resting	1-7[b-d]	1200-1450[b-d]	40-61[b,c,l]	?
Plaque fluid	(60-70)[e]	30-40[h]	?	2-3[h,m]
Gingival exudate	(0.2-1)[f]	30-50[j]	?	4-5[j,m]

[a]Assayed with ABTS [2,2'-azino-di-(3-ethyl-benzthiazoline-6-sulphonic acid)] as a substrate using bovine milk LP as a standard. The values indicate the range of enzyme concentrations found in various samples. The reported enzyme activities were converted to pure bovine LP concentrations using the conversion factor 25 mU/ml = $\mu g/ml$.
[b]From Ref. 81.
[c]From Ref. 116.
[d]From Ref. 114.
[e]Estimated from Ref. 14. The ABTS units were obtained by dividing pyrogallol units by 0.017.
[f]Estimated from Ref. 52. The ABTS units were obtained by dividing guaiacol units by 8.
[g]From Ref. 90.
[h]From Ref. 109.
[i]From Ref. 102.
[j]From Ref. 3.
[k]From Ref. 122.
[l]From Ref. 80.
[m]From Ref. 110.

(highest activity 3.8 ± 2.4 days before ovulation, n = 12), the individual variations are so large that peroxidase assay was concluded not to be a reliable marked for ovulation in individual samples (112). This area clearly requires further investigations since in rats, estradiol-17β seems to increase peroxidase activities both in uterus and in parotid and submandibular glands (113).

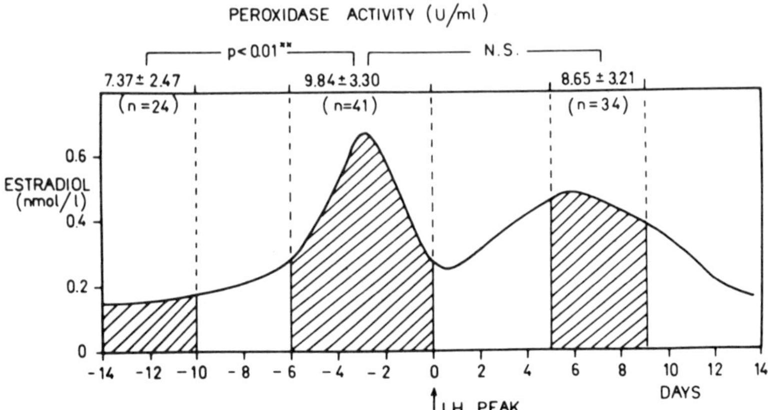

Figure 1 Variation in salivary peroxidase activity during menstrual cycles of 12 women. All samples from the periods with different levels of serum estrogen (hatched area) were analyzed and compared with each other. The estradiol curve is a reference curve obtained and used at the Unversity Central Hospital in Turku, Finland. Peroxidase activity is expressed as guaiacol units (53). (From Ref. 112.)

3. Adsorption of Salivary Peroxidase

Morrison and Steele (66) first demonstrated that LP binds to streptococci in an enzymatically active form. Later, detailed studies showed that the bound LP is slowly degraded or desorbed as the bacteria stand in saline suspension (79) and that increasing concentrations of phosphate desorbed LP effectively (103). In vitro, LP is readily adsorbed also by glass surfaces (29,80), synthetic hydroxyapatite (105), human enamel powder (78), and human salivary sediment (105). In all cases, the enzyme is bound in active form and retains its ability to inhibit hexokinase activity (78) and plaque acid production (105) as well as to produce $OSCN^-$ ions (108).

Recent studies have shown that in the human mouth the peroxidase is concentrated in dental plaque (14) and that the major part of the total activity in plaque is bound to plaque bacteria (109). Pruitt and Adamson (78) showed that the adsorption of LP to enamel may produce a 40% or greater increase in the concentration of LP in the enamel surface phase as compared with its concentration in liquid phase. Plaque fluid peroxidase activities are significantly higher in plaque of adults as compared with those of children (14).

Since many oral bacteria excrete peroxide, adsorption of salivary peroxidase to bacterial cells or tooth surfaces should be regarded as a favorable phenomenon for antibacterial effects. This binding would place the enzyme at the site of highest peroxide concentration, thus kinetically favoring the generation of antimicrobial oxidation products of SCN$^-$ (79). Similarly, the antimicrobial agents (OSCN$^-$ and others) generated by cell-bound peroxidase (108) would be at their greatest concentration in the immediate vicinity of their targets. Furthermore, bound peroxidase is more resistant to external inactivating factors than free peroxidase (111).

The current information suggests that adsorption of peroxidase to surfaces is simply a consequence of physicochemical forces between charged groups (77). However, recent findings of the binding of LP to immunoglobulins, especially to IgA (117), may indicate an additional, more complex adsorption phenomenon. Immunoglobulin A is frequently detected in pellicle (72) and in plaque (100), and it may act as a "carrier" for salivary peroxidase (or vice versa). So far, there is no evidence of the existence of IgA-LP complexes in vivo.

B. Thiocyanate, SCN$^-$

Thiocyanate, a detoxification product of cyanide, was long regarded as metabolically inert. However, the high concentration of SCN$^-$ ions in body fluids was later connected with metabolic events in the thyroid gland. The SCN$^-$ concentration in body fluids is related to the diet and to smoking habits. It is derived both endogenously during the detoxification reaction between thiosulfates and cyanide and exogenously after ingestion of the anion, its esters, and other precursor compounds such as nitriles and isothianates (131). Excessive amounts of ingested SCN$^-$ are rapidly excreted, at a rate corresponding to a half-life of 2-5 days (131).

Thiocyanate is present in parotid and whole saliva (90) and gingival exudate (3). The salivary concentrations show a wide range (Table 2), mainly because of elevated levels of SCN$^-$ in human secretions as a result of smoking (131). In whole saliva, the concentration of SCN$^-$ ions seems to correlate positively with the number of daily cigarettes (102). With heavy smokers, the salivary concentration of SCN$^-$ may be as high as 6 mM.

In the gingival exudate there is a tendency toward higher levels of SCN$^-$ in smokers compared with nonsmokers (3). Gingival inflammation also slightly increases the crevicular concentration of SCN$^-$ ions.

Azen (5) and Shannon et al. (90) have found a slight negative correlation between parotid saliva flow rate and SCN$^-$ concentration (stimulation by sour-lemon candies), whereas expectoration resulted in slightly positive correlation, probably due to the contribution of SCN$^-$ present in oral debris and exfoliated cells (116). Stimulation of salivary flow by lemon-flavored candies has resulted in a decrease of SCN$^-$ concentration also in whole saliva (81). Azen (5) also reported a slight positive correlation between salivary SCN$^-$ concentration and age. All evidence suggests that there is some active trapping of SCN$^-$

in human salivary glands because the saliva/plasma ratio is usually
above 1 (131). Because many bacteria possess rhodanese activity
(cyanide sulfurtransferase, E.C. 2.8.1.1),

$$S_2O_3{}^{2-} + CN^- \xrightarrow{\text{rhodanese}} SCN^- + SO_3{}^2$$

it is possible that such bacteria are present also in human oral flora
and generate small amounts of SCN^-.

C. Iodine, I_2, and Iodide, I^-

It has been known for many years that the salivary glands secrete
iodine in the saliva at a considerably higher (20- to 100-fold) concentration than is found in the plasma (87). The average iodine concentration in human parotid saliva is about 1-2 μM (90) and in stimulated
whole saliva about 10 μM (102) Table 2). Although it is known that
iodide ions can replace SCN^- in the LP-antimicrobial system in vitro
(40), it has been thought that the in vivo concentration of I^- ions in
all body fluids is too low to inhibit bacteria together with peroxidase
and H_2O_2 (42).

The form of iodide present in human saliva has been a matter of
controversy. Peroxidases in the presence of H_2O_2 or peroxide-generating systems are capable of iodinating tyrosine and different proteins. Human salivary peroxidase is also able to catalyze the oxidation
of iodide to iodine, the iodination of tyrosine, and the iodination of
proteins (101,106,127). Human salivary proteins, especially α-amylase
and albumin, are susceptible to iodination in vitro by human salivary
peroxidase (86,104),and extrathyroidal biosynthesis of the thyroid
hormone has been proposed to occur in human saliva (21,69). However, most investigators think that the iodine in human saliva is not
organically bound (46,59,110), although some have reported findings
of small amounts of protein bound iodine (9).

Recent studies have failed to demonstrate any iodinated proteins
or iodinated tyrosine derivatives in human whole saliva (110). On
the other hand, salivary sediment seems to contain free I^- ions, loosely
bound iodine (released by washings with saline), and strongly bound
iodine (released by sonication, detergent, and acid hydrolysis). Thus,
bacterial uptake of iodide seems to occur in human saliva, but the possible role of peroxidases in this process is still unknown. Klebanoff
(41) has shown that many bacteria could be iodinated in the presence
of peroxidase and H_2O_2. It is proposed that peroxidase-catalyzed oxidation of I^- yields I_2, which reacts with bacterial components to yield
the oxidized components and I^- (121). The I^- that is released can be
reoxidized and participate again in the oxidation of bacterial components,
and in this way I^- acts as a cofactor in the peroxidase-catalyzed oxidation of bacterial components.

Why is no organic iodine detected in human saliva in spite of the presence of all the necessary components for the in vivo iodination of proteins? The reason for this is probably the presence of relatively high concentrations of SCN^-. Thiocyanate ions inhibit the uptake of iodide by the thyroid and salivary glands (69), the oxidation of guaiacol catalyzed by thyroid peroxidase (31), the oxidation of iodide to iodine, and the iodination of tyrosine catalyzed by LP (101,107). Iodide oxidation and tyrosine iodination are inhibited due to the competitive action of SCN^- ions (107). Inhibition of tyrosine iodination is not affected by pH, and SCN^- ions are even able to deiodinate monoiodotyrosine (107). The average salivary SCN^- concentration (1 mM) almost totally inhibits the oxidation of I^- and the iodination of tyrosine in vitro (107). Therefore, iodine metabolism in saliva does not seem to be possible in the presence of the usual concentrations of SCN^- ions. However, this is not the situation in some other species. In the saliva of macaque monkeys, the amount of SCN^- ions is very low (0-9 μM), whereas peroxidase activity is much higher than in humans (54). In this species salivary oxidation of the I^- ion may occur. In dog saliva more than 50% of total salivary iodine is protein bound, and the form of iodine is primarily monoiodo- or diiodotyrosine (8). Rabinowitz (82) found considerable amounts of both thyroxine and triiodothyronine in the sublingual glands of thyroidectomized dogs, and Chatterjee et al. (10) have recently purified a protein containing triiodothyronine and thyroxine from goat submandibular gland.

D. Hydrogen Peroxide, H_2O_2

Peroxide generation is discussed in detail in Chap. 9.

E. Hypothiocyanite, $OSCN^-$

The antimicrobial activity of the human salivary peroxidase system is due to peroxidase-catalyzed oxidation of SCN^- by H_2O_2-yielding antimicrobial agents, of which hypothiocyanite ($OSCN^-$) and hypothiocyanous acid (HOSCN) have been clearly identified (see Chap. 3). Human whole saliva contains detectable amounts of $OSCN^-$ (122). Furthermore, whole saliva contains all the components required to continue to produce $OSCN^-$ during incubation in vitro. Thomas et al. (123) fractionated human saliva and demonstrated that the required components for $OSCN^-$ production were (a) peroxidase activity and SCN^- ion, (b) the saliva sediment, which produced H_2O_2 in the presence of oxygen and a divalent cation, and (c) heat-stable factors of the saliva supernatant. The supernatant factors comprised carbohydrate, glycoprotein, and protein components. Glucosamine and N-acetylglucosamine were the most effective, whereas neutral sugars, such as sucrose, were less effective in stimulating H_2O_2 production by saliva sediment.

General agreement exists that H_2O_2 is a limiting factor for the antimicrobial efficiency of the human salivary peroxidase system (30, 80,103,123). Indeed, attempts to prevent dental caries and plaque formation by means of H_2O_2-generating enzymes have led to reduction of caries both in rats and in human beings (44). However, Mühlemann et al. (68) were unable to reproduce the effect in rats (see Chap. 11). Supplementation of human saliva with H_2O_2 results in significant increase in $OSCN^-$ levels (80) (Fig. 2). With excess SCN^-, the most effective H_2O_2 concentration was near 700 μM (final concentration). However, SCN^- ions can be limiting also when saliva is supplemented with H_2O_2 (80). A combination of H_2O_2 (700 μM) and SCN^- (10 mM) resulted in a severalfold increase in salivary $OSCN^-$ levels both in vitro and in vivo (80). In contrast to expectations, supplementation of saliva with excess LP resulted in decreased generation of $OSCN^-$ ions.

Addition of H_2O_2 to saliva sediment rapidly generates $OSCN^-$, but also the decomposition of $OSCN^-$ is fast (108). Iodide ions present in saliva competitively inhibit $OSCN^-$ formation by salivary peroxidase (108).

The reported average concentrations of $OSCN^-$ in whole saliva range from 10 to 58 μM (80,114,122). Thomas et al. (122), using expectoration to collect saliva, determined an average whole saliva concentration of 10 μM, whereas Pruitt and coworkers determined the respective value for unstimulated whole saliva to be 40-58 μM (80,114). Further studies revealed that stimulation (expectoration) of salivary flow rate results in a rapid decrease in $OSCN^-$ concentration, whereas SCN^- concentration and peroxidase activity are increased (116). The decrease in $OSCN^-$ levels is greater than could be accounted for by dilution of whole saliva volume. Thus, the decrease in $OSCN^-$ may be due in part to decrease production of $OSCN^-$ or to elimination of $OSCN^-$ by possible reducing agents released into expectorated saliva. On the other hand, stimulation of salivary flow by lemon-flavored lozenges results in a net increase in the total production (nmol/min) of $OSCN^-$, although the actual concentrations in stimulated whole saliva remain lower than in resting whole saliva (81). Supplementation of saliva with H_2O_2 and SCN^- resulted in increase of $OSCN^-$ levels both in resting and expectorated saliva (116).

Surprisingly, $OSCN^-$ has been detected also in parotid and submandibular saliva (58a,81,118). This finding was surprising because there is no apparent source of H_2O_2 in pure saliva that does not contain significant concentrations of bacteria and where the concentration of leukocytes is very low (97). Therefore, the source of H_2O_2 is probably in eukaryotic cells. Molecular oxygen (O_2) may be reduced to superoxide anion (O_2^-) by numerous biological mechanisms (42). The oxygen tension in pure parotid saliva is relatively high, from 20 to 140 mmHg (24), which may favor this type of reaction. Superoxide anions may produce H_2O_2 either via spontaneous dismutation

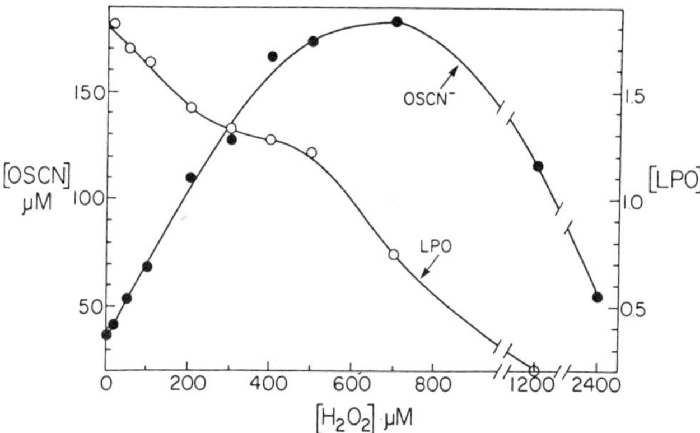

Figure 2 Effect of H_2O_2 addition on the generation of OSCN⁻ ions and on the activity of peroxidase in human whole saliva during a 5-min incubation at +37°C. The concentration of SCN⁻ was 0.55 mM. Peroxidase activity (LPO), assayed with the pyrogallol method (79), is expressed as $\Delta A_{400} \times ml^{-1} \times min^{-1}$. (From Ref. 80.)

$$O_2^{\cdot -} + O_2^{\cdot -} + 2H^+ \longrightarrow O_2 + H_2O_2$$

(a relatively slow reaction at neutral pH), or via catalysis by the enzyme superoxide dismutase that is present in the mitochondria of mammalian cells.

Other metabolic routes for intracellular generation of H_2O_2 also exist. Amino acid oxidases, which are present in most mammalian tissues, can catalyze the oxidative deamination of amino acids to form corresponding keto acids, ammonia, and H_2O_2 (42). However, no evidence of extracellular excretion and accumulation of H_2O_2 from eukaryotic cells (except leukocytes) exists. In salivary glands the SCN⁻ ions are concentrated from blood by the striated duct epithelial cells and subsequently secreted at relatively high concentrations (131). Because active oxidative metabolism with enhanced O_2 uptake occurs in these cells during secretion (88), it may be possible for SCN⁻ and H_2O_2 to react intracellularly with further catalysis by peroxidase in the ducts. This enhanced O_2 uptake resembles the metabolic burst in leukocytes during phagocytosis that results in significant production of both $O_2^{\cdot -}$ and H_2O_2 and in the extracellular release of myeloperoxidase (42). In salivary glands, the oxidative metabolic activity has been found to be higher in the ductal cells than in the acini (88). Exfoliated ductal cells frequently exist in parotid secretions (97).

III. THE PEROXIDASE SYSTEM IN HUMAN MILK

A. Milk Peroxidase

Extensive research has been carried out on the LP system in bovine
milk [see reviews by Reiter (83,84)], but only a few communications
have dealt with peroxidase in human milk. Human milk was first analyzed for peroxidase by Gothefors and Marklund (25); they estimated
the peroxidase level at about 5% of that in bovine milk. Several reports have shown that, in contrast to bovine milk, the peroxidase activity in human milk is highest in early milk (colostrum) but declines
rapidly after delivery (25,57,60,84). Over 50% of mature milk samples
(taken 10 days postpartum and later) are totally peroxidase negative
(57,84).

Recently, Moldoveanu et al. (60) studied the immunologic and
chromatographic behavior of human milk peroxidase. Antiserum to
bovine LP (developed in rabbit) gave reactions of identity in double
immunodiffusion tests between the immunogen and bovine milk and a
reaction of partial identity between immunogen and human parotid
saliva (Fig. 3). However, no precipitation was found with the extract
of PMN leukocytes, human colostrum, or mature milk. Staining of the
plates with peroxidase substrate revealed that all samples contained
peroxidase activity. In molecular exclusion chromatography, the
human colostral peroxidase activity behaved similarly to that of PMN
leukocytes, and was clearly different from that of bovine milk, purified bovine LP, or human parotid saliva peroxidase. Furthermore,
total colostral peroxidase activity seemed to increase as a function of
the number of cells. Histochemical staining revealed that peroxidase-
positive granules were numerous in colostral cells. All this evidence
suggests that there is no LP in human milk and that all the peroxidase
activity is derived from milk leukocytes, especially PMNs, which are
abundant in early milk. Macrophages may also be numerous in human
colostrum, but these cells are rarely peroxidase positive (16).

There seems to be a wide variation of peroxidase activity in human
milk with a range from 0 to 970 mU/ml when assayed with ABTS (see
Table 2) as a substrate (60,84,96). Several factors may affect the
actual levels of peroxidase in milk (e.g., the cell content of the milk
and the manner in which it is treated and stored). The cell count in
human colostrum and milk is highest in early milk and drops sharply
during the postpartum period (27). The same pattern is observed for
human milk peroxidase activity. The high peroxidase levels reported
for Gambian mothers (84) might be due to infections (high PMN counts?)
or due to less gentle treatment of milk under field conditions with a
corresponding increase in cell lysis and peroxidase release. Nutritional
status might also have some influence (84).

It should be emphasized that supplementation of human milk with
peroxidase cofactors, SCN$^-$ and H_2O_2, results in bactericidal action

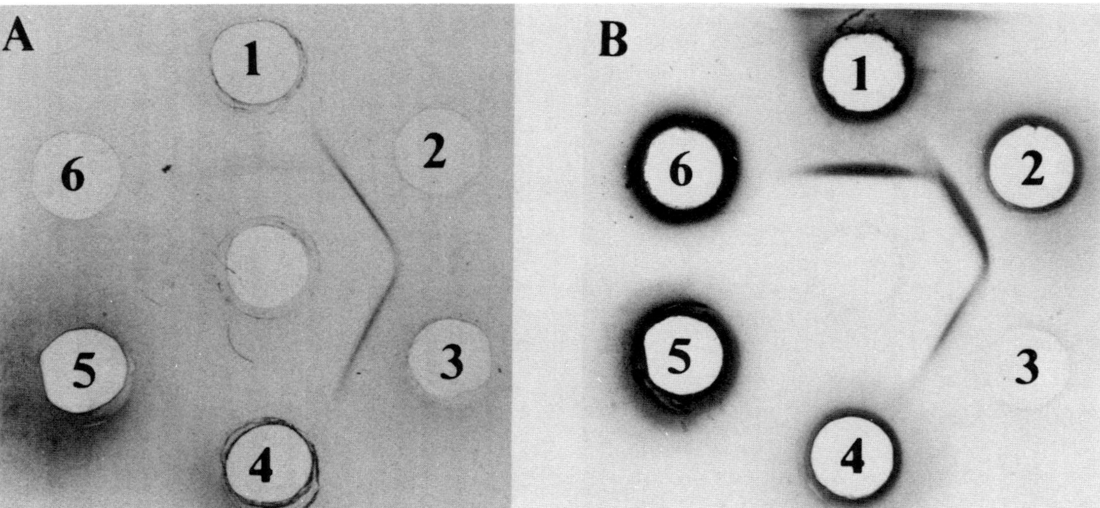

Figure 3 Double immunodiffusion tests with rabbit antiserum to bovine LP. Antiserum to LP (central well) was obtained from two rabbits immunized with commercial bovine milk LP. The wells contained (1) human parotid saliva, (2) purified bovine LP, (3) centrifuged raw bovine milk, (4) human colostral whey, (5) lysate of human colostral cells, and (6) lysate of human PMN leukocytes. Panel A: precipitin lines were stained with 1% thiazine red. Panel B: precipitin lines stained for peroxidase activity. (From Ref. 60.)

against *Escherichia coli* (84) and *Salmonella typhimurium* (47), supporting the presence of peroxidase-mediated antimicrobial system in human milk. Human milk peroxidase has been shown to remain active in human gastric juice (25).

B. Milk Thiocyanate, Iodide, and Chloride

The concentration of SCN^- is approximately the same both in bovine and human milk. Values ranging from 10 to 200 μM have been reported in cow's milk, but the concentration depends largely on the feeding regime (83). In human milk, Gothefors and Marklund (25) could not determine the exact level of SCN^- but reported it to be low (less than 80 μM). Mäkinen and Tenovuo (57) measured the SCN^- concentration in mature milk to be about 120 μM. In the stomach, SCN^- appears to be actively secreted (by the parietal cells which secrete HCl?) because in some cases it may exceed the salivary SCN^- concentration (7).

The iodide concentration in mature human milk is quite low, approximately 2 μM (57), but the chloride level is much higher, about 1.3 mM (37). This means that because there is leukocyte peroxidase (myeloperoxidase) rather than LP in human milk the oxidation of chloride is also possible (LP does not catalyze the oxidation of Cl^-) (61). In conclusion, it seems evident that myeloperoxidase-mediated antimicrobial system (Cl^- and/or SCN^- as a substrate) may function in early human milk, thus protecting the newborn from infections. Measurements of hypothiocyanite or hypochlorite levels have not been reported.

C. Peroxidase in Breast Cancer

As stated on page 104, peroxidases may serve as indicators or estrogen responsiveness in various tissues (36). It has been clearly shown that administration of estrogen to rats increases uterine peroxidase activity and that the effect is strictly limited to those rat tissues whose growth is affected by steroids (50). Peroxidase activity has been detected in the carcinogen DMBA (7,12-dimethylbenz(a)anthracene) induced rat mammary tumors and in human breast carcinomas (18,50), and peroxidase activity has been suggested to be a useful marker for estrogen-stimulated growth of cancer (50,51). However, the postulated relationship between peroxidase content and hormone dependence in these tumors is a matter of controversy. Although positive correlation has been reported in some studies (51,74), many others have failed to find such correlation (15,19) or have even reported a negative correlation (48). Part of the controversy may be explained by the lack of correlation between biochemical and histochemical assessments of peroxidase activity in mammary tumors (75). Rat mammary tumor peroxidase has been purified and characterized and has many similarities to rat uterine peroxidase (17).

The origin of human breast cancer peroxidase is unknown. Some of the activity may be derived from contaminating leukocytes or induced by other hormones. No significant purification of this enzyme has been achieved, and this area clearly warrants further studies.

IV. THE PEROXIDASE SYSTEM IN HUMAN LACRIMAL FLUID

The information on human lacrimal peroxidase is very scarce; for example, Gachon et al. (23), in an extensive review on human tear proteins, do not even mention the presence of peroxidase. Peroxidase has been demonstrated in the lacrimal gland of cows and steers (65), rats (35), and monkeys (54). Peroxidase has been suggested to act as an antiinfectious agent since SCN^- and endogenous H_2O_2 are also present in conjunctival secretions (35). Peroxidase activity has been detected also in human tears (125), but no purification or characterization of the enzyme has been done. Preliminary data from the author's laboratory indicate that peroxidase activity in human tears is very high (5- to 10-fold compared with saliva), and the enzyme has a molecular weight of approximately 90,000 and pI values of 5.6-5.8 and 6.2-6.4. Thiocyanate ions are present in human tear fluid, but the concentration is very low, only about 20 μM (125). However, human tears are rich in Cl^- (130-150 mM) (unpublished data).

This limited information on the human tear peroxidase system does not allow any strong statements on the nature and function of this enzyme, but clearly indicates the need of further investigation on this topic.

V. THE PEROXIDASE SYSTEM IN THE HUMAN UTERUS

Peroxidase activity has been found in human endometrium (49,50) and cervical mucus (28,92), and the enzyme from cervical mucus has been isolated and characterized (92). Electrophoretic examinations showed this enzyme to be a major component of the soluble proteins of cervical mucus. Chemical and physical properties show that the enzyme is similar to a classic peroxidase. The purified enzyme had a well-defined pH maximum at 4.45 with ABTS as a donor.

Unlike peroxidase activity in the rat uterus, human peroxidase from premenopausal endometrium (28) and endocervical epithelium (124) does not increase with plasma estrogen levels. It was recently found that peroxidase from human uterine epithelium is inhibited in vitro by estrogens, especially catecholestrogens (124). In addition, the peroxidase activity in human cervical mucus has been reported to decrease 20- to 100-fold in the middle of the menstrual cycle as compared with other times of the cycle (124). This drop in peroxidase activity coincided with the peak of plasma estrogens and may be causally related to them.

At present, no exact knowledge of the physiological function of
uterine peroxidase exists. In rats, the uterine peroxidase activity is
estrogen dependent, possibly antimicrobial, and may participate in
protein crosslinking reactions (36). It seems possible that also in
human beings, peroxidase may protect vaginal mucosa from infective
agents, but further studies are required to verify this presumption.
Interestingly, uterine fluid when combined with H_2O_2 and either
iodide or thiocyanate is toxic to sperm, as measured by a loss of
motility or a decrease in pyruvate oxidation (42). Physical properties
of cervical mucus (e.g., viscosity) change drastically at midcycle (20),
and decreased peroxidase activity may be related to decreased crosslinking of mucus proteins during ovulation.

VI. SUMMARY

Lactoperoxidase (LP) has been proposed to act as an antimicrobial enzyme in human saliva, milk, and tears. However, LP has never been
satisfactorily purified and characterized from any of these human
secretions. Recently, it was reported that there is no detectable LP in
human milk, but all the activity is probably derived from milk leukocytes. On the other hand, in human saliva the peroxidase enzyme is
very similar, but not identical, to that found in bovine milk. Thus, the
name salivary peroxidase would be more appropriate than lactoperoxidase for the human salivary enzyme. By further analogy, the name
lacrimal peroxidase would be appropriate for the peroxidase in human
tear fluid.

The cofactors required to produce antimicrobial agents by peroxidase-catalyzed oxidation reactions have been detected in all above-
mentioned secretions. The likely donor in saliva is SCN^-, in milk Cl^-
and/or SCN^-, and in tears Cl^-. So far, the antimicrobial oxidation
product, hypothiocyanite ion ($OSCN^-$), has been detected only in
saliva.

In addition to the antimicrobial properties, the lactoperoxidase
system may exert also other biological functions in vivo. Among these
are degradation of mutagenicity of various carcinogens (132), which
has been reported to occur in human saliva (71), and protection of
human cells from the toxicity of hydrogen peroxide. The myeloperoxidase system, which may also be effective in various human secretions,
is known to inactivate leukocyte chemoattractants (12) and to inhibit
neutrophil motility and lymphocyte transformation to mitogens (120),
thus regulating cellular immune functions. However, further studies
are required to show whether these interesting activities exist in vivo.

The following areas warrant further investigations: (a) purification and chemical characterization of peroxidases from human saliva,
milk, mammary tumors, and tears; (b) studies of estrogen-dependence
of human peroxidases; (c) evaluation of possible in vivo complexes of

salivary peroxidase with other oral proteins, especially with immunoglobulins; (d) detection and analysis of antimicrobial oxidation products of SCN⁻ and Cl⁻ in milk and tears, and (e) development of techniques to increase the amount of antimicrobial oxidation products in vivo.

REFERENCES

1. Alexander, N. M., and Corcoran, B. J., *J. Biol. Chem. 237*: 243 (1962).
2. Allen, P. Z., and Morrison, M., *Arch. Biochem. Biophys. 102*: 106 (1963).
3. Anttonen, T., and Tenovuo, J., *Proc. Finn. Dent. Soc. 77*: 318 (1981).
4. Azen, E. A., *Biochem. Genet. 15*:9 (1977).
5. Azen, E. A., *Arch. Oral Biol. 23*: 801 (1978).
6. Banerjee, R. K., and Datta, A. G., *Acta Endocrinol. 96*: 208 (1981).
7. Boulos, P. B., Dave, M., Whitfield, P. F., and Hobsley, M., *Gut 18*: A946 (1977).
8. Burgen, A. S. V., and Emmelin, N. G., *Physiology of the Salivary Glands*, Edward Arnold, London (1961).
9. Carlström, A., *Acta Chem. Scand. 23*: 171 (1969).
10. Chatterjee, D. K., Banerjee, R. K., and Datta, A. G., *Biochim. Biophys. Acta 612*: 29 (1980).
11. Christensen, T. G., and Hayes, J. A., *Am. Rev. Respir. Dis. 125*: 341 (1982).
12. Clark, R. A., and Szot, S., *J. Immunol. 128*: 1507 (1982).
13. Cockle, S. M., and Harkness, R. A., *Br. J. Obstet. Gynaecol. 85*: 776 (1978).
14. Cole, M. F., Hsu, S. D., Baum, B. J., Bowen, W. H., Sierra, L. I., Aquirre, M., and Gillespie, G., *Infect. Immun. 31*: 998 (1981).
15. Collings, J. R., and Savage, N., *Br. J. Cancer 40*: 500 (1979).
16. Crago, S. S., Prince, S. J., Pretlow, T. G., McGhee, J. R., and Mestecky, J., *Clin. Exp. Immunol. 38*: 585 (1979).
17. DeSombre, E. R., and Lyttle, C. R., *Cancer Res. 38*: 4086 (1978).
18. Duffy, M. J., and Duffy, G., *Biochem. Soc. Trans. 5*: 1738 (1977).
19. Duffy, M. J., and O'Connell, M., *Eur. J. Cancer 17*: 711 (1981).
20. Elstein, M., *Br. Med. Bull. 34*: 83 (1978).
21. Evans, E. S., Schooley, R. A., Evans, A. B., Jenkins, C. A., and Taurog, A., *Endocrinology 78*: 983 (1966).

22. Floche, L., Schaich, E., Voelter, W., and Wendell, A., *Hoppe Seylers Z. Physiol. Chem. 352*: 170 (1971).

23. Gachon, A. M., Verrelle, P., Betail, G., and Dastugue, B., *Exp. Eye Res. 29*: 539 (1979).

24. Globerman, D. Y., and Kleinberg, I., In *Proceedings Saliva and Dental Caries*, Kleinberg, I., Ellison, S. A., and Mandel, I. D. (Eds.), Sp. Suppl. Microbiol. Abstr., pp. 275-292 (1979).

25. Gothefors, L., and Marklund, S., *Infect. Immun. 11*: 1210 (1975).

26. Hanssen, F. S., *Br. J. Exp. Pathol. 5*: 271 (1924).

27. Ho, F. C. S., Wong, R. L. C., and Lawton, J. W. M., *Acta Pediatr. Scand. 68*: 389 (1979).

28. Holinka, C. F., and Gurpide, E., *Am. J. Obstet. Gynecol. 138*: 599 (1975).

29. Honka, E., Ohlsson, P. I., and Paul, K. G., *Acta Chem. Scand. B36*: 273 (1982).

30. Hoogendoorn, H., *The Effect of Lactoperoxidase-Thiocyanate-Hydrogen Peroxide on the Metabolism of Cariogenic Microorganisms in Vitro and in the Oral Cavity*. Mouton, Den Haag, The Netherlands (1974).

31. Hosoya, T., *J. Biol. Chem. (Tokyo) 53*: 381 (1963).

32. Iwamoto, Y., and Matsumura, T., *Arch. Oral Biol. 11*: 667 (1966).

33. Iwamoto, Y., Nakamura, R., Tsunemitsu, A., and Matsumura, T., *Arch. Oral Biol. 13*: 1015 (1968).

34. Iwamoto, Y., Nakamura, R., Watanabe, T., and Tsunemitsu, A., *J. Dent. Res. 15*: 503 (1972).

35. Iwata, T., Ohkawa, K., and Uyama, M., *Invest. Ophthalmol. 15*: 40 (1976).

36. Jellinck, P. H., Newcombe, A., and Keeping, H. S., *Adv. Enzyme Regul. 17*: 325 (1979).

37. Jennes, R., *Semin. Perinatol. 3*: 225 (1979).

38. Kataoka, K., *Histochemie 26*: 319 (1971).

39. Keenan, E. J., Bacon, D. R., and Garrison, L. B., *Proc. West. Pharmacol. Soc. 22*: 227 (1979).

40. Klebanoff, S. J., and Luebke, R. G., *Proc. Soc. Exp. Biol. Med. 118*: 483 (1965).

41. Klebanoff, S. J., *J. Exp. Med. 126*: 1063 (1967).

42. Klebanoff, S. J., and Clark, R. A., *The Neutrophil: Function and Clinical Disorders*, North-Holland, Amsterdam (1978).

43. Klinkhamer, J. M., and Mitchell, M. D., *J. Dent. Res. 58*: 531 (1979).

44. Koch, G., and Strand, G., *Swed. Dent. J. 3*: 9 (1979).

45. Kowolik, M. J., and Grant, M., *Arch. Oral Biol. 28*: 293 (1983).

46. Kumlien, A., *Acta Endocrinol. 70*: 239 (1972).

47. Laven, G. T., Pruitt, K. M., and Smith, J. C., personal communication (1982).

48. Levy, J., Liel, Y., Feldman, B., Aflallo, L., and Glick, S. M., *Eur. J. Cancer Clin. Oncol. 17:* 1023 (1981).

49. Lucas, F. V., Carens, V. M., Schmidt, H. J., Sipes, D. R., and Hall, D. G., *Am. J. Obstet. Gynecol. 88:* 965 (1964).

50. Lyttle, C. R., and DeSombre, E. R., *Nature (Lond.) 268:* 337 (1977).

51. Lyttle, C. R., Thorpe, S. M., DeSombre, E. R., and Daehnfeldt, J. L., *J. Natl. Cancer Inst. 62:* 1031 (1979).

52. Mäkinen, K. K., and Tenovuo, J., *Acta Odontol. Scand. 34:* 141 (1976).

53. Mäkinen, K. K., Tenovuo, J., and Scheinin, A., *J. Dent. Res. 55:* 652 (1976).

54. Mäkinen, K. K., Bowen, W. H., Dalgard, D., and Fitzgerald, G., *J. Nutr. 108:* 779 (1978).

55. Mäkinen, K. K., Tenovuo, J., and Bowen, W. H., *Acta Chem. Scand. B32:* 387 (1978).

56. Mäkinen, K. K., Kölling, D., and Söderling, E., *Int. J. Vit. Nutr. Res. 50:* 79 (1980).

57. Mäkinen, J., and Tenovuo, J., *Nutr. Rep. Int. 22:* 793 (1980).

58. Mäkinen, K. K., Näsi, M., and Alaviuhkola, T., *Nut.. Rep. Int. 23:* 793 (1981).

58a. Mandel, I. D., Behrman, J., Levy, F., and Weinstein, D., *J. Dent. Res. 62:* 922 (1983).

59. Mason, D. K., Harden, R. M., and Alexander, W. D., *Br. Dent. J. 122:* 485 (1967).

60. Moldoveanu, Z., Tenovuo, J., Mestecky, J., and Pruitt, K. M., *Biochim. Biophys. Acta 718:* 103 (1982).

61. Moldoveanu, Z., Tenovuo, J., Pruitt, K. M., Månsson-Rahemtulla, B., and Mestecky, J., in *Secretory Immune System*, McGhee, J. R., and Mestecky, J. (Eds.), Ann. N.Y. Acad. Sci. New York, Vol. 409, p. 848 (1983).

62. Morrison, M., Hamilton, H. B., and Stotz, E., *J. Biol. Chem. 228:* 767 (1957).

63. Morrison, M., and Allen, P. Z., *Biochem. Biophys. Res. Commun. 13:* 490 (1963).

64. Morrison, M., Allen, P. Z., Bright, J., and Jayasinghe, W., *Arch. Biochem. Biophys. 111:* 126 (1965).

65. Morrison, M., and Allen, P. Z., *Science 152:* 1626 (1966).

66. Morrison, M., and Steele, W. F., in *Biology of the Mouth*, Person, P. (Ed.), American Association for Advancement of Science, Washington, D.C., p. 89 (1968).

67. Mosimann, W., and Sumner, J. B., *Arch. Biochem. Biophys. 33:* 487 (1951).

68. Mühlemann, H. R., Schmid, R., and Firestone, A. R., *Caries Res. 15:* 46 (1981).

69. Myant, N. B., *Ann. N.Y. Acad. Sci. 85*: 208 (1960).
70. Nickerson, J. F., Kraus, F. W., and Perry, W. I., *Proc. Soc. Exp. Biol. Med. 95*: 405 (1957).
71. Nishioka, H., Nishi, K., and Kyokane, K., *Mutation Res. 85*: 323 (1981).
72. Ørstavik, D., and Kraus, F. W., *Scand. J. Dent. Res. 82*: 202 (1974).
73. Paul, K. G., Ohlsson, P. I., and Henriksson, A., *FEBS Lett. 110*: 200 (1980).
74. Penney, G. C., Scott, K. M., and Hawkins, R. A., *Br. J. Cancer 41*: 648 (1980).
75. Penney, G. C., and Hawkins, R. A., *Histochem. J. 13*: 983 (1981).
76. Pilz, H., O'Brien, J. S., and Heipertz, R., *Clin. Biochem. 9*: 85 (1976).
77. Pruitt, K. M., *Swed. Dent. J. 1*: 225 (1977).
78. Pruitt, K. M., and Adamson, M., *Infect. Immun. 17*: 112 (1977).
79. Pruitt, K. M., Adamson, M., and Arnold, R., *Infect. Immun. 25*: 304 (1979).
80. Pruitt, K. M., Tenovuo, J., Fleming, W., and Adamson, M., *Caries Res. 16*: 316 (1982).
81. Pruitt, K. M., Månsson-Rahemtulla, B., and Tenovuo, J., *Arch. Oral. Biol. 28*: 517 (1983).
82. Rabinowitz, J. L., *J. Dent. Res. 57*: Spec. Issue A., abstr. 1184 (1978).
83. Reiter, B., *Ann. Rech. Vet. 9*: 205 (1978).
84. Reiter, B., in *Immunological Aspects of Infection in the Fetus and Newborn*, Lambert, H. P., and Wood, C. B. S. (Eds.), Academic Press, London, p. 155-195 (1981).
85. Revis, G. J., *Arch. Oral Biol. 22*: 155 (1977).
86. Sarimo, S. S., and Tenovuo, J., *Biochem. J. 167*: 23 (1977).
87. Schiff, L., Stevens, C. D., Molle, W. E., Steinberg, H., Kumpe, C. W., and Stewart, P., *J. Natl. Cancer Inst. 7*: 349 (1947).
88. Schneider, R. M., and Person, P., *Ann. N.Y. Acad. Sci. 85*: 201 (1960).
89. Schultz, J., and Kaminker, K., *Arch. Biochem. Biophys. 96*: 465 (1962).
90. Shannon, I. L., Suddick, R. P., and Dowd, Jr., F. J., *Monographs in Oral Science*, vol. 2, S. Karger, Basel (1974).
91. Shindler, J. S., and Bardsley, W. G., *Biochem. Biophys. Res. Commun. 67*: 1307 (1975).
92. Shindler, J. S., Childs, R. E., and Bardsley, W. G., *Eur. J. Biochem. 65*: 325 (1976).
93. Slowey, R. R., Eidelman, S., and Klebanoff, S. J., *J. Bacteriol. 96*: 575 (1968).

94. Smith, D. C., and Klebanoff, S. J., *Biol. Reprod.* 3: 229 (1970).

95. Stelmaszynska, T., and Zgliczynski, J. M., *Eur. J. Biochem.* 19: 56 (1971).

96. Stephens, S., Harkness, R. A., and Cockle, S. M., *Br. J. Exp. Pathol.* 60: 252 (1979).

97. Syrjänen, S. M., and Syrajänen, K. J., *Proc. Finn. Dent. Soc.* 77: 283 (1981).

98. Tabak, L., Mandel, I. D., Herrera, M., and Baurmash, H., *J. Oral Pathol.* 7: 91 (1978).

99. Taichman, N. S., Tsai, C.-C., Baehni, P. S., Stoller, N., and McArthur, W. P., *Infect. Immun.* 16: 1013 (1977).

100. Taubman, M. A., *Arch. Oral Biol.* 19: 439 (1974).

101. Taurog, A., Dorris, M. L., and Lamas, L., *Endocrinology* 94: 1286 (1974).

102. Tenovuo, J., and Mäkinen, K. K., *J. Dent. Res.* 55: 661 (1976).

103. Tenovuo, J., and Knuuttila, M. L. E., *J. Dent. Res.* 56: 1608 (1977).

104. Tenovuo, J., and Sarimo, S. S., *Scand. J. Dent. Res.* 85: 355 (1977).

105. Tenovuo, J., Valtakoski, J., and Knuuttila, M. L. E., *Caries Res.* 11: 257 (1977).

106. Tenovuo, J., *Arch. Oral Biol.* 23: 253 (1978).

107. Tenovuo, J., *Arch. Oral Biol.* 23: 899 (1978).

108. Tenovuo, J., *Caries Res.* 13: 137 (1979).

109. Tenovuo, J., and Anttonen, T., *Caries Res.* 14: 269 (1980).

110. Tenovuo, J., Söderling, E., and Anttonen, T., *Scand. J. Dent. Res.* 88: 430 (1980).

111. Tenovuo, J., and Kurkijärvi, K., *Arch. Oral Biol.* 26: 309 (1981).

112. Tenovuo, J., Laine, M., Söderling, E., and Irjala, K., *Biochem. Med.* 25: 337 (1981).

113. Tenovuo, J., and Laine, M., *J. Dent. Res.* 60: Spec. Issue A., abstr. 1380 (1981).

114. Tenovuo, J., Månsson-Rahemtulla, B., Pruitt, K. M., and Arnold, R., *Infect. Immun.* 34: 208 (1981).

115. Tenovuo, J., *Arch. Oral Biol.* 26: 1051 (1981).

116. Tenovuo, J., Pruitt, K. M., and Thomas, E. L., *J. Dent. Res.* 61: 982 (1982).

117. Tenovuo, J., Moldoveanu, Z., Mestecky, J., Pruitt, K. M., and Månsson-Rahemtulla, B., *J. Immunol.* 128: 726 (1982).

118. Tenovuo, J., Pruitt, K. M., and Månsson-Rahemtulla, B., *ORCA Abstr.* No. 29 (1982).

119. Theorell, H., and Åkesson, A., *Arkiv. Kemi Mineral. Geol.* 16A: 1 (1942).

120. Theron, A., Anderson, R., Grabow, G., and Meiring, J. L.,
     Clin. Exp. Immunol. 44: 295 (1981).
121. Thomas, E. L., and Aune, T. M., *Antimicrob. Agents Chemo-
     ther. 13:* 1000 (1978).
122. Thomas, E. L., Bates, K. P., and Jefferson, M. M., *J. Dent.
     Res. 59:* 1466 (1980).
123. Thomas, E. L., Bates, K. P., and Jefferson, M. M., *J. Dent.
     Res. 60:* 785 (1981).
124. Tsibris, J. C. M., Thomason, J. L., Kunigk, A., Khan-
     Dawood, F. S., Kirschner, C. V., and Spellacy, W. N., *Con-
     traception 25:* 59 (1982).
125. Van Haeringen, N. J., Ensink, F. T. E., and Glasius, E.,
     Exp. Eye Res. 28: 343 (1979).
126. Venkatachalam, M. A., Saltani, M. H., and Fahimi, H. D.,
     J. Cell Biol. 46: 168 (1970).
127. Virion, A., Pommier, J., Deme, D., and Nunez, J., *Eur. J.
     Biochem. 117:* 103 (1981).
128. Watanabe, K., *Acta Histochem. Cytochem. 11:* 151 (1978).
129. Watanabe, K., *Ann. Otol. 89:* 241 (1980).
130. Wever, R., Hamers, M. N., Weening, R. S., and Roos, D.,
     Eur. J. Biochem. 108: 491 (1980).
131. Wood, J. L., in *Chemistry and Biochemistry of Thiocyanic
     Acid and its Derivatives*, Newman, A. A. (Ed.), Academic
     Press, London, p. 156 (1975).
132. Yamada, M., Tsuda, M., Nagao, M., Mori, M., and Sugimura,
     T., *Biochem. Biophys. Res. Commun. 90:* 769 (1979).

7

The Lactoperoxidase System of Bovine Milk

BRUNO REITER / *University of Oxford, John Radcliffe Hospital, Headington, Oxford and National Institute for Research in Dairying,* Shinfield, Reading, England*

I. INTRODUCTION

The history of the lactoperoxidase system (LPS) is intimately associated with the antibacterial activity of bovine milk. This activity was recognized at about the same time as that of blood, but until recently attracted only limited attention. Epidemiologists investigated whether milk could be a vehicle for the spreading of cholera bacillus, *Salmonella typhosa* (13,16), or scarlet fever streptococci (70). Veterinarians

---

*Retired

tried to answer the question of whether or not the in vitro antistrepto-
coccal activity of milk contributes to the defense of the bovine udder
against infection (20,21), a problem which remains unsolved (27,50,
62). Dairy research workers were interested in the inhibition of lactic
acid streptococci that are used in the manufacture of most cheese var-
ieties (44,46,47,71). More recently, it was found that LPS could be
used to suppress gram negative organisms such as pseudomonads that
spoil milk on prolonged storage at refrigeration temperatures (6,7,49,
57). LPS is being used to preserve milk without cooling in developing
countries (8,14). Also, LPS can kill potential intestinal pathogens
such as coliforms, salmonellae, shigellae, including multiple antibiotic-
resistant strains in vitro and in vivo (51-55,58). It is now evident
that LPS is part of the immune system of milk, consisting of immunoglobulins, complement, lysozyme, lactoferrin, and leukocytes, that
protects the neonate against intestinal infections until it can build up
its own defense systems. The total effect is greater than the sum of
the individual components (60) and, if we accept that leukocytes are
the primary defense against invading organisms, we could regard
colostrum (and milk) as liquid leukocytes because so many of the
antimicrobial factors are common to both (56).

II. THE COMPONENTS OF LPS AND THEIR INTERACTION

Hanssen (13) was first to suggest that the bactericidal activity of raw
bovine milk against *Bacillus typhosa* and *B. paratyphosa* was associated with the oxidases and peroxidases occurring in milk. He based
his findings on the concurrent destruction of the bactericidal activity
and the reaction of the milk with paraphenylenediamine by time and
temperature combinations such as 75°C, 15 min. Wright and Tramer
(71), working with group N streptococci (lactic acid streptococci),
came to the same conclusion. The inhibition occurred only under
aerobic conditions and could be reversed by reducing agents, confirming the findings of Jones and his collaborators (20,21). Moreover,
Wright and Tramer (71) suggested also that the inhibition could only
be caused by an oxidation product formed by LP in the presence of
H_2O_2—the latter being a metabolic end product of the streptococci
under aerobic conditions. In the meantime, Morrison et al. (35) had
published an easy method for the isolation and purification of LP by
ion-exchange chromatography that enabled Portman and Auclair (43) to
demonstrate conclusively the role of LP. They succeeded in restoring
the inhibitory activity of heated milk through the addition of a purified
preparation of LP. The role of H_2O_2 was substantiated by Jago and
Morrison (19) when they showed that the inhibition of streptococci
could be prevented by the addition of catalase, albeit at very high,
hence unphysiological, concentrations that do not occur in milk or
other biological fluids. The same authors disputed, however, the in-

volvement of a third component. The necessity of a third component
became evident when it was found (44,46) that dialyzed milk became
noninhibitory, and the inhibition could be restored by the addition of
the dialysate. Naturally occurring, oxidizable substrates in milk such
as iodide and indican (indoxyl sulfuric acid) could replace the dialysate but only at unphysiological concentrations. Furthermore, the
oxidation product of these substrates did not inhibit the lactic acid
streptococci temporarily as in raw milk, but killed them. The third
factor that fulfilled all the required characteristics was identified as
thiocyanate, inhibiting temporarily some strains of lactic acid streptococci, whereas others were resistant (38,39,46). (See Chap. 8.)

III. CONCENTRATIONS OF THE COMPONENTS OF LPS

A. Lactoperoxidase

Lactoperoxidase is the most abundant enzyme in bovine milk, constituting about 1% of the whey proteins (total protein less casein) or 10-30
μg/ml of milk. Unfortunately, the data in the literature are difficult
to compare because of the various chromogens used [e.g., p-phenel-
enediaminechloride (24), o-dianisidine (38) and pyrogallol (12)]. The
most sensitive method yet devised is by Shindler et al. (65) oxidizing
2,2'-azino-di(3-ethylbenzthiazoline-6-sulfonic acid) (ABTS).

LP occurs in the whey of all cow's milk, varying slightly between
individuals and possibly breeds. Feeding is supposed to influence the
level (23), and high cell count is reported to increase the LP level
both in bovine and human milk (12); however, this is disputed by
Korhonen (26) for bovine milk. Moldoveanu et al. (34) came to the
conclusion that human milk does not contain any LP, and all the peroxidative activity is derived from leukocytes, the enzyme thus being
myeloperoxidase (MPO). This is an important finding because thiocyanate, bromide, and iodide are oxidized by both LP and MPO, but chloride
only by MPO. A total cell count cannot be strictly correlated with
enzyme activity, because only polymorphonuclear leukocytes (PMN)
possess MPO and can excrete MPO during phagocytosis. In milk,
phagocytosis is not only induced by bacteria but also by casein and
fat (see under H_2O_2, Sec. III.C). Bovine and human milk seem to
have different cell populations. Lee et al. (29), using electron micro-
scopy and staining, found in bovine colostrum the predominant cell
type to be PMN (50-80%) but macrophages in midlactation milk (69-88%),
the total count being 6×10^6/ml in colostrum and 1×10^6 in milk. In
humans (33) the colostrum was reported to contain 10% PMN and milk
30%, 4-14 days postpartum, the total being, respectively, 2.1×10^6/ml
and 1.5×10^6/ml. The "reservoir" or cell-bound LP is therefore not
inconsiderable and needs to be reinvestigated separately assaying LP
and MPO activity (oxidation of Cl^-) before and after lysing the cells;
the initial values must be obtained immediately without storage of the
milk.

Bovine LP behaves differently from other protective proteins (immunoglobulins, lysozyme, lactoferrin, and so on). Its concentration is low in the bovine colostrum and increases rapidly to reach a peak at 4-5 days postpartum. It declines rapidly afterwards to reach a constant, rather high, plateau during the lactation. Human peroxidase is highest in colostrum and declines rapidly within 1 week (12,24). If we accept the identification of the cells by Mohr et al. (33) and the fact that only PMN possess MPO, a rapid fall in peroxidative activity should not occur. Obviously, clarification is needed. Human milk peroxidase (20 mu/ml ABTS units) in the presence of added thiocyanate and peroxide has been shown to kill *Escherichia coli* (60). Björck (7) arrived at a limit of 0.5 μg/ml for LP in a synthetic medium that is far below the average of 10-30 μg/ml, present in bovine milk.

The comparative data are based on ABTS units in Table 1 and show that guinea pig milk is far richer in LP than even cow's milk.

LP concentration in bovine milk may also be influenced by estrogen. Kern et al. (22) reported that peroxidative activity of the milk varied periodically in nonpregnant but not in pregnant cows. The milk of cows in estrus showed increased LP activity that became normal only after ovulation. However, Linford (30) could not detect such variation in the milk but found that the LP concentration in cervical mucus. dropped to very low levels in 6 out of 7 animals 2 days before ovulation. Estrus induced in two ovariectomized heifers by intramuscular injection

Table 1 Peroxidase Activity (mu/ml) Assayed with ABTS as Electron Donor

Source (n)	Mean	Range	Ref. no.
Bovine (11) (3-30 weeks)	1422	738-3889	69
Human[a]			
1 day (4)	700	519-970	60
2-10 days (21)	314	60-970	
Guinea pig (73)	22,000	4569-54,500	69
Sow (2)	1700		Unpublished
Goat (2)	2550		
Rabbit (1)	800		
Mouse (1)	2000		

[a]Milk samples obtained through courtesy of the Pediatric Department, Cardiff Hospital, Cardiff, England.
Source: Ref. 65.

of 400 g estradiol benzoate mimicked the natural estrus, LP activity
being reduced. The finding that LP concentrations are low at ovulation is of some interest because LPS inhibits the motility and penetration of cervical mucus by bovine spermatozoa (15,25,45).

In summary, it is important to consider that peroxidase concentrations in human milk are lower than in bovine milk. However, the
salivary peroxidase levels in babies is high from birth, whereas the
calf is born with little or no LP in its saliva (12,36). In this context,
it is also interesting that the milk of the guinea pig contains the highest
levels of LP as yet observed.

B. Thiocyanate

Thiocyanate is a ubiquitous anion in animal tissue and secretions. It
occurs in the mammary, salivary and thyroid glands, in the stomach,
kidney, and fluids such as synovial, cerebral, spinal, lymph, and
plasma.

Cows on natural pastures containing clover and other nongrasses
give milk with higher concentrations of thiocyanate, particularly at
the height of the summer (up to 15 ppm), than cows on winter feed on
ley pastures (9,28), the latter consisting of grasses only. Direct
feeding of sodium cyanate to cows has also been shown to increase the
level (42). The health of the udder also seems to influence the level of
thiocyanate. Milk containing less than 5×10^5/ml leukocytes—a guide
for an apparently disease-free udder—contained less thiocyanate than
milk from apparently infected udders with above 5×10^5/ml leukocytes.
Obviously, the increase is derived from the blood plasma.

C. H_2O_2

Peroxide is generally assumed to be absent from milk. This is difficult
to understand, considering the very high metabolic activity of a secretory tissue such as the mammary gland. Theoretically H_2O_2 could
also be generated by xanthine oxidase, Cu^{2+}, ascorbic acid, and sulfhydryl oxidase, always assuming the presence of free O_2. However,
milk contains not only peroxidase and catalase, but also superoxide
dismutase (18). Hence, the full gambit of protective enzymes against
the toxicity of H_2O_2 is present in milk. Any H_2O_2 generated would be
either bound to LP or reduced by catalase. It is therefore essential
that these enzymes are inactivated before any analysis for H_2O_2 is
made. It was, for instance, possible to determine nanomolar concentrations of H_2O_2 for leukocytes suspended in milk when the enzymes
were inactivated by sodium azide; 10^6 leukocytes per ml generated
up to 26 nM H_2O_2 in the resting state, but 250 times as much when they
ingested casein micelles (27; Korhonen and Reiter, unpublished data).
Besides such an exogenous supply of H_2O_2, streptococci can themselves
produce H_2O_2, provided the udder is not anaerobic. Peroxide generated

in this way could activate LPS against other organisms. We have good
evidence that this happens in the intestinal tract. Lactobacilli colonizing the intestine were found to activate LPS, thus killing catalase-
positive organisms such as *E. coli* (see Sec. IV.D).

IV. BIOLOGICAL SIGNIFICANCE OF LPS

Immunity is generally defined as resistance to infection through the
presence of cellular and noncellular antibody systems. However, it has
become increasingly evident that nonantibody factors (see Chap. 1)
contribute to immunity, either to augment antibody and leukocyte action or promote protection before specific antibody responses become
effective. The question arises, therefore, whether the presence of
LPS is designed to be one of the factors that protect the newborn
against intestinal infection at the same time as providing nourishment.

A. The Mammary Gland

The bovine udder is known to be very sensitive to bacterial infection.
Infusions of extremely small numbers of pathogens (as few as 10 organisms) are capable of setting up a chronic or even acute mastitis. Since
milk is such a good medium for the multiplication of bacteria, certain
mastitic organisms can kill a cow within days. So far, in the udder,
the only proven effective defense against bacterial infection is phagocytosis (17,37,48,50,63). There is some circumstantial evidence that
the failure of *Streptococcus uberis* to infect the bovine udder is due
to LPS (48). More recently, attempts are being made to breed mastitis-
resistant herds by selecting heifers that give milk with high levels of
LP (5).

The bovine udder is not the only mammary gland susceptible to infection. The incidence of mastitis is high in rabbits (1), and the mammary glands of mice are easily infected (3). Considering the very high
levels of LP in guinea pig milk, this animal might be usefully employed
in mastitis research. To elucidate the role of LPS, a good approach
might be to add LP antiserum continuously by means of an intravascu-
lar drop. Similar experiments were successfully done to elucidate
the role of phagocytes in the bovine udder, using antileukocyte serum
(63).

The hypothesis that leukocytes could provide H_2O_2 for extracellular activation of LPS has an interesting analogy. Phagocytizing leukocytes of patients suffering from chronic granulomatous disease (PMN,
monocytes, and macrophages) ingest pathogens but do not kill catalase-
positive organisms because the leukocytes are unable to generate H_2O_2.
Such patients, however, do not suffer from streptococcal and pneumo-
coccal infection because catalase-negative organisms release H_2O_2 and

in this way aid their own destruction through the rest of the killing
mechanisms (31).

Summing up, the case for LPS protecting the mammary gland is
not proven. It will be necessary to establish whether or not aerobiosis
exists in the gland, and further investigations seem to be warranted.

B. LPS and the Newborn

At birth the intestinal tract is sterile, but within hours becomes colon-
ized with coliforms and clostridia that are eventually suppressed by
lactobacilli and bacteroides which become the dominant flora (66). It
is generally recognized that natural feeding—suckling the dam—promotes the establishment of such desirable flora and helps to suppress
potential pathogens.

Some strains of *E. coli* were found to be pathogenic for piglets when
they possessed certain antigens (K_{87} and K_{88}) that were genetically
transmissible (40,41,68). Such antigens are responsible for the
attachment to the epithelial surface of the intestines (4) and the production of enterotoxins that cause diarrhea in piglets, calves, and
lambs (67,68). These plasmid-controlled colonization factors are not
restricted to strains affecting animals but are also found in human
beings (10).

A useful method for studying attachment in vitro was developed
by Selwood et al. (64) who showed that *E. coli* possessing K_{88} antigen
attached to brush-border cells isolated from pig intestines. The addition of specific secretory IgA to K_{88} antigen largely prevented the
attachment, confirming the role of this antigen. A similar phenomenon
was observed with porcine and bovine strains of *E. coli*: when these
strains were exposed to LPS, attachment was appreciably inhibited
(56,60).

There is no immediate explanation for these findings, unless it can
be shown that motility of *E. coli* is vital for attachment. LPS had
previously been shown to inhibit the motility of spermatozoa (45) and
not surprisingly was found to inhibit the motility of *E. coli*. At present,
however, it has only been shown that motility can be regarded to be a
virulence factor for *Vibrio cholerae* (2), which enables the organisms
to transverse the continuous mucous blanket covering the intestinal
villi and become attached to the epithelial cells. The bactericidal activity of LPS may therefore not be the only biological role of LPS, but
the interference with attachment could be equally important, if proven
in vivo. Thus, LP would either support the role of sIgA in colostrum
and milk or replace it when absent.

C. The Calf as an Experimental Animal

There are several advantages to using the calf as an experimental animal. It can be separated from the dam without ill effect within 1 hr after

birth or before it starts to suck. It can then be fed controlled amounts
of colostrum and milk, thus making such "artificial" feeding equal to
nursing by the dam, a procedure which is difficult or impossible to
achieve with other experimental animals. Also, the milk can be mani-
pulated or heat treated whenever required and used as control feed.
The feeding of host-specific milk avoids the nutritional and digestive
complications arising from feeding nonspecific milk for formula feeds
based on bovine milk. The results of the experiments obtained with
calves can be extrapolated because the calf remains monogastric (abomasum), albeit with some reservations, as long as it is only fed milk
without access to roughage (straw, hay, grass) which develops the
rumen. The main reservation is that bovine milk is clotted in the abomasum by a unique enzyme, rennin, not possessed by many animals.
Since LP is the dominant protective protein in bovine milk, the calf
is suitable for the study of LPS, particularly as saliva can contribute
LP only during feeding because it is diverted to the undeveloped rumen
at other times.

D. In Vivo Experiments

Cannulated calves (in the abomasum or upper duodenum) were fed 2.2
l portions of milk twice daily. During the fasting periods, the pH of
abomasal fluid is 4 and below, but is increased to ~6 after feeding
because of the great buffering capacity of bovine milk. Since the acid
barrier, the most important defense against intestinal infections (11),
is neutralized by the ingestion of milk, only the antibacterial properties
of the milk protect the newborn. Heat-treated or powdered milk provide little protection but do neutralize the acid barrier. The feeding
of these preparations may aid the passage of potential pathogens.

The LP concentration of the abomasal fluid is almost completely
derived from the milk because any LP of the calf's saliva can only enter
the abomasum during feeding. It gradually diminishes and reaches a
very low level before feeding (Table 2). In mammals other than ungul-
ates, saliva containing LP would enter the stomach continuously. It
must, therefore, be assumed that LP levels are maintained, for instance,
in the human infant, although there are no data available.

In contrast, the thiocyanate content of abomasal fluid is very high
during the fasting periods and actually decreases after feeding, since
it is diluted by the milk (Table 2). Obviously, the thiocyanate concentration of the milk itself is relatively unimportant.

Hydrogen peroxide, the third factor for the activation of LPS, was
provided experimentally by the addition of glucose oxidase/glucose,
magnesium peroxide (which hydrolyzes at pH 6 and below, releasing
active H_2O_2), or biologically by feeding an H_2O_2-producing strain of
Lactobacillus casei (NCDO 820). This strain was found to be resistant
to LPS.

Table 2 Concentration of SCN⁻ and LP Activity in Calf Abomasal Fluid Before and After Feeding Raw Milk[a]

	Before feeding	Time of sampling, after feeding		
		30 min	60 min	120 min
SCN⁻ concentration (mM)	0.45 ± 0.14 (17)	0.15 ± 0.08 (30)	0.15 ± 0.08 (37)	0.20 ± 0.09 (38)
LP concentration u/ml	0.009 ± 0.004 (75)	1.4 ± 9.7 (20)	1.14 ± 0.88 (18)	1.09 ± 0.68 (19)

[a]Mean values with standard deviation are shown. Figure in parenthesis is sample size. Four calves were sampled over a period of 50 days. The milk feeds contained 1.9 ± 0.85 u/ml (n = 11), assay method of Shindler et al. (65). At 5 hr no LP was detected.
Source: Ref. 58.

To establish the in vivo activity of LPS, calves were first fed 200 ml of heated milk containing ~10^6 cfu/ml of *E. coli* 0111 [$K_{58}(B_4)H^-$, NCTC 9703], followed by 2000 ml of raw milk containing one of the sources of H_2O_2. The abomasal samples taken immediately after feeding and periodically thereafter contained very few viable coliforms (10^2 cfu/ml is the limit of the assay used) (32). The original inoculum had been reduced by at least 99.9%. However, nearly all the inoculated organisms could be recovered on addition of a reducing agent, thus confirming that the reduction in numbers was due to LPS. Essentially, the same results were obtained with any of the three sources of H_2O_2 used with similar concentrations of thiocyanate and LP.

The use of lactobacilli as source of H_2O_2 is of considerable interest, pointing to a novel function of the much researched and maligned lactobacilli. That they did not produce an antibiotic or bactericidal concentration of H_2O_2 can be attributed to the in vivo activation of LPS. The strain of *L. casei* has an interesting history because it was originally isolated from a cheese, probably made with dried calf stomach, as a source of rennin in the Jura. Table 3 shows that H_2O_2-producing lactobacilli are common in abomasal fluid (58), the esophagus, and upper duodenum (unpublished). Also more recently, *L. casei* was isolated and identified from calf's abomasum (Marshall, personal communication). Unfortunately, there is only indirect evidence of H_2O_2 in the abomasum because the assays of the turbid fluid are rather dubious (0.002-0.007 mM). Nevertheless, there is also some indirect evidence that naturally colonizing lactobacilli (or rather lactic acid bacteria) can produce sufficient H_2O_2 to activate LPS as previously suggested (52) (Fig. 1). When calves were given *E. coli* (10^7 cfu/ml) orally and fed raw milk without the addition of a source of H_2O_2 (Fig. 2), the abomasal fluid showed an appreciable reduction of the inoculum (>99% at 1 hr). However, when *heated* milk, in which LP was inactivated, was fed, nearly all the inoculum was recovered. Feeding raw milk with an H_2O_2-generating system (glucose oxidase/glucose or magnesium peroxide) was, of course, more effective. Nevertheless, these experiments proved that the natural intestinal flora can contribute H_2O_2, albeit at limiting concentrations, to activate LPS. Thus, LPS may be regarded as a natural antibiotic system.

Similar experiments were attempted with piglets, but the results varied greatly, due to many piglets dying of severe dehydration by diarrhea. The artificial feed based on cow's milk often formed a bolus that distended the stomach up to 3 times its normal size (unpublished data). Further work is required to determine whether or not LPS plays a role in the protection of piglets.

Table 3 Percentage of Peroxidogenic Lactobacilli in Abomasal Fluid[a]

	Days						
	4-7	8-14	15-21	22-28	29-35	36-42	43-49
Log_{10} cfu/ml lactobacilli	6.5	6	5.85	6.35	6	7	7.2
Range	5.8-7.3	4.3-6.95	3.7-7	6-6.7	5.5-6.8	6-8	6.3-7.9
Percentage that produce H_2O_2	57	56	45	56	57	62	58
Range	19-87	0-85	0-82	9-93	25-92	52-68	32-90
Number of samples counted	4	7	7	8	8	5	5

[a]Means and range of log_{10} cfu/ml are shown. Samples of abomasal fluid were taken from three calves.
Note: one calf was monitored beyond 49 days: between 57 and 70 days the percentage H_2O_2-producing lactobacilli was 87% (range 72-94%).
Source: Ref. 58.

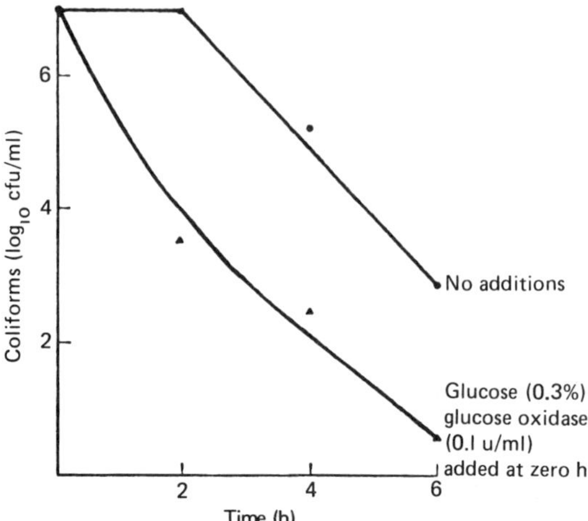

Figure 1 Bactericidal activity of abomasal fluid containing indigenous H_2O_2-producing lactobacilli (10^7 cfu/ml) (58). Abomasal fluid was withdrawn from the fistula of a 12-week-old calf 45 min after feeding raw milk. The fluid was adjusted to pH 5 and inoculated with *E. coli* (8×10^6 cfu/ml). (From Ref. 58.)

V. PRACTICAL APPLICATIONS OF LPS

A. Calf Trials

Based on the in vivo results, it was found in four trials (>200 animals) that LPS was growth promoting. Calves are liable to scour (diarrhea) early in life, particularly when they are transferred while still quite young to large calf units. Scouring is either dietary when milk replacers are used or caused by infection with *E. coli* or viruses. Depending on the severity and period of infection, afflicted animals lose weight or grow less rapidly. Some mortality also occurs. It was shown in these trials (61) that in the case of high incidence of scouring in the control calves (no LPS) the benefit of feeding milk plus LPS was the greatest, the LPS-treated animals showing the best live-weight gains in a given period (Fig. 3).

B. Preservation of Milk

In Western countries milk is cooled and stored for increasingly long periods because of working and distribution circumstances. After 2 days such milk can deteriorate through the multiplication of psychrotrophic organisms (mainly pseudomonads), which produce extremely heat-resistant lipases, and proteases, which survive pasteurization. These

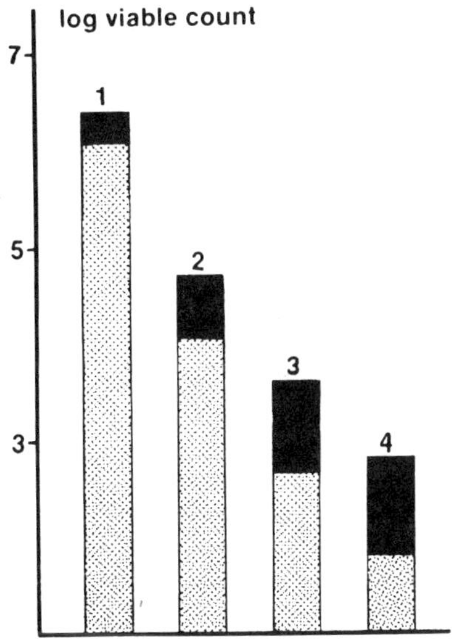

■ 30 min. sample;

▧ 1 h sample

Figure 2 Bactericidal activity of abomasal fluid after feeding *E. coli* NCTC 9703 (0111) (approximately 10^7 cfu/ml) in 200 ml of heated milk (90°C/10 min) followed by feeding 2000 ml of: (1) heated milk, (2) raw milk, (3) raw milk + glucose (0.3%)/glucose oxidase (0.1 U/ml), and (4) raw milk + MgO_2 (1 mM). (From Ref. 59.)

enzymes can make the milk unpalatable or spoil dairy products such as butter and cheese. Milk does not normally contain, under present feeding conditions, sufficient thiocyanate for LPS, and it must be added at the same time as a source of H_2O_2. Figure 4 (6) shows the effect on *Pseudomonas fluorescens* after such supplements were added; the number of organisms growing out afterwards are not resistant to LPS because the same rate of kill under the given conditions (concentration of thiocyanate and H_2O_2) could be achieved when the residual bacteria were allowed to reach maximum growth and were repeatedly exposed to the LPS. The spoilage effect of the heat-resistant enzymes can be clearly seen in Table 4. Undue multiplication of *P. fluorescens* resulted in the production of an unpalatable, rancid cheese, although the organisms were killed by heat prior to the manufacture of the cheese. Activating LPS reduced the number of organisms sufficiently to produce an acceptable cheese without rancidity.

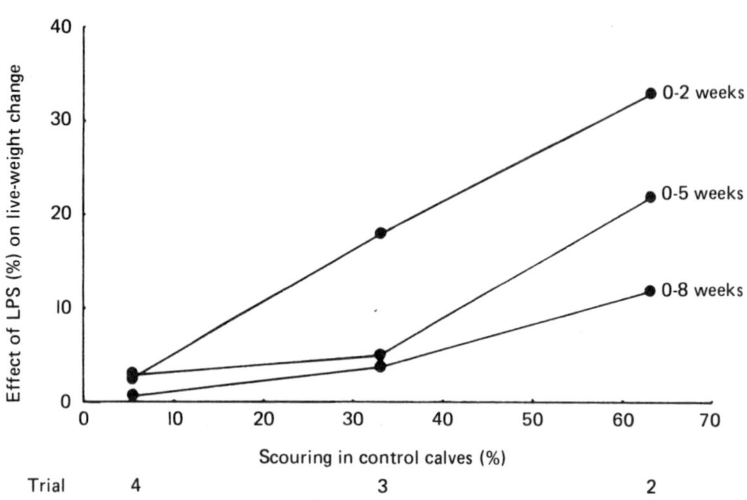

Figure 3 Relationships between the effect of the LPS (%) on live-weight change and the level of scouring (%) in calves given whole milk only. (From Ref. 61.)

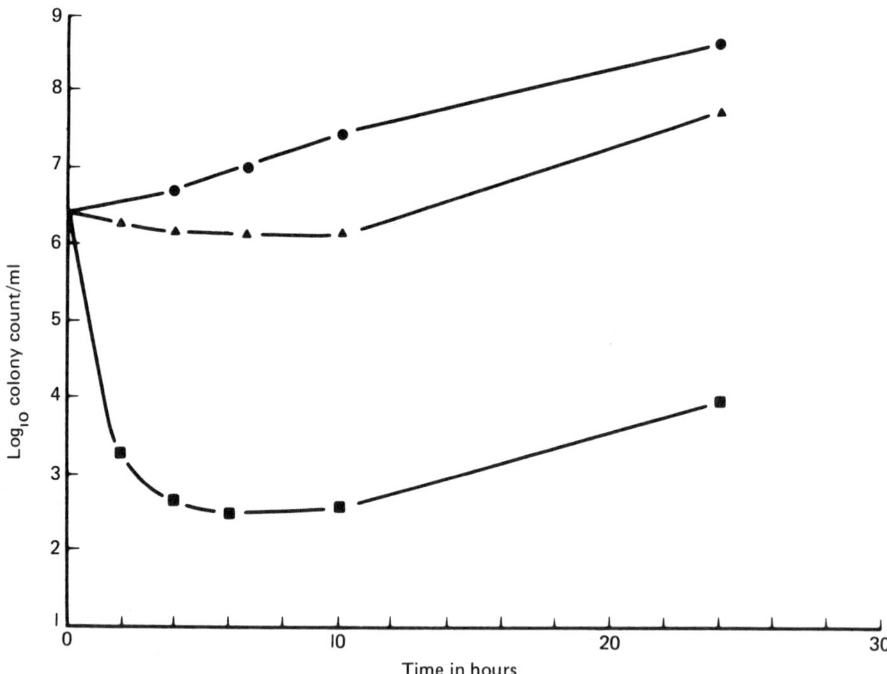

Figure 4 *Pseudomonas fluorescens* EF 1998 in raw milk containing 0.085 mM SCN⁻. Supplements: ●, none; ▲, 0.1 U/ml of glucose oxidase and 0.3% glucose; ■, 0.1 U/ml of glucose oxidase, 0.3% glucose, and 0.083 mM SCN⁻. (From Ref. 6.)

Table 4 Effect of LP System on Multiplication of *Ps. fluorescens* and Cheese Quality

Treatment of milk	No. of *Ps. fluorescens* (cfu ml^{-1} × 10^4) in milk stored at 5°C for (d)				Cheese quality at 4 months	
	0	1	2	3	FFA (μmol 10 g^{-1})	Flavor assessment
None	15	29	150	1400	248	Rancid
LP system	21	1.1	0.2	0.1	50	Normal

Source: Ref. 57.

LPS can also be employed to prevent the spoilage of uncooled raw milk at ambient temperatures of up to 30°C and above. In many developing countries, raw, uncooled milk is taken to collecting centers, also without cooling facilities, and transported for many hours to the creameries. Depending on the original hygienic quality, ambient temperatures, and distance from the collecting center, a high proportion of the milk becomes unfit for further handling, distribution as liquid milk, or for manufacture. The addition of thiocyanate and sodium percarbonate, as a source of H_2O_2 (hydrolyzing at the normal pH of milk, 6.5-6.6), increases the shelf life of milk sufficiently to be acceptable even after transporting it for many hours at high ambient temperatures. Figure 5 (14,59) demonstrated (in Sri Lanka) how well milk can be preserved; the test used (dye reduction) estimates approximately the number of organisms, depending on their metabolic activity. The raw milk flora are dominated by lactic acid bacteria. Therefore, the activation of LPS not only prevents the multiplication of gram-negative organisms, but also inhibits lactic acid bacteria (44,59), which are the main producers of lactic acid. Similarly successful trials have been made in Kenya (8) and Mexico (Härnulv, Alfa-Laval AB, Sweden, personal communication). Food spoilage is as great a problem as adequate

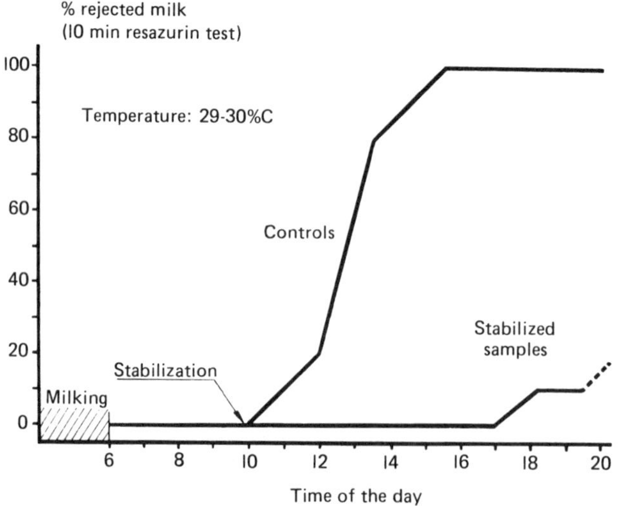

Figure 5 Effect of stabilization of raw milk by activation of its LPS. Results from Narahenpita Collection Centre, Sri Lanka. Additions: 20 ppm of sodium thiocyanate and sodium percarbonate to generate approximately 8.5 ppm of H_2O_2. (From Ref. 14.)

food production in many developing countries, and it appears that enhancement of LPS may help to prevent milk spoilage and encourage dairy farming under otherwise adverse circumstances.

REFERENCES

1. Adlam, C., and Ward, P. D., *Infect. Immunol. 17*: 250 (1977).
2. Allweiss, B., Dostal, J., Carey, K. E., Edwards, T. F., and Freter, R., *Nature (Lond.) 266*: 448 (1977).
3. Anderson, J. C., *Br. Vet. J., 135*: 163 (1979).
4. Arbuckle, J. B. R., *J. Med. Microbiol. 3*: 333 (1970).
5. Bassalik-Chabialska, L., in *Symposium on Mastitis Control*, Bassalik-Chabialska, L. (Ed.), Jablonna, Poland, p. 212 (1982).
6. Björck, L., Rosén, C-G., Marshall, V. M. E., and Reiter, B., *Appl. Microbiol. 30*: 199 (1975).
7. Björck, L., *J. Dairy Res. 45*: 109 (1978).
8. Björck, L., Claesson, O., and Schulthess, W., *Milchwissenschaft 34*: 726 (1979).
9. Boulangé, M., *Completes Rendues Séances de la Société de Biologie Paris 153*: 2019 (1959).
10. Evans, D. G., Silver, R. P., Evans, D. J., Jr., Chese, D. G., and Gorbach, S. L., *Infect. Immun. 12*: 656 (1975).
11. Giannella, R. A., Broitman, S. H., and Samcheck, *Ann. Intern. Medicine 78*: 271 (1973).
12. Gothefors, S. L., and Marklund, S., *Infect. Immun. 11*: 1210 (1975).
13. Hanssen, F. S., *Br. J. Exp. Pathol. 5*: 271 (1924).
14. Hänulv, B. G., and Kandasamy, C., *Milchwisseuschaft. 37*: 454 (1982).
15. Hehn, S., *Andrologia 7*: 255 (1975).
16. Hesse, W., *Zeitschrift für Hygiene und Infections–Krankheiten 17*: 238 (1894).
17. Hill, A. W., Shears, A. L., and Hibbitt, K. G., *Res. Vet. Sci. 25*: 89 (1978).
18. Hill, R. D., *Aust. J. Dairy Technol. 30*: 26 (1975).
19. Jago, G. R., and Morrison, M., *Proc. Soc. Exp. Biol. Med. 111*: 585 (1962).
20. Jones, F. S., and Little, R. B., *J. Exp. Med. 45*: 319 (1927).
21. Jones, F. S., and Simms, H. F., *J. Exp. Med. 51*: 135 (1930).
22. Kern, V. R., Wildbrett, G., and Kiermeier, F., *Zeitschrift Naturforschung 18*: 1082 (1963).
23. Kiermeier, F., and Kayser, C., *Zeitschrift für Lebensmittel Untersuchung und–Forschung 112*: 481 (1960).
24. Kiermeier, F., and Kuhlmann, H., *Münch. Med. Wochenschr. 114*: 2144 (1972).

25. Klebanoff, S. J., and Smith, D. C., *Gynecol. Invest. 1*: 21 (1970).
26. Korhonen, H., *Untersuchungen zur Bakterizidie der Milch und Immunisierung der Bovinen Milchdruse*, Dissertation, Helsinski, p. 88 (1973).
27. Korhonen, H., in *Symposium on Mastitis Control* Bassalik-Chabialska, L. (Ed.) Jablonna, Poland, p. 421 (1982).
28. Lawrence, A. J., The thiocyanate content of milk, in *XVIIIth International Dairy Congress*, vol. 1E, p. 94 (1970).
29. Lee, C. S., Wooding, F. B. P., and Kemp, P., *J. Dairy Res. 47*: 39 (1980).
30. Linford, E., *J. Reprod. Fertil. 87*: 239 (1974).
31. Mandel, G. L., and Hook, E. W., *J. Bacteriol. 100*: 531 (1969).
32. Miles, A. A., and Misra, S. S., *J. Hygiene 38*: 732 (1938).
33. Mohr, J. A., Leu, R., and Mabry, S., *J. Surg. Oncol. 2*: 163 (1970).
34. Moldoveanu, Z., Tenovuo, J., Mestecky, J., and Pruitt, K. M., *Biochim. Biophys. Acta 718*: 103 (1982).
35. Morrison, M. H., Hamilton, B., and Stotz, E., *J. Biol. Chem. 228*: 767 (1957).
36. Morrison, M. H., and Steele, W. F., in *Biology of the Mouth*, Person, P. (Ed.), American Society for Advancement of Science, pp. 89-110 (1968).
37. Newbould, F. H. S., and Neave, F. K., *J. Dairy Res. 32*: 171 (1965).
38. Oram, J. D., and Reiter, B., *Biochem. J. 100*: 373 (1966).
39. Oram, J. D., and Reiter, B., *Biochem. J. 100*: 382 (1966).
40. Ørskov, I., Ørskov, F., Sojka, W. J., and Leach, J. N., *Acta Pathol. Microbiol. Scand. 79*: 142 (1961).
41. Ørskov, I., Ørskov, F., Smith, H. W., and Sojka, W. J., *Acta Pathol. Microbiol. Scand. B83*: 31 (1975).
42. Piironen, C., and Virtanen, A. I., *Zeitschrift fur Ernährungswissenschaften 3*: 140 (1963).
43. Portman, A., and Auclair, J. E., *Le Lait 39*: 1 (1959).
44. Reiter, B., Pickering, A., Oram, J. D., and Pope, G. S., *J. Gen. Microbiol. 33*: xii (1963).
45. Reiter, B., and Gibbons, R. A., *Annual Report of the National Institute for Research in Dairying*, p. 87 (1964).
46. Reiter, B., Pickering, A., and Oram, J. D., in *Microbial Inhibitors in Food*, 4th International Symposium on Food Microbiology, pp. 297-305 (1964).
47. Reiter, B., and Oram, J. D., *Nature (Lond.) 216*: 328 (1967).
48. Reiter, B., Sharpe, M. E., and Higgs, T. M., *Res. Vet. Sci. 11*: 18 (1970).
49. Reiter, B., Björck, L., Marshall, V. M. E., Longman, A. G., and Cousins, C. M., *Annual Report of the National Institute for Research in Dairying*, p. 98 (1973/74).

50. Reiter, B., and Bramley, A. J., in *Proceedings of Seminar on Mastitis Control*, Dodd, F. H., Griffin, T. K., and Kingwill, R. G. (Eds.), pp. 210-222 (1975).

51. Reiter, B., and Marshall, V. M. E., *Annual Report of the National Institute for Research in Dairying*, p. 90 (1975/76).

52. Reiter, B., Marshall, V. M. E., Björck, L., and Rosén, C.-G., *Infect. Immun. 13*: 800 (1976).

53. Reiter, B., in *Inhibition and Inactivation of Vegetative Microbes*, Skinner, E. A., and Hugo, W. B. (Eds.), Academic Press, New York, pp. 31-60 (1976).

54. Reiter, B., *Ann. Recherches Vet. 9*: 205 (1978).

55. Reiter, B., *J. Dairy Res. 45*: 131 (1978).

56. Reiter, B., in *Oxygen Free Radicals and Tissue Damage*, Ciba Foundation Symposium 65 (new series), Excerpta Medica, pp. 285-294 (1979).

57. Reiter, B., and Marshall, V. M., in *Cold Tolerant Microbes in Spoilage and the Environment*, Russel, A. D., and Fuller, R. (Eds.), Academic Press, New York, pp. 153-164 (1979).

58. Reiter, B., Marshall, V. M., and Philips, S. M., *Res. Vet. Sci. 28*: 116 (1980).

59. Reiter, B., and Härnulv, B. G., *Dairy Industries Int. 47*: 13 (1982).

60. Reiter, B., in *Immunological Aspects of Infection in the Fetus and Newborn*, Lambert, H. P., and Wood, C. B. S. (Eds.), The Beecham Colloquium 1979, Academic Press, New York, pp. 115-195 (1981).

61. Reiter, B., Fulford, R. J., Marshall, V. M. E., Yarrow, N., Ducker, M. J., and Knutsson, M., *Anim. Prod. 32*: 297 (1981).

62. Reiter, B., in *Symposium on Mastitis Control*, Bassalik-Chabialska, L. (Ed.), Jablonna, Poland, p. 351 (1982).

63. Schalm, O. W., Lasmanis, A., and Jain, N. C., *Am. J. Vet. Res. 37*: 835 (1976).

64. Selwood, R., Gibbons, R. A., Jones, G. H., and Rutter, J. M., *J. Med. Microbiol. 8*: 405 (1975).

65. Shindler, J. S., Childes, R. E., and Bardsley, W. G., *Eur. J. Biochem. 65*: 325 (1976).

66. Smith, H. W., *Ann. N.Y. Acad. Sci. 176*: 110 (1971).

67. Smith, H. W., and Linggwood, M. A., *J. Med. Microbiol. 5*: 243 (1972).

68. Sojka, W. J., *Review Series No. 7*, Commonwealth Bureau of Animal Health, Weybridge, England (1965).

69. Stephens, S., Harkness, R. A., and Cockle, S. M., *Br. J. Pathol. 60*: 252 (1979).

70. Wilson, A. T., and Rosenblum, H., *J. Exp. Med. 95*: 20 (1952).

71. Wright, R. C., and Tramer, J., *J. Dairy Res. 25*: 104 (1958).

8

Biochemistry of Peroxidase System: Antimicrobial Effects

KENNETH M. PRUITT* and BRUNO REITER† / *University of Oxford, John Radcliffe Hospital, Headington, Oxford, England*

Current affiliations:

*Department of Biochemistry, The University of Alabama at Birmingham, Birmingham, Alabama

†National Institute for Research in Dairying, Shinfield, Reading, England (Retired)

I. INTRODUCTION

Peroxidase enzymes catalyze the oxidation of electron donors by peroxide to generate highly reactive products with a wide range of antimicrobial properties. The actual structures of these products and
the chemistry of their reactions depend upon the specific peroxidase-
electron donor pair. The details of the antimicrobial effects vary
from organism to organism. The chemistry of peroxidase systems are
described in Chap. 3. Human secretory peroxidase systems are considered in Chap. 6, and the bovine lactoperoxidase system in Chap. 7.
In the present chapter, we review the reactions of the human salivary
peroxidase system and the bovine system with specific microorganisms.
We will discuss the cellular components affected by the products of
these systems and will consider the mechanisms that render some organisms less susceptible or resistant to peroxidase system antimicrobial
effects. We conclude with some theoretical interpretations of bacterial
dose-response curves.

The following abbreviations will be employed: LP, bovine lactoperoxidase; SP, human salivary peroxidase; LPS and SPS, bovine and
salivary peroxidase systems, respectively (the system is composed of
the appropriate enzyme, hydrogen peroxide, and an electron donor);
LPS-SCN and LPS-I, the bovine lactoperoxidase system with the thiocyanate ion and the iodide ion, respectively, as electron donors; and
SPS-SCN and SPS-I, the salivary peroxidase system with the specified
donor.

A. System Components

SP is secreted into saliva by the salivary glands, whereas LP is a
product of the mammary glands and is found in high concentrations in
bovine milk. Antibodies raised against LP will cross react with SP, but
the structures of these two enzymes are not identical. Although both
SP and LP will utilize Br^-, I^-, and SCN^- as electron donors, the two
enzymes differ significantly in stability and in kinetic properties (60).
Human salivary peroxidase has been called *lactoperoxidase*. This nomenclature is inaccurate.

Hydrogen peroxide is excreted by many species of commensal
lactobacilli and streptococci (Chap. 9), as well as by activated leukocytes (49). The consistently observed presence of the hypothiocyanite
ion (the principal product of the SPS-SCN) in human saliva (109,114)
implies a continuous source of hydrogen peroxide in the human mouth.
Apparently there is a source of H_2O_2 in addition to commensal bacteria
and leukocytes because hypothiocyanite is a normal component of parotid saliva collected directly from the Stensen's duct of healthy parotid
glands (84).

The electron donor that is most significant in vivo is the thiocyanate
ion. It is a normal component of human saliva and bovine milk and is

derived from the diet (Chaps. 6 and 7). The iodide and bromide ions
are not present in high enough concentrations in milk and in saliva to
be of biological significance, but are included for historical and theoretical reasons.

B. System Products

The major product of the LPS-SCN and the SPS-SCN at neutral pH is
the hypothiocyanite anion ($OSCN^-$), which is in equilibrium with hy-
pothiocyannous acid (HOSCN, pK 5.3) (111). There are other products of the LPS-SCN and the SPS-SCN that are generated in small
amounts and are relatively unstable at neutral pH compared with hypothiocyanite (8,13,32,85,86). These minor products may have even
more potent antimicrobial properties than does hypothiocyanite (13,
107). The end products of the reaction (SO_4^{2-}, CO_2, NH_4^+) are not
inhibitory (74). For the LPS-I and the SPS-I, the major product is
iodine (I_2) (Chap. 3).

C. Reactive Microbial Components

The major cellular components that react with $OSCN^-$ or with HOSCN
are sulfhydryl groups (9) and reduced nicotinamide nucleotides (33,
75,95).

The sulfhydryl groups may be the cysteine residues of specific
proteins, free cysteine itself, or reduced glutathione. Sulfhydryl
groups are oxidized to disulfides (-S-S-), sulfenyl thiocyanates
(-S-SCN⁻), and sulfinic acids (-S-OH) (9). Disulfides, sulfenyl thiocyanates, and sulfiniuc acids are easily converted back to sulfhydryls
by an excess of reducing agents such as cysteine, glutathione, mercaptoethanol, dithiothreitol, and sodium hydrosulfite.

The nucleotides NADH and NADPH are oxidized to NAD^+ and
$NADP^+$, and this reaction is also reversible.

Hypothiocyanite does not react with tyrosine or tryptophan and
reacts with histidine only at high histidine concentrations (10). However, modification of aromatic amino acids was observed when the
reactants were combined with the LPS-SCN⁻ (10). This observation
suggests the formation of highly reactive, transient intermediates by
the LPS-SCN⁻, as discussed in the previous section. Histidine gave a
major derivative that incorportated both carbon and sulfur atoms of
the SCN⁻, suggesting the formation of an aryl thiocyanate. However,
there was a preferential incorporation of the carbon atom of the SCN⁻
into tyrosine and tryptophan that could be the result of further oxidation of aryl thiocyanates (10). These oxidations of aromatic amino
acids by the LPS-SCN occur only when the active products of the LPS-
SCN are generated in the presence of the reactants and in excess over
any -SH compounds which may also be present. The oxidations of

tyrosine, tryptophan, and histidine by the LPS-SCN are not reversible by addition of excess thiol compounds.

Iodine oxidizes the same components as hypothiocyanite but, after sulfhydryls are oxidized, tyrosine and histidine residues are iodinated (18). Tryptophan may also be oxidized (5). These iodination reactions with aromatic amino acids are not reversible by excess thiol compounds.

II. EFFECTS ON MICROORGANISMS

A. General Observations

The data in the Appendix shows that the SPS and LPS can kill or inhibit the growth and metabolism of many different species of microorganisms. For any particular organism, the antimicrobial effects depend upon the reaction conditions.

Although there are structural and biochemical differences between SP and LP, both enzymes are effective at very low concentrations when combined with SCN^- or I^- and H_2O_2. LP is catalytically effective at concentrations as low as 0.5 µg/l (79). This corresponds to a concentration of 6.5×10^{-12} M (assuming a molecular weight of 77,500 daltons). SP has been only partially purified (39,60,100). However, the enzyme activity in resting human whole saliva is equivalent to the activity of an LP solution with a concentration of 26×10^{-9} M (84), and human saliva diluted 10-fold retains its peroxidase-dependent capacity for inhibiting bacterial metabolism (27). Both enzymes remain catalytically active when adsorbed to bacterial cell surfaces. LP is effective when fewer than 100 molecules are adsorbed per cell of *Streptococcus mutans* (79).

Peroxidase enzyme concentration is not a limiting factor for LPS or SPS antibacterial activity in bovine milk or in human saliva. The SCN^- concentration is a limiting factor in milk and sometimes in saliva, but usually it is the availability of H_2O_2 that determines the magnitude of antibacterial activity of peroxidase systems (87) (for details see Chaps. 6 and 7).

In vitro, at concentrations high enough to produce significant antibacterial effects, no qualitative differences have been reported between results obtained with SP or with LP as catalyst. When adequate concentrations of either enzyme are provided, microbicidal effects are greather with I^- rather than SCN^- as electron donor, at low temperatures (0°-5°C), at low pH (5 or less), and in the absence of reducing agents.

Under otherwise identical conditions, the effectiveness of the LPS or SPS may vary with the medium in which the test is carried out. For example, small molecular weight components present in brain-heart infusion broth interfere with the antimicrobial action of the LPS (36).

A given quantity of hydrogen peroxide is more effective when it is supplied by the metabolism of the cells or by continuous generation with glucose/glucose oxidase than when it is added separately.

When the components of the LPS or SPS are brought together in the presence of the target cells, killing or inhibition is more effective than if the cells are added after the components are combined.

When microorganisms are exposed to the LPS or the SPS in experiments using otherwise identical reaction conditions, the results obtained will depend upon the state of the cells. In general, resting cells or cells in the stationary growth phase are more susceptible to killing or inhibition than are metabolically active or growing cells. Bacteria grown anaerobically are more susceptible to the LPS than are those grown aerobically (17).

Increased permeability of the cell envelope is associated with increased susceptibility to LPS antibacterial effects (88).

Target cells bearing catalytically active peroxidase adsorbed to the cell surface are more readily inhibited by the SPS or the LPS than are cells exposed to systems where the products are generated exclusively in the fluid phase. For a given concentration of enzyme, peroxide, and electron donor, the LPS is more effective at low cell densities than at high cell densities (92,112,115).

Lactoperoxidase interacts with other components of milk and saliva, and this interaction may be significant in vivo. In vitro experiments have shown that LP binds to secretory IgA, IgM, myeloma IgA_1, and myeloma IgA_2 (108). No binding was observed with IgG or with lactoferrin (70). The interactions between LP and the immunoglobulins were nonspecific. The LP-Ig complex was more stable than the free enzyme.

In the presence of 20 μM hypothiocyanite, the glucose-stimulated acid production of *S. mutans* was reduced 50% (108). When S-IgA was present, 20 μM hypothiocyanite completely inhibited acid production. The effect was not dependent on *S. mutans*-specific antibodies. Similar results were obtained when lactoferrin replaced S-IgA (70). Neither S-IgA nor lactoferrin alone inhibited acid production.

B. Effects on Specific Microorganisms

1. Viruses

With halides (I^-,Br^-) as electron donors, the LPS was able to kill both an RNA (poliovirus) and a DNA (vaccina) virus (11). Optimum killing was observed at pH 4.5. These particular viruses are more resistant than are most others to the effects of drying, heat, and disinfectants. These results illustrate the theoretical range and potency of the antimicrobial effects of the LPS even on the most primitive life forms.

2. Mycoplasmas

There has been only one report (90) of the killing of mycoplasma by the LPS. However, the killing of *Mycoplasma pneumoniae* by the horseradish peroxidase (HRP)/H_2O_2/I^- system has been described (42).

Since the HRP system generates the same products as the LPS when I^-
is the electron donor (see Chap. 3), it seems reasonable to assume
that the LPS and the SPS would have general mycoplasmacidal activity.

3. Gram-Positive Bacteria

Metabolic activities of most strains of lactobacilli and streptococci
can be inhibited by the LPS and the SPS. However, the sensitivity
varies from strain to strain, and some strains are not inhibited. For
the common oral streptococci, the relative resistance of the cells to
inhibition is in the order *S. mitis* > *S. sanguis* > *S. mutans* > *S. naes-
lundi* > *S. salivarius*. This is also the relative order of H_2O_2-excreting
capacity for these cells. Different strains of the oral pathogen (28)
S. mutans vary in their peroxidogenic capacity and, generally, the
greater the peroxidogenicity, the more resistant is the cell to LPS/
SPS inhibition. However, all strains of *S. mutans* thus far tested can
be inhibited by the LPS under appropriate conditions (see Sec. IV.).
Many strains of *S. cremoris* are resistant to the LPS. Serological
groups A, F, and G were most sensitive, whereas some group N strains
were not affected (95). Strains of *S. agalactiae* (group B) also varied
in their sensitivity to LPS inhibition (67), whereas strains of *S. dys-
galactiae* (group C) are resistant. Reasons for variations in resistance
to the LPS are discussed later.

Exposure of susceptible cells to the LPS or the SPS results in a
rapid (less than 1 min) inhibition of metabolism and, within minutes,
leakage of amino acids and potassium. Carbohydrate transport and
utilization, oxygen uptake, amino acid and purine transport (hence,
nucleic acid and protein syntheses), production and excretion of extracellular products (e.g., lactic acid, H_2O_2, collagenase), and growth
may be inhibited. Many species recovery spontaneously from inhibition
when they are exposed to low concentrations of I_2 or $OSCN^-$ for short
periods of time. The inhibition of cells by the LPS or the SPS can be
blocked by the presence of reducing compounds (glutathione, cysteine,
mercaptoethanol, or dithiothreitol). When an excess of these compounds
is added to inhibited cells, there may be a rapid and complete recovery
of activity.

4. Gram-Negative Bacteria

The earliest reports of the effect of the LPS on gram-negative
bacteria were those of Hesse (31) and Hanssen (30). These reports
are not listed in the Appendix because they are difficult to interpret.
These authors found that gram-negative, catalase-positive species of
Vibrio and *Salmonella* were killed in raw milk. No additions of peroxide or peroxide-generating substances were made. Therefore, we must
assume that the milk contained a source of peroxide. Contaminants of
peroxidogenic lactic acid bacteria are likely candidates. Also, the
inoculum may have transferred sufficient xanthine or hypoxanthine to

serve as a substrate for the milk xanthine oxidase, with resultant generation of H_2O_2 (50,94). Another possibility is the generation of H_2O_2 by the metal-catalyzed (Cu^{2+}) reaction of O_2 and ascorbic acid (50). These same comments apply to the reports of the killing of *Escherichia coli* by guinea pig milk in the absence of a specified source of H_2O_2 (102).

Most of the general comments made above regarding LPS and SPS effects on gram-positive bacteria apply also to the gram-negative species, but there are significant differences. Gram-negative bacteria seem to be more easily killed than are gram-positive cells by extended incubation with $OSCN^-$ in excess of 100 µM, especially at low temperatures. The dependence of killing on pH seems to be greater for gram-negative species. When SCN^- is the electron donor, *E. coli* and *S. typhimurium* are difficult to kill when incubation is carried out at pH 7 or above and at temperatures of 20°C or more. Under these same conditions, I^- as electron donor will produce killing. Both SCN^- and I^- promote killing by the LPS when incubated with bacteria at pH 5.5 or less and at 0-5°C. *E. coli* recover much more readily from LPS treatment when they are subsequently incubated anaerobically rather than aerobically (2). The inner membrane of gram-negative bacteria appears to be more extensively damaged by LPS treatment than is that of gram-positive species (64). In contrast to what was observed with gram-positive bacteria and with some strains of *E. coli*, two strains of *S. typhimurium* were found to be more easily killed by the LPS when they were treated in exponential phase of growth than when treated in lag phase of growth (88).

5. Fungi

Candida tropicalis were killed by the LPS when I^- was used as electron donor (29). In this interesting study, H_2O_2 was supplied by a strain of peroxidogenic oral streptococci (*S. mitis*) inoculated into the test medium along with the *C. tropicalis*. The antifungal properties of the LPS and the SPS probably extended beyond this particular organism. Lehrer (56) found that several strains of *C. albicans* as well as species of *Saccharomyces*, *Rhodotorula*, *Geotrichum*, and *Aspergillus* were killed by the myeloperoxidase/H_2O_2/I^- system. Candida strains were also killed when horseradish peroxidase was substituted for MP. Since MP, HRP, and LP generate the same products when I^- is the electron donor (Chap. 3), the LPS would probably also kill the fungi studied by Lehrer.

6. Parasites

There have been no reports of the effects of the LPS or the SPS on parasites. However, several studies have been made utilizing eosinophil peroxidase (EP). These studies are relevant in the present context because the biochemistry of the EP-catalyzed oxidation of halides and thiocyanate is similar to that found with SP or LP as catalysts (46, Chap. 3). The major difference is that EP will utilize Cl^- as an electron donor, but LP and SP will not. The bactericidal effects of the EP system on *E. coli* are similar to those of the LPS (46).

Trypomastigotes of *Trypanosoma cruzi* were killed by the EP system with Cl^-, Br^-, or I^- as electron donors (73). The enzyme was bound to the surface of these parasites, and these EP-coated organisms could be killed by the addition of H_2O_2 and halides. These authors did not report any studies with LP or SCN^-. However, LP utilizes both Br^- and I^- as electron donors and also binds in a catalytically active form to the surface of microorganisms (78,101,103,110). These similarities suggest that LP could substitute for EP in killing experiment with *T. cruzi*.

Myeloperoxidase from human neutrophils was found to be toxic for *T. dionisii* in the presence of H_2O_2 (116). The electron donor was probably Cl^-. This organism is closely related to *T. cruzi*, which was killed by the EP system with Cl^-, Br^-, or I^- as electron donors (73). Since LP can utilize both Br^- and I^- as electron donors to generate the same products as the EP system (Chap. 3), we suggest that *T. dionisii* would be killed by the LPS with either Br^- or I^- as electron donor.

The $EP/H_2O_2/Cl^-$ system was shown to kill newborn larvae of *Trichinella spiralis* (16). By the same reasoning as previously, we predict that the $LP/H_2O_2/I^-$ system would kill this organism.

7. Human Oral Flora

Activation of the salivary peroxidase system by mouth rinses or dentifrices that generate peroxide has been shown to reduce the formation of dental plaque and to decrease caries and gingivitis (38,52,53, 97). These studies are discussed in detail in Chap. 11. The results of these clinical tests are consistent with the in vitro findings. The data in the Appendix show that most species of oral microorganisms which have been tested are susceptible to inhibition by the SPS or LPS.

Human dental plaque is a mixture of many different species of microorganisms. The glucose-stimulated metabolism of plaque is inhibited in vitro by human saliva (107). The inhibition depends critically on the hypothiocyanite concentration in the saliva. When this concentration is elevated above 100 μM by addition of SCN^- and H_2O_2, the glucose-stimulated plaque acid production is almost completely inhibited. The concentration of hypothiocyanite in normal, unstimulated human whole saliva is just below the threshold level required for inhibition of plaque acid production. Thus, it would be expected that any measures that elevate hypothiocyanite concentration in saliva above 100 μM should reduce plaque formation and its consequences to oral health. Such an elevation has been attained with a simple mouth rinse (0.5% citrate, pH 5.5, 4 mM H_2O_2, 1 mM SCN^-) (62). The hypothiocyanite concentration is unstimulated whole saliva was 65 ± 24 μM (n = 13), whereas the concentration in the expectorate collected after subjects had rinsed for 2 min with 5 ml of the solution was 132 ± 37 μM (n = 15).

III. CELLULAR SYSTEMS ALTERED

A. Outer Membrane

In addition to the cytoplasmic (inner) membrane, the cell envelopes of gram-negative bacteria have a lipopolysaccharide-containing outer membrane. This membrane serves, among other functions, as a permeability barrier (21). There is no evidence that peroxidase systems or their products alter the function of the outer membrane. That the outer membrane offers some protection against the antibacterial effects of peroxidase systems can be deduced from the experiments with *S. typhimurium* mutants (so-called rough strains). These strains have lost the capacity to synthesize the complete lipopolysaccharide chain. They were much more sensitive to the LPS-SCN or to $OSCN^-$ prepared from $(SCN)_2$ than was the parent strain (so-called smooth strain) with an intact outer membrane (88,118).

Treatment of *E. coli* by techniques that removed lipopolysaccharide from the outer membrane (112) increased the killing by the LPS-I by a factor greater than 10^3 (ratio of viable counts in intact cells to that in treated cells). When SCN^- rather than I^- was the electron donor, killing was the same for the intact cells and the treated cells. Apparently, in this case, the outer membrane is able to interfere with the action of I_2 on the cells but not with that of $OSCN^-$. Similar results were obtained with spheroplasts that had had their cell walls as well as outer membranes removed (112). These results suggest that the target for the products of the LP system is in the cytoplasmic membrane or the cytoplasm and that the cell wall and outer membrane may partially limit accessibility but do not totally exclude the products of the LPS-SCN from the cell interior.

B. Cell Wall

The cell wall of *E. coli* may also be altered by exposure of cells to the LPS-SCN. After more than 1-hr exposure, electron micrographs revealed damaged and lysed cells (89-91). However, these effects are probably a consequence of damage to the cytoplasmic membrane rather than a direct attack on the cell wall.

C. Cytoplasmic Membrane

Marshall and Reiter (64) found evidence that the cytoplasmic membrane is altered by hypothiocyanite. They prepared hypothiocyanite by adding H_2O_2 to mixtures of SCN^- and sepharose-bound LP until the SCN^- concentration reached a minimum. Treatment of *E. coli* suspensions with these solutions led to extensive leakage of [^{14}C]amino acids and [42]K within 10 min but less so with *S. lactis*. Such leakage would have been prevented by an intact cytoplasmic membrane. Damage to the inner membrane of *E. coli* was also suggested by the increase in hydrogen ion permeability of cells treated with the LPS-SCN (55). It would appear that the cell wall of gram-positive bacteria is a greater barrier to the products of the LPS than is the cell wall of gram-negative bacteria.

There is abundant evidence that the cytoplasmic membrane of gram-positive bacteria is also altered by the LP system. The data in the Appendix show that treatment with the LP system or with hypothiocyanite inhibits amino acid tranport in *Lactobacillus acidophilous* (19,100) and *S. aureus* (29), sugar transport in *S. agalactiae* (68), and glucose and oxygen uptake in numerous species. These various effects suggest damage to the cytoplasmic membrane where systems associated with these processes are found.

Mickelson found that the glucose transport system of *S. agalactiae* was inhibited by the LPS-SCN (68). The inhibition could be reversed with reducing agents. Thus, for this bacterium, the LPS apparently inhibits the glucose transport system by modification of essential membrane sulfhydryl groups of that system. In other studies, Mickelson showed (69) that the LPS incorporated $S^{14}CN^-$ into bacterial protein, and the incorporated label could be released by treatment with reducing agents. When the cytoplasmic membrane was altered by detergents, the amount of incorporated label increased 30-fold. Thus, there are reactive cytoplasmic components in this species that are, at least somewhat, shielded from the LP system by the cytoplasmic membrane.

Marshall and Reiter (64) found that $OSCN^-$ produced some leakage of ^{14}C-labeled amino acids and [41]K from cells of *S. lactis*, suggesting damage to the cytoplasmic membrane. This leakage was much less than that found for *E. coli*.

D. Transport Systems

The LPS-SCN inhibited the active tranport of glutamic acid, lysine, valine, and phenylalanine in *L. acidophilous* (19,100). Saliva could substitute for LP. There was no loss of cell viability. Since the transport of glutamic acid by this organism requires the presence of glucose, the inhibition of transport by the LPS-SCN may be due to inhibition of glucose metabolism or to direct alteration of components of the glutamic acid transport system or to a combination of these effects.

The SPS-SCN has been shown to completely inhibit glucose transport in *S. agalactiae* (68). Transport was also inhibited by p-chloromercuribenzoate (pCMB) and N-ethylmaleimide (NEM). The inhibition by any of these agents could be reversed by dithiothreitol (DTT).

These results suggest that the LPS-SCN oxidizes -SH groups, which
are essential for the transport system, in the cytoplasmic membrane.
This organism also has an active phosphoenol pyruvate-dependent
phosphotransferase system (PTS) (98). The PTS was inhibited by
pCMB and NEM, and the inhibition could be reversed by DTT. However, the PTS was only slightly inhibited by treatment with LPS-SCN.
Thus, the complete inhibition of glucose transport in *S. agalactiae*
by the LPS-SCN cannot be due entirely to effects of the PTS system.

In contrast to the results obtained with *S. agalactiae*, the PTS of
S. mutans (99) was completely inhibited by treatment with the LPS-
SCN (34). The PTS in starved cells was more easily inhibited than
that in active cells. When separated from the LPS-SCN, inhibited cells
recovered PTS activity. The phosphorylation of glucose by hexokinase
and ATP was also inhibited in LPS-SCN-treated cells (34).

E. Glycolytic Enzymes

Several glycolytic enzymes are inhibited by the products of the LPS.
In one type of experiment, cells were treated with the LP-SCN or with
OSCN$^-$, and the activity of the enzyme in question in extracts from the
treated cells and from untreated controls was compared. Hexokinase
and aldolase activities in extracts from LPS-SCN-treated *S. cremoris*
were significantly reduced (74,75). Some inhibition was also found for
6-phosphogluconate dehydrogenase and for glucose-6-phosphate dehydrogenase.

Similar results were obtained with *S. mutans* (34). Extracts from
treated cells had significantly lowered pyruvate kinase, hexokinase,
and aldolase activities. Levels of enolase phosphoglycerate kinase and
phosphoglycerate mutase were reduced to a lesser extent. When cells
were treated with the LPS-SCN in the presence of glucose, the inhibition of glycolytic enzymes in the cellular extracts was much less than
that obtained for cells treated in the absence of glucose (34).

In another type of experiment, enzymes were extracted from nontreated cells, and the effect of LPS-SCN on the extracted enzymes in
vitro was studied. For *S. mutans*, the extent of inactivation of pyruvate kinase, hexokinase, aldolase, and enolase was similar for both
types of experiments (34). Hexokinase from *S. cremoris* was inactivated to the same extent (80-100%) in both types of experiments. However, the activity of LPS-SCN treated hexokinase could not be restored
by the addition of reducing agents, although similar treatment of inhibited cells of *S. cremoris* restored metabolic activity as well as hexokinase activity in subsequent cell extracts. Hexokinase from yeast cells
was inhibited by the LPS-SCN (3).

Glyceraldehyde-3-phosphate dehydrogenase activity in extracts of
S. pyogenes was totally inhibited by LP/H_2O_2 mixtures in the absence
of SCN$^-$ (67). Much less inhibition was observed when SCN$^-$ was added.
These results would be expected if the LP/H_2O_2 complex (compound I)

were attacking the glyceraldehyde phosphate dehydrogenase molecule directly by using available -SH groups as donors. In the presence
of SCN⁻, the extent of this reaction might be reduced because of competition between SCN⁻ and -SH groups for the available compound I.
However, it has been shown that OSCN⁻ can directly oxidize glyceralde-
hyde-3-phosphate dehydrogenase (17). Treatment of cell extracts of
this enzyme (NAD linked) from *S. mitis*, *S. sanguis*, *S. mutans*, and
S. salivarius with OSCN⁻ solutions resulted in complete inhibition of
enzyme activity (17). The concentration required for complete inhibition varied from organism to organism. The NADP-linked glyceraldehyde phosphate dehydrogenase from *S. mitis* was not inhibited by
OSCN⁻. However, the same enzyme extracted from *S. sanguis*, *S.
mutans*, and *S. salivarius* was inhibited 60-90%.

F. Nucleic Acids

Mutagen-sensitive strains (6) of *Salmonella typhimurium* were exposed
to high concentrations of OSCN⁻ (118). Although the cells were *killed*
at concentrations above 10 μM, no *mutagenic* effects were observed for
any concentration of OSCN⁻. The viability of a strain of *Saccharomyces cerevisiae* commonly used as a test cell for evaluating the potential of a compound to produce gene conversion was unaffected by concentrations of OSCN⁻ in excess of 800 μM. Calf thymus deoxyribonucleic acid (DNA) was not oxidized by OSCN⁻. These results indicate
that neither bacterial nor mammalian DNA is altered by OSCN⁻.

IV. MICROBIAL RESISTANCE TO PEROXIDASE SYSTEMS

A. Resistant Strains of *S. cremoris*

Several strains of *S. cremoris* showed little susceptibility to inhibition
or killing by the LPS-SCN (95). Extracts from a resistant strain were
able to reverse the inhibition of a susceptible strain. The data suggested that the resistant strains utilize an NADH₂-oxidizing enzyme
to catalyze the oxidation of NADH₂ by OSCN⁻ (74). Presumably this
reaction kept the concentration of OSCN⁻ generated by the LPS-SCN
below inhibitory levels.

B. Resistant Strains of *S. agalactiae*

Mickelson found that certain strains of *S. agalactiae* developed, under
conditions of aerobic growth, a cyanide-sensitive respiratory system
that was not inhibited by the LPS-SCN (67). This LPS-SCN-resistant
system may utilize the PTS for glucose transport since that system in
S. agalactiae was resistant to LPS-SCN inhibition (68).

C. Resistance of Oral Streptococci

Carlsson et al. (17) found that *S. mitis* and *S. sanguis*, but not *S. salivarius* and *S. mutans*, had a high capacity for recovering from inhibition by $OSCN^-$. They found an enzyme that catalyzed the reduction of $OSCN^-$ to SCN^-. The activity of this NAD(P)H-OSCN oxidoreductase was much higher in *S. mitis* and *S. sanguis* than in *S. salivarius* and *S. mutans*. The relative resistance of these organisms to $OSCN^-$ may be due to relative difference in activity of this oxidoreductase enzyme. This enzyme may serve the same function in oral streptococci as the $NADH_2$-oxidizing enzyme that Oram and Reiter (74) extracted from resistant strains of *S. cremoris*.

The potential importance of NADPH in *S. mutans'* resistance to the LPS-SCN has also been pointed out by Hoogendoorn (35). His hypothesis is that inhibited cells recover by utilizing NADPH to reduce compounds that have been oxidized by $OSCN^-$. When the supply of NADPH is exceeded by the level of H_2O_2 (from which $OSCN^-$ is generated), cells are unable to reverse the effects of the LPS-SCN. This hypothesis has some similarity to the one suggested by Thomas et al. (115), which is discussed below.

Månsson-Rahemtulla (58) and Månsson-Rahemtulla et al. (63) reported that the resistance of strains of oral bacteria to $OSCN^-$ inhibition was correlated with peroxidogenicity. The more resistant strains were more peroxidogenic. Germaine and Tellefson (27) studied the inhbition of *S. mitis* and *S. mutans* by saliva. They found that *S. mitis* was more resistant to inhibition by saliva than was *S. mutans* and that the *S. mitis* strain also produced more peroxide.

Peroxide-generating strains of *S. mutans* were studied in great detail by Thomas et al. (115). They identified three major types of *S. mutans*: class I (OMZ-176, FA-1, and BHT) produced large amounts of peroxide, class II (Ingbritt, B-13) moderate amounts; and class III (GS-5, HS-6, AHT, LM-7, OMZ-175, and 6715-15) produced little or none. Class I and class II strains were subject to autoinhibition as a result of utilization of the peroxide that they produce by LP-SCN to generate $OSCN^-$. For class I and class II, peroxide and $OSCN^-$ accumulation increased with culture age. Detectable peroxide was excreted by class III cells but did not accumulate due to the high levels of peroxide-reducing enzymes present in these strains. Cells of all classes were inhibited by the LPS-SCN when peroxide was added exogenously. These authors did not observe any direct relationship of resistance to the LPS-SCN with peroxidogenicity. They did find that resistance was correlated with a number of other factors, and it may be that correlations with peroxidogenicity reported by others are indirect.

Plots of lactate production as a function of added peroxide (in the presence of active cells and LP-SCN) showed that in all cases a threshold amount of peroxide had to be added before any inhibition was ob-

served (115). As the amount of added peroxide increased beyond the
threshold level, lactate production fell sharply. Since the curves were
nearly symmetrical, they could be conveniently characterized by the
quantity of peroxide that had to be added to give 50% inhibition of lactate production (ED_{50}). When peroxide was added in the absence of
LP and SCN^-, the ED_{50} values were 20 and 30 times higher than in the
presence of LP and SCN^-. Thus, $OSCN^-$ (or other products of the
LPS-SCN) is 20 to 30 times more effective than peroxide as an inhibitor.
The relative resistance of the strains as measured by ED_{50}s were correlated with a number of factors. Lower ED_{50}s were observed at low
pH and with cells from stationary phase. Preincubation of cells with
glucose led to accumulation of stores of intracellular carbohydrate
polymers and increased resistance to inhibition. However, the LPS-
SCN could also inhibit the metabolism of these reserves as well as the
utilization of extracellular glucose.

The increased resistance associated with increased stores of internal polysaccharides was not directly proportional to the level of these
reserves (115). However, the length of time during which cells were
able to maintain resistance was determined by the level of internal
reserves. Thus, resistance may be determined by the amounts of substances generated by the metabolism of these reserves. Attractive
candidates are NADH and NADPH, which could reduce $OSCN^-$. Resistance was found to be associated with the ability to eliminate $OSCN^-$ by
reducing it to SCN^- (115).

Preincubation of cells with glucose and with certain sulfhydryl compounds led to increased cell sulfhydryl content and to increased resistance (115). These observations were used to construct an attractive
hypothesis for explaining LPS-SCN resistance (115). The first part of
this hypothesis postulates a reductase-dependent NADPH generation of
sulfhydryl compounds from intracellular disulfides. In the second step,
these sulfhydryl compounds rapidly reduce $OSCN^-$ to SCN^- in an en-
zyme-independent reaction. The net result is an NADPH-dependent
reduction of $OSCN^-$ to SCN^- with conservation of intracellular sulfhydryl concentration.

V. THEORETICAL INTERPRETAITON OF HYPOTHIO-
CYANITE-INHIBITION CURVES

Plots of the degree of inhibition of various microbial activities as a
function of hypothiocyanite concentration (or of peroxide concentration
when it is the limiting factor for activity of the LPS-SCN) are characteristically S shaped (58,59,115). There is a threshold concentration
of the limiting component that must be reached before any significant
inhibition is observed. Once the threshold is attained, the degree of
inhibition rises sharply with increasing concentration and rapidly
reaches the final limiting value (usually 100% inhibition). The shapes

of these curves suggest that a critical number of cellular components
must be oxidized before inhibition occurs (81,83).

Plots of the percent lysis of sensitized red cells as a function of
the volume of complement added have shapes (65) similar to those of
hypothiocyanite-inhibition curves.

Lysis curves obey the von Krogh equation (117)

$$\ln V = \ln V_{1/2} + m \ln \left[\frac{Y}{1-Y} \right] \tag{1}$$

where V is the volume of complement added to the system, $V_{1/2}$ is
the volume of complement that gives 50% lysis, Y is the fraction of
cells lysed, ln is the natural logarithm, and m is a factor which determines the symmetry of the Y versus V curve. A plot of lnV versus
ln [(Y/(1 − Y)] is linear, and $V_{1/2}$ may be estimated from the inter-
cept. Hypothiocyanite-inhibition curves obey a similar equation (83)

$$\ln C = \ln C_{1/2} + m \ln \left[\frac{Y}{1-Y} \right] \tag{2}$$

where C is the concentration of hypothiocyanite or of the limiting LPS-
SCN factor and Y is degree of inhibition. For example, if respiration
is measured, then Y is the respiration at a given hypothiocyanite concentration divided by the respiration in the absence of hypothiocyanite.
From the linear plots of data transformed in this way, $C_{1/2}$ and m may
be estimated. The significance of the $C_{1/2}$ was recognized by Thomas
et al. (115) and was called the 50% effective dose (ED_{50}). However,
these authors did not represent their data in the form of Eq. (2).
The point to be made is that for both lysis and hypothiocyanite-inhibition curves, the shape of the curves is determined by only two parameters that have similar interpretations in both types of experiments.

These similarities may be a consequence of the qualitive similarities
of the underlying molecular events. For sensitized red cells a minimum
number of complement lesions must be formed before the cells lyse, and
for hypothiocyanite inhibition a minimum number of cellular components
must be oxidized before the cells will be inhibited. Only a single complement lesion is required to lyse a sensitized red cell (66). However,
probably a large number of groups must be oxidized in order to inhibit
bacterial metabolism. From the data of Thomas and Aune (112), intact
cells of *E. coli* can be estimated to have 5×10^7 -SH groups per cell.
About one-half to one-third of these groups were oxidized by the LPS-
SCN (113). From Thomas et al. (115) *S. mutans* can be estimated to
have approximately 1×10^7 -SH groups per cell. Of course, these
numbers vary greatly with the metabolic state of the cell and with other
factors. However, if the oxidation of one-half of the cellular -SH groups
produced inhibition, the number oxidized would be very large.

Whenever a very large number of critical targets must be hit in
order to have an effect on a cell, the theoretical curves of the degree of

lysis or of inhibition as a function of the extent of reaction show very
sharp transitions at the point of inflection (4). In other words, a
very slight increase in the extent of reaction will produce a very large
increase in effect. This is precisely what is observed for hypothiocyanite-inhibition curves, and the similarity offers further support
for the hypothesis that a minimum threshold number of cellular components must be oxidized in order for any inhibition to occur (83).

VI. SUMMARY

Lactoperoxidase and salivary peroxidase catalyze the oxidation of the
thiocyanate and iodide ions to generate highly reactive oxidizing agents.
These products have a broad spectrum of antimicrobial effects. They
can kill viruses, gram-positive and gram-negative bacteria, fungi,
and probably also mycoplasmas and parasites. The molecular components of cells that are oxidized are sulfhydryl groups, NADH, NADPH,
and under some conditions aromatic amino acid residues. Oxidation of
these molecular components alters the functions of cellular systems.
The cytoplasmic membrane, sugar, and amino acid transport systems,
and glycolytic enzymes may be damaged. The result of such damage
may be cell death or inhibition of growth, respiration, active transport,
or other vital metabolic functions. The major products responsible for
these effects are the hypothiocyanite ion ($OSCN^-$), hypothiocyanous
acid (HOSCN), and iodine (I_2). However, minor products are also
generated. These minor products are highly reactive and short-
lived but have even more potent antimicrobial properties. Microorganisms show great variability in their response to peroxidase systems.
Killing of cells is usually greater at low pH, low temperature, and with
I^- as the electron donor. Gram-negative bacteria are more susceptible
to killing and to cytoplasmic membrane damage than are gram-positive
species. However, the killing of both species requires long incubation
periods (on the order of an hour) and high concentrations ($[OSCN^-]$) >
10 µM at pH 7) of the active products. Some species of bacteria are
able to resist the antibacterial effects by generating substances that
reduce $OSCN^-$ to SCN^-. These same reducing agents can also enable
cells to recover from inhibition by reversing the oxidation of sulfhydryl
groups of cellular components caused by peroxidase system products.
Plots of the degree of inhibition of cell metabolism as a function of hypothiocyanite concentration show that a threshold concentration of hypothiocyanite is required before significant inhibition is observed. Once
the threshold concentration is attained, inhibition rises very rapidly
with only small increases in hypothiocyanite concentration. These results suggest that a critical number of cellular components must be oxidized before any inhibition can be obtained. For bacteria, this critical
number may be of the order of 10^5-10^7 sulfhydryl groups per cell.

Appendix The Effects of the Lactoperoxidase and Salivary Peroxidase Systems on Bacteria

Microorganism	Peroxidase source/donor	H_2O_2 source	Test medium	Biological effects		Inhibited functions	Comments	Reference
				K^a	Other			
Actinomyces naeslundi	Saliva/SCN⁻	Reagent[d]	Saliva		Rev.[b]	Acid production	Effective [OSCN⁻] < 100 µM	58
A. viscous	Saliva/SCN⁻	Reagent	Saliva		Rev. Pre.[c]	Glucose uptake		26,27
Bacillus cereus	LP/SCN⁻	Reagent	Buffer			Growth and collagenase production	Effective [OSCN⁻] = 200 µM	106
B. megatherium	LP/SCN⁻	Reagent	Buffer		Pre.	Growth		50
Lactobacillus acidophilus	Saliva	Bacteria[e]	Saliva	X		Growth		20
	Saliva	Bacteria	Medium	X			pH 5.5; more than 2 logs killing; growing cells more sensitive than resting cells	122
	Saliva/ SCN⁻, LP/I⁻	Bacteria	Saliva, buffer		Pre.	Growth		50,51,121
	Saliva, LP/SCN⁻	Bacteria, reagent	Saliva, buffer			Amino acid accumulation		19
	SP,LP/SCN⁻	Bacteria	Buffer			Growth and lysine accumulation	SP inhibitors found in saliva	100
L. casei	Saliva/SCN⁻	Bacteria	Saliva, buffer			Growth		22,23
	Saliva/I⁻	Reagent	Saliva			Growth		41

Appendix (Continued)

Microorganism	Peroxidase source/donor	H_2O_2 source	Test medium	K^a	Other	Inhibited functions	Comments	Reference
	LP/SCN⁻	Bacteria	Medium			Inhibition zones around agar wells		36
	SP/SCN⁻	Bacteria	Buffer			Growth		40
L. planatarum	SP/SCN⁻	Bacteria	Buffer			Growth		39
	LP/SCN⁻	Reagent	Medium			Inhibition zones around agar wells		36
L. bulgaricus, L. helveticus, L. jugurti	LP/SCN⁻	Bacteria	Milk			Acid production		77
Sarcina lutea	LP/SCN⁻	Reagent	Buffer	X	Pre.		White mutant strain was killed, but wild pigmented strain was not	89
Staphylcocci								
Staphylococcus albus	LP/SCN⁻	Reagent	Medium			Growth		50
S. aureus	LP/I⁻	*S. mitis*	Buffer	X			More than 3 logs killing	29
	LP/SCN⁻	*S. mitis*	Medium			Growth and amino acid uptake		29
	Saliva/SCN⁻	Reagent	Saliva		Pre.	Glucose uptake		26
Streptococci								
Serological groups of streptococci								
A	Milk	?	Milk	X			All strains killed, aerobiosis necessary	119,95

B,C,D,E	Milk	?	Milk	Rev.	Growth		119
F,G,H,K,L	Milk	?	Milk		Growth	Some strains resistant; strains F, G most susceptible	119,95
Streptococcus cremoris	Milk	?	Milk		Acid production, growth	Some strains resistant; aerobiosis necessary for inhibition	120
	LP	?	Milk		Acid production	No inhibition with horse-radish peroxidase (HRP)	76
	LP	Bacteria	Milk, medium		Acid production, growth	Both HRP and catalase blocked LP inhibition	43
	Milk, LP/SCN$^-$	Bacteria, reagent	Milk, medium		Acid production, growth, O$_2$ uptake, glycolysis	Strain 972 inhibited, strain 803 resistant; cell extract of strain 803 reversed strain 972 inhibition; SCN$^-$ shown to be required; O$_2$ uptake stopped in less than 1 min by LPS-SCN; Oxidation of NaDH and SCN$^-$ by LPS also rapid; inhibition due to intermediate oxidation products of SCN$^-$; final products not inhibitory; LP adsorbed to cells	95,96
	LP/SCN$^-$	Bacteria, reagent	Medium	Rev.	Growth, O$_2$ uptake, glycolysis	Strain 972 inhibited; Strain 803 resistant but was inhibited in absence of energy source; resistance due to NaDH$_2$-oxidizing enzyme which catalyzed reduction of intermediate oxidation products; this enzyme found in all	74,75

Appendix (Continued)

| Microorganism | Peroxidase source/donor | H$_2$O$_2$ source | Test medium | Biological effects | | Inhibited functions | Comments | Reference |
				K^a	Other			
							resistant strains but not in susceptible strains; hexokinase of all strains inhibited by LPS in non-metabolizing suspensions; inhibiting product of LPS similar to sulfur dicyanide	
	LP/SCN$^-$	Reagent	Medium			Growth	LP bound to cells in active form; pig LP more effective than bovine LP; inhibition reaction rapid; cells recovered when separated from LPS	72
	LP/SCN$^-$	Bacteria, reagent	Medium			Growth	LP bound to cells in active form; inhibition more effective at pH 6.6 than at 7.3	101
	LP/SCN$^-$	Reagent	Buffer			Oxygen uptake and acid production	Inhibition more effective at pH 4.5 than 7	32
S. lactis	LP/SCN$^-$	Reagent	Medium				About 4 hr inhibition by 20 μM OSCN$^-$; OSCN$^-$ prepared with sepharose-bound LP; 25 μM OSCN$^-$ produced some leakage of ^{42}K$^+$ and ^{14}C amino acids in 30 min	64

Organism	System	Enzyme source	Test medium		Treatment	Parameter measured	Comments	Ref.
S. pyogenes	Whey		Whey, medium	X			Killing required several hours incubation, probably to give time for bacterial H_2O_2 generation	45
	LP		Milk	X				76
	Milk, LP/SCN$^-$	Bacteria	Milk, medium	X		Acid production in medium	Killing in milk	95
	LP/SCN$^-$	Bacteria	Medium		Pre.	Growth	Glyceraldehyde phosphate dehydrogenase inhibited	67
S. agalactiae	Milk		Milk			Acid production		44
	Milk/SCN$^-$	Bacteria	Milk			Acid production	Inhibition blocked by cysteine	15
	LP/SCN$^-$	Reagent	Medium			Growth	S^{14}CN$^-$ incorporated into cell proteins by LPS and released by thiols; LP cell-bound in catalytically active form	69
	LP/SCN$^-$	Reagent	Medium		Rev. Pre.	Sugar transport and utilization, and lactic acid formation		68
	LP/SCN$^-$	Bacteria	Medium		Pre.		Several strains tested; some had alternative oxidative pathway and were not inhibited by LPS	67
S. fecalis	LP/SCN$^-$	Reagent	Medium			Growth		50
S. mitior (*mitis*)	Saliva/SCN$^-$	Reagent	Saliva			Glucose uptake		26
	Saliva/SCN$^-$	Bacteria	Saliva		Pre.		*S. mitis* more resistant to LPS than *S. mutans*	27

Appendix (Continued)

Microorganism	Peroxidase source/donor	H_2O_2 source	Test medium	Biological effects		Inhibited functions	Comments	Reference
				K^a	Other			
	LP/SCN$^-$	Reagent	Buffer			H_2O_2 excretion, oxygen uptake, acid production	Spontaneous recovery from inhibition; *S. mitis* recovered more easily than *S. mutans*	17
	Saliva/SCN$^-$	Reagent	Saliva			Acid production	Inhibition occurred when OSCN$^-$ generated in presence of saliva and bacteria, but not when cells were added after OSCN$^-$ generation	58
S. mutans	LP/SCN$^-$	Reagent, bacteria	Buffer, medium			Growth, acid production	Spontaneous recovery from inhibition; effectiveness of LPS varies with medium	36
	LP/SCN$^-$	Reagent, bacteria	Buffer, medium				Higher [H_2O_2] required for inhibition if added exogeneously, compared to endogenously generated; length of inhibition depends on [H_2O_2]; cells more difficult to inhibit in presence of glucose	34
	LP/SCN$^-$	Reagent	Buffer		Rev.	Acid production	Effective [OSCN$^-$] = 70 μM	35
	LP/SCN$^-$	Reagent	Buffer		Pre.		OSCN$^-$ prepared from (SCN)$_2$ and from LPS-SCN gave some inhibitory effects on acid production; Effective [OSCN$^-$] = 40 μM	37

System	Source	Medium			Parameter	Comments	Ref.
LP/SCN⁻	Reagent	Medium				Cells recovered spontaneously from growth inhibition	104
SP,LP/SCN⁻	Reagent	Medium				SP and LP adsorbed to cells and released with phosphate	105
LP/SCN⁻	Reagent	Buffer	Rev.		Acid production	Instantaneous inhibition when all LPS components present; instant recovery when mercaptoethanol added; enzyme adsorbed to cells in active form; fewer than 100 enzyme molecules/cell were effective	79
Human MP/SCN⁻	Reagent	Buffer		X	Acid production	Cells killed at pH 5 but not at pH 7	47
Saliva/SCN⁻	Bacteria	Saliva	Pre.		Glucose uptake		26,27
LP/SCN⁻	Bacteria, reagent	Buffer			Glucose uptake and lactate production	Cells depleted of CHO reserves and -SH compounds are more easily inhibited; inhibition more effective at pH 5 than at pH 7; effective [OSCN⁻] = 10-20 μM	115
LP/SCN⁻	Reagent	Buffer			Oxygen uptake and acid production		17
Saliva/SCN⁻	Reagent	Saliva			Acid production	Inhibition more effective when OSCN⁻ generated in presence of bacteria	61

Appendix (Continued)

Microorganism	Peroxidase source/donor	H_2O_2 source	Test medium	Biological effects		Inhibited functions	Comments	Reference
				K^a	Other			
	Saliva, LP/SCN⁻	Reagent	Saliva, buffer			Acid production	OSCN⁻ prepared from (SCN₂) gave similar results to LPS when OSCN⁻ was generated in absence of cells; effective [OSCN⁻] = 15 μM	58
	LP, saliva/SCN⁻	Bacteria, reagent	Buffer		Rev.	Acid production, rapidly (less than 15 sec)	Spontaneous recovery; depends on growth phase; growing cells recover more rapidly	1
	LP, saliva/SCN⁻	Reagent	Buffer		Rev.	Glucose consumption, lactate production, acid production	Metabolism of stored internal polysaccharides inhibited; resting cells irreversibly inhibited; active cells reversibly inhibited	24,25
S. salivarius	Saliva/SCN⁻	Reagent	Saliva			Acid production	Cells very sensitive, more sensitive than *S. mutans*, *S. sanguis*, or *A. naeslundi*; greater inhibition when saliva supplemented in presence of bacteria; effective [OSCN⁻] = 5-10 μM	58
	LP/SCN⁻	Reagent	Buffer			Acid production, O_2 uptake	*S. salivarius* more sensitive to LPS than *S. mutans*, *S. mitis*, *S.*	17

Organism	System				Effect	Comments	Ref.
						mitior and also re-covered more slowly from inhibition; effective $[OSCN^-]$ = <30 μM	
S. sanguis	LP/SCN⁻	Bacteria, reagent	Medium, buffer		Growth and acid	Cells revovered spontaneously with low H_2O_2	36
	Saliva/SCN⁻	Bacteria	Saliva		Glucose uptake	*S. sanguis* more sensitive than *S. mutans* but less than *S. mitis* to LPS	26
	Saliva/SCN⁻	Reagent	Saliva		Acid production	*S. sanguis* more sensitive than *S. mitior* but less than *S. mutans*	58
	LP/SCN⁻	Reagent	Buffer		Oxygen uptake and acid production	*S. sanguis* and *S. mitis* had greater capacity to recover from inhibition than did *S. mutans* and *S. salivarius*; inhibition was 100% for acid production and for oxygen uptake within less than 1 min after activation of LPS by addition of H_2O_2 (Conc. = 150 μM); acid production recovered in 20 min and oxygen consumption in 10 min	17

Gram-Negative Bacteria

Organism	System				Effect	Comments	Ref.
Escherichia coli	LP/SCN⁻	Reagent	Medium		Growth, in trypticase soy broth but not in brain heart infusion	Dialysis of BHI removed the factors responsible for blocking inhibition	50
	LP/I⁻	Reagent	Buffer	X		Complete killing in acetate buffer pH 5; aerobic incubation, 37°C 30 min;	48

167

Appendix (Continued)

Microorganism	Peroxidase source/donor	H_2O_2 source	Test medium	Biological effects		Inhibited functions	Comments	Reference
				K^a	Other			
							optimum killing required cells to be in presence of LPS during activation; iodine incorporated into treated cells; killing pH dependent; no killing above pH 6.5. Maximum iodination at and below pH 5.5. Minimum pH 8; killing and iodination blocked by reducing agents	
LP/I⁻	S. mitis	Glucose	X				Killing produced by incubation at 37°C, pH 6.5, for 60 min	29
LP/SCN⁻	S. mitis	Buffer				Acid uptake and growth		29
Saliva/SCN⁻	S. mitis	Saliva	X			Growth, amino acid uptake		29
Whey/SCN⁻	glu/GO^f	Whey	X					14
LP/SCN⁻	glu/GO	Medium	X	Pre.			Over 3 logs kill in 4 hr; killing greater at low pH and depended on cell density	92
LP/I⁻	Reagent	Medium	X	Rev.			Little killing at 25°C, much killing at 0-5°C; exposure to DTT gave	112

						partial recovery; cells with altered envelopes more easily killed	
LP/SCN⁻	Reagent	Medium	X	Rev.		Only cells with altered envelopes killed; par-partial recovery of viability with DTT	112
LP/SCN⁻	Reagent	Buffer	X	Rev.		Respiration inhibited by $OSCN^-$ in dose-dependent way; rate of recovery also dose-dependent; no recovery from cells incubated with excess $OSCN^-$ for 1 hr; differences between SCN^- and I^- as electron donors; (a) higher $[SCN^-]$ than of $[I^-]$ required for antibacterial effects; (b) I_2 could oxidize all bacterial -SH(3) I_2 reaction irreversible	113
Guinea pig milk/SCN⁻	?	Guinea pig milk		Rev.	Growth, by milk 10 or more days postpartum		102
LP/SCN⁻	Reagent	Medium	X			Three logs kill in 2 hr at 37°C, pH 5.5; $OSCN^-$ generated with sepharose-bound LP; 25 μM $OSCN^-$ caused loss of $[^{14}C]$amino acids and $^{42}K^+$ within 10 min; uptake of $[^{14}C]$ leucine blocked by $OSCN^-$; effective $[OSCN^-]$ = 5 μM	64

Appendix (Continued)

Microorganism	Peroxidase source/donor	H_2O_2 source	Test medium	Biological effects		Inhibited functions	Comments	Reference
				K^a	Other			
	LP/SCN⁻	?	Abomasum fluid	X	Rev.		Bacteria inoculated into abomasum fluid killed rapidly	93
	LP/SCN⁻	glu/GO	Abomasum fluid	X	Rev.		Calves fed milk inoculated with *E. coli* and with *S. lactis* had abomasum fluid which killed *E. coli*; natural flora also provided enough H_2O_2	93
	LP/SCN⁻	Reagent	Medium	X			Cells incubated 2 hr at 37°C, pH 6.7; complete killing not obtained even at highest [OSCN⁻], suggesting some recovery; killing reduced when long time elapsed after OSCN⁻ generation before inoculating reaction mixture with cells; effective [OSCN⁻] = 40-70 µM	13
	LP/SCN⁻	Reagent	Medium	X	Rev.	Growth	OSCN⁻ generated from (SCN)₂; added to cells; some conditions as above; no killing; effective [OSCN⁻] = 70 µM or less	13
	Saliva/SCN⁻	Reagent	Saliva		Pre.	Glucose uptake, when peroxide		26

					added to saliva-bacteria mixture		
	LP/SCN⁻	Reagent	Buffer		LDH activity	In addition to killing, LPS prevented cells from forming pH gradient	55
	LP/SCN⁻	Reagent	Medium			Exponentially growing cells treated with LPS; over 3 logs kill in 2 hr at 37°C; plating and subsequent aerobic incubation gave only slight recovery, but very good recovery of viability obtained with anaerobic incubation; bacteriostatic effect also observed	2
	LP/SCN⁻	Reagent	Human milk	X		Cells killed at 21°-23°C and 4°C; LP, SCN⁻, peroxide added to human milk	54
	LP/SCN⁻	Reagent	Medium		Growth	Spontaneous recovery	80
Legionella pneumophila	MP/Cl	Reagent	Buffer	X		Cells also killed by xanthine oxidase system	57
Multiple antibiotic-resistant strains of *E. coli*, *Klebsiella aerogenes*, and *Salmonella typhimurium* isolated from infant feces	LP/SCN⁻	Reagent		X			89

Appendix (Continued)

Microorganism	Peroxidase source/donor	H_2O_2 source	Test medium	Biological effects K^a	Other	Inhibited functions	Comments	Reference
Salmonellae								
S. typhimurium	LP/SCN⁻	glu/GO	Medium	X			Over 2 logs kill in 4 hr	92
	LP/SCN⁻	Reagent	Human milk	X			LP, SCN⁻, peroxide added to human milk; no killing at 21°-23°C; killing at 4°C	54
	LP/SCN⁻	Reagent	Buffer	X			Cell wall-defective mutants more easily killed than parents strain; same results obtained with OSCN⁻ from $(SCN)_2$; effective $[OSCN^-] = 10$ μM or greater	118
	LP/SCN⁻	Reagent	Buffer, medium	X		Acid production of all strains	Both bacteriostatic and bactericidal effects observed; more permeable cells more easily killed; growth phase had no effect on bacteriostatic effects; log phase bacteria more sensitive to killing than stationary phase cells; inhibition of acid production not reversed with thiols, but cells were viable	88

Pseudomonads

P. fluorescens	Bovine milk/SCN⁻	glu/GO	Bovine milk	X	Pre.	Over 3 log killing in 6 hr at 30°C	14
	Bovine milk/SCN⁻	Reagent	Bovine milk	X		Killing more effective at 5°C than at 30°C	12
P. aeruginosa	LP/SCN⁻	glu/GO	Medium	X		Over 2 log killing in 4 hr	92
	LP/SCN⁻	Reagent	Medium, buffer	X		MSH added after treatment with OSCN⁻; partial recovery; 30 min incubation required for significant killing; better killing in acid solution; no difference in mucoid, non-mucoid strains; effective [OSCN⁻] = 100 μM	82

aKilling.
bInhibition reversed by addition of excess thiol compounds or other reducing agents to inhibited cells.
cInhibition blocked by presence of excess thiol compounds during exposure to LPS or SPS.
dPeroxide added from stock dilution of commercial H_2O_2.
ePeroxide generated by cells themselves.
fPeroxide generated by glucose-glucose oxidase system.

REFERENCES

1. Adamson, M., "Interactions of Lactoperoxidase and its Sub-
    strates with *Streptococcus mutans*" Dissertation, Department
    of Biochemistry, University of Alabama in Birminghan (1980).
2. Adamson, M., and Carlsson, J., *Infect. Immun. 35*: 30 (1982).
3. Adamson, M., and Pruitt, K. M., *Biochim. Biophys. Acta 658*:
    238 (1981).
4. Alberty, R. A., and Baldwin, R. L., *J. Immunol. 66*: 725
    (1951).
5. Alexander, N. M., *J. Biol. Chem. 249*: 1946 (1974).
6. Ames, M. N., McCann, J. T., and Yamasaki, E., *Mut. Res. 31*:
    347 (1975).
7. Austin, L. B., and Zeldow, B. J., *Proc. Soc. Exp. Biol. Med.
    107*: 406 (1961).
8. Aune, T. M., and Thomas, E. L., *Eur. J. Biochem. 80*: 209
    (1977).
9. Aune, T. M., and Thomas, E. L., *Biochemistry 17*: 1005 (1978).
10. Aune, T. M., Thomas, E. L., and Morrison, M., *Biochemistry
    16*: 4611 (1977).
11. Belding, M. E., Klebanoff, S. J., and Ray, G. C., *Science
    167*: 195 (1970).
12. Björck, L., *J. Dairy Res. 45*: 109 (1978).
13. Björck, L., and Claesson, O., *J. Dairy Sci. 63*: 919 (1980).
14. Björck, L., Rosén, C.-G., Marshall, V., and Reiter, B.,
    Appl. Microbiol. 30: 199 (1975).
15. Brown, R. W., and Mickelson, M. N., *Am. J. Vet. Res. 40*:
    250 (1979).
16. Buys, J., Wever, R., vanStigt, R., and Ruitenberg, E. J.,
    Eur. J., Immunol. 11: 843 (1981).
17. Carlsson, J., Iwami, Y., and Yamada, T., *Infect. Immun.
    40*: 70 (1983).
18. Cohen, L. A., *Ann. Rev. Biochem. 37*: 695 (1968).
19. Clem, W. H., and Klebanoff, S. J., *J. Bacteriol. 91*: 1848
    (1966).
20. Clough, O. W., Bibby, B. G., and Berry, G. P., *J. Dent.
    Res. 17*: 493 (1938).
21. Costerton, J. W., Ingram, J. M., and Cheng, K. J., *Bacter-
    iol. Rev. 38*: 87 (1974).
22. Courant, P., *Odontol. Revy 18*: 251 (1965).
23. Dogon, I. L., Kerr, A. C., and Amdur, B. H., *Arch. Oral
    Biol. 7*: 81 (1962).
24. Edelen, C., "The Effects of the Lactoperoxidase System on
    Streptococcus mutans Metabolism" thesis, Department of Oral
    Biology, University of Louisville, Louisville, Ky. (1983).
25. Edelen, C., Adamson, M., and Arnold, R. R., *J. Dent. Res.
    62*: 217 (1983).

26. Germaine, G. R., and Tellefson, L. M., *Infect. Immun. 31*:
     598 (1981).
27. Germain, G. R., and Tellefson, L. M., *Infect. Immun. 38*:
     1060 (1982).
28. Hamada, S., and Slade, H. D., *Microbiol. Rev. 44*: 331 (1980).
29. Hamon, C. B., and Klebanoff, S. J., *J. Exp. Med. 137*: 438
     (1973).
30. Hanssen, F. S., *Br. J. Exp. Pathol. 5*: 271 (1924).
31. Hesse, W., *Zeitschrift fur Hygiene und Infections Krankheiten
     17*: 238 (1894).
32. Hogg, D. McC., and Jago, G. R., *Biochem. J. 117*: 779 (1970).
33. Hogg, D. McC., and Jago, G. R., *Biochem. J. 117*: 791 (1970).
34. Hoogendoorn, H., "The Effect of Lactoperoxidas-Thiocyanate-
     Hydrogen Peroxide on the Metabolism of Cariogenic Microorgan-
     isms in vitro and in the Oral Cavity" thesis, Delft, Mouton,
     The Haag, Netherlands (1974).
35. Hoogendoorn, H., *Microbial Aspects of Dental Caries, Sp. Supp.
     Microbiol. Abstr.*, p. 353 (1976) Information Retrieval, Inc.,
     New York, NY.
36. Hoogendoorn, H., and Moorer, W. R., *Odontol. Revy 24*: 355
     (1973).
37. Hoogendoorn, H., Piessens, J. P., Scholtes, W., and Stoddard,
     L. A., *Caries Res. 11*: 77 (1977).
38. Hugoson, A., Koch, G., Thilander, H., and Hoogendoorn, H.,
     Odontal. Revy 25: 69 (1974).
39. Iwamoto, Y., and Matsumura, T., *Arch. Oral Biol. 11*: 667
     (1966).
40. Iwamoto, Y., Nakamura, R., Watanabe, T., and Tsunemitsu,
     A., *J. Dent. Res. 51*: 503 (1972).
41. Iwamoto, Y., Tsunemitsu, A., and Okuda, K., *J. Dent. Res.
     51*: 877 (1972).
42. Jacobs, A. A., Low, I. E., Paul, B. B., Strauss, R. R., and
     Sbarra, A. J., *Infect. Immun. 5*: 127 (1972).
43. Jago, G. R., and Morrison, M., *Proc. Soc. Exp. Biol. Med.
     111*: 585 (1962).
44. Janota-Bassalik, L., Zajac, M., Pietrassek, A., and Piotrowska,
     E., *Acta Microbiol. Pol. 26*: 413 (1977).
45. Jones, F. S., and Simms, H. S., *J. Exp. Med. 51*: 327 (1930).
46. Jong, E. C., Henderson, W. R., and Klebanoff, S. J., *J.
     Immunol. 124*: 1378 (1980).
47. Kersten, H. W., Moorer, W. R., and Wever, R., *J. Dent.
     Res. 60*: 831 (1981).
48. Klebanoff, S. J., *J. Exp. Med. 126*: 1063 (1967).
49. Klebanoff, S. J., *Semin. Hematol. 12*: 117 (1975).
50. Klebanoff, S. J., Clem, W. H., and Luebke, R. G., *Biochim.
     Biophys. Acta 117*: 63 (1966).

51. Klebanoff, S. J., and Luebke, R. G., *Proc. Soc. Exp. Biol. Med. 118:* 483 (1965).
52. Koch, G., Edlund, K., and Hoogendoorn, H., *Odontol. Revy 24:* 367 (1973).
53. Koch, G., and Strand, G., *Swed. Dent. J. 3:* 9 (1979).
54. Laven, G. T., and Pruitt, K. M., *Fed. Proc. 42:* 1328, Abstr. 6075 (1983).
55. Law, B. A., and John, P., *FEMS Microbiol. Lett. 10:* 67 (1981).
56. Lehrer, R. I., *J. Bacteriol. 99:* 361 (1969).
57. Lochner, J. E., Friedman, R. L., Bigley, R. H., and Iglewski, B. H., *Infect. Immun. 39:* 487 (1983).
58. Månsson-Rahemtulla, B., "Hypothiocyanite - A Regulatory Factor in Oral Biology" thesis, Department of Oral Biology, School of Dentistry, University of Alabama in Birmingham (1982).
59. Månsson-Rahemtulla, B., and Pruitt, K. M., *Caries Res. 17:* 166, Abstr. 30 (1983).
60. Månsson-Rahemtulla, B., Rahemtulla, F., Pruitt, K. M., and Harrington, P. G., in *Protides of the Biological Fluids,* XXXI in press (1985).
61. Månsson-Rahemtulla, B., Pruitt, K. M., Tenovuo, J., and Adamson, M., in *Basic Concepts of Streptococci and Streptococcal Disease,* Holm, S. E., and Christensen, P. (Eds.), Reedbooks, Chertsey, England, pp. 118-119 (1982).
62. Månsson-Rahemtulla, B., Pruitt, K. M., Tenovuo, J., and Le, T. M., *J. Dent. Res. 62:* 1062 (1983).
63. Månsson-Rahemtulla, B., Tenovuo, J., and Pruitt, K., *J. Dent. Res. 61:* 257 (1982).
64. Marshall, V. M. E., and Reiter, B., *J. Gen. Microbiol. 120:* 513 (1980).
65. Mayer, M. M., in *Experimental Immunochemistry,* Kabat, E., and Mayer, M. M. (Eds.), Charles C Thomas, Springfield, Ill., pp. 133-240 (1971).
66. Mayer, M. M., *Immunochemistry 7:* 485 (1970).
67. Mickelson, M. N., *J. Gen. Microbiol. 43:* 31 (1966).
68. Mickelson, M. N., *J. Bacteriol. 132:* 541 (1977).
69. Mickelson, M. N., *Appl. Environ. Microbiol. 38:* 821 (1979).
70. Moldoveanu, Z., Tenovuo, J., Pruitt, K. M., Månsson-Rahemtulla, B., and Mestecky, J., *Ann. N.Y. Acad. Sci. 409:* 848 (1983).
71. Moldoveanu, Z., Tenovuo, J., Mestecky, J., and Pruitt, K. M., *Biochim. Biophys. Acta 718:* 103 (1982).
72. Morrison, M., and Steele, W. F., *Lactoperoxidase, the Peroxidase in the Salivary Gland,* Sump. Washington Mtg. Am. Assoc. Adv. Sci., Publication #89, Person, P. (Ed.) American Association for the Advancement of Science, Washington, DC. (1966).
73. Nogueira, N. M., Klebanoff, S. J., and Cohn, Z. A., *J. Immunol. 128:* 1705 (1982).

74. Oram, J. D., and Reiter, B., *Biochem. J. 100*: 373 (1966).

75. Oram, J. D., and Reiter, B., *Biochem. J. 100*: 382 (1966).

76. Portmann, A., and Auclair, J. E., *Lait 39*: 147 (1959).

77. Portmann, A., Gate, Y., and Auclair, J., *Sixteenth International Dairy Congress*, vol. B Copenhagen, Denmark (1962).

78. Pruitt, K. M., and Adamson, M., *Infect. Immun. 17*: 112 (1977).

79. Pruitt, K. M., Adamson, M., and Arnold, R., *Infect. Immun. 25*: 304 (1979).

80. Pruitt, K. M., DeMuth, R. E., and Turner, M. E., Jr., *Growth 43*: 19 (1979).

81. Pruitt, K. M., Månsson-Rahemtulla, B., and Smith, J. C., *Caries Res. 17*: 173, Abstr. 49 (1983).

82. Pruitt, K. M., Hansen, J., and McDanal, C., unpublished results (1983).

83. Pruitt, K., Smith, J. Hazelrig, J., and Månsson-Rahemtulla, B., in *Protides of the Biological Fluids*, XXXII in press (1985).

84. Pruitt, K. M., Månsson-Rahemtulla, B., and Tenovuo, J., *Arch. Oral Biol. 28*:517 (1983).

85. Pruitt, K. M., and Tenovuo, J., *Biochim. Biophys. Acta 704*: 204 (1982).

86. Pruitt, K. M., Tenovuo, J., Andrews, R. W., and McKane, T., *Biochemistry 21*: 562 (1982).

87. Pruitt, K. M., Tenovuo, J., Fleming, W., and Adamson, M., *Caries Res. 16*: 315 (1982).

88. Purdy, M. A., Tenovuo, J., Pruitt, K. M., and White, W. E., Jr., *Infect. Immun. 39*: 1187 (1983).

89. Reiter, B., *Ann. Rech. Vet. 9*: 205 (1978).

90. Reiter, B., in *Immunological Aspects of Infection in the Fetus and Newborn*, Lambert, H. P., and Wood, C. B. S. (Eds.), Academic Press, New York, pp. 155-195 (1981).

91. Reiter, B., in *Oxygen Free Radicals and Tissue Damage*, Ciba Foundation Series 65, p. 285 Elsevier, Amsterdam (1979).

92. Reiter, B., Marshall, V. M. E., Björck, L., and Rosen, C.-G., *Infect. Immun. 13*: 800 (1976).

93. Reiter, B., Marshall, V. M., and Philips, S. M., *Res. Vet. Sci. 28*: 116 (1980).

94. Reiter, B., and Oram, J. D., *Nature 216*: 328 (1967).

95. Reiter, B., Pickering, A., and Oram, J. D., *Microbial Inhibitors in Food*, 4th Int. Symp. on Food Microbiol. p. 297 Almqvist and Wiksell, Stockholm (1964).

96. Reiter, B., Pickering, A., Oram, J. D., and Pope, G. S., *J. Gen. Microbiol. 33*: 12 (1963).

97. Rotgans, J., and Hoogendoorn, H., *Caries Res. 13*: 144 (1979).

98. Saier, M. H., Jr., *Bacteriol. Rev. 41*: 856 (1977).

99. Schachtele, C. F., and Mayo, J. A., *J. Dent. Res. 52*: 1209 (1973).

100. Slowey, R. R., Eidelman, S., and Klebanoff, S. J., *J. Bacteriol. 96*: 577 (1968).
101. Steele, W. F., and Morrison, M., *J. Bacteriol. 97*: 635 (1969).
102. Stephens, S., Harkness, R. A., and Cockle, S. M., *Br. J. Exp. Pathol. 60*: 252 (1979).
103. Tenovuo, J., *Caries Res. 13*: 137 (1979).
104. Tenovuo, J., and Knuuttila, M. L. E., *J. Dent. Res. 56*: 1603 (1977).
105. Tenovuo, J., and Knuuttila, M. L. E., *J. Dent. Res. 56*: 1608 (1977).
106. Tenovuo, J., and Mäkinen, K. K., *Scand. Assoc. Dent. Res.* Aug., Abstr. (1983).
107. Tenovuo, J., Månsson-Rahemtulla, B., Pruitt, K. M., and Arnold, R., *Infect. Immun. 34*: 208 (1981).
108. Tenovuo, J., Moldoveanu, Z., Mestecky, J., Pruitt, K. M., and Månsson-Rahemtulla, B., *J. Immunol. 128*: 726 (1982).
109. Tenovuo, J., Pruitt, K. M., and Thomas, E. L., *J. Dent. Res. 61*: 982 (1982).
110. Tenovuo, J., Valtakoski, J., and Knuuttila, M. L. E., *Caries Res. 11*: 257 (1977).
111. Thomas, E. L., *Biochemistry 20*: 3273 (1981).
112. Thomas, E. L., and Aune, T. M., *Antimicrob. Agents Chemother. 13*: 261 (1978).
113. Thomas, E. L., and Aune, T. M., *Infect. Immun. 20*: 456 (1978).
114. Thomas, E. L., Bates, K. P., and Jefferson, M. M., *J. Dent. Res. 59*: 1466 (1980).
115. Thomas, E. L., Pera, K. A., Smith, K. W., and Chwang, A. K., *Infect. Immun. 39*: 767 (1983).
116. Thorne, K. J. I., Svvennsen, R. J., and Franks, D., *Infect. Immun. 21*: 798 (1978).
117. Von Krogh, M., *J. Infect. Dis. 19*: 452 (1916).
118. White, W. E. Jr., Pruitt, K. M., and Månsson-Rahemtulla, B., *Antimicrob. Agents Chemother. 23*: 267 (1983).
119. Wilson, I. R., and Rosenblum, H., *J. Exp. Med. 95*: 25 (1952).
120. Wright, R. C., and Tramer, J., *J. Dairy Res. 25*: 104 (1958).
121. Zeldow, B. J., *J. Immunol. 90*: 12 (1963).
122. Zeldow, B. J., *J. Dent. Res. 40*: 446 (1961).

9

Bacterial Hydrogen Peroxide Production

EDWIN L. THOMAS / *St. Jude Children's Research Hospital, Memphis, Tennessee*

I. INTRODUCTION

Production of hydrogen peroxide (H_2O_2) and other "activated" forms
of oxygen is ubiquitous in biological systems exposed to air. In prin-
ciple, the oxidation of any reduced substance by dioxygen (O_2) may
yield H_2O_2. The transfer of 1 electron (e^-) from the reduced substance to O_2 yields superoxide (represented as $O_2^- \cdot$ or O_2^-), which
rapidly undergoes a "dismutation" reaction that yields H_2O_2

$$1e^- + O_2 \longrightarrow O_2^-$$

$$2O_2^- + 2H^+ \longrightarrow H_2O_2 + O_2$$

The transfer of 2 electrons to O_2 yields H_2O_2 directly.

$$2e^- + 2H^+ + O_2 \longrightarrow H_2O_2$$

The interior of living cells is rich in reduced substances, whereas
the extracellular environment usually contains O_2 and catalysts that
facilitate the transfer of electrons to O_2. Also, many cells make use of
such catalysts in the form of enzymes. When O_2 enters the cell and
reacts with reduced substances in the presence of appropriate catalysts,
H_2O_2 may be formed.

However, there are other pathways of O_2 reduction that do not
yield H_2O_2. For example, one or both of the atoms of O_2 may be incorporated into the reduced substance. Also, the four-electron reduction of O_2 to water can occur when O_2 is bound to a catalyst in such a
way that O_2^- and H_2O_2 are not released as intermediates.

$$4e^- + 4H^+ + O_2 \longrightarrow 2H_2O$$

Oxidation of reduced substances and reduction of O_2 to water are
part of the controlled burning process by which aerobic organisms
liberate the energy required for growth, mobility, and maintenance of
structure. The released energy is conserved in the form of ion gradi-
ents across biological membranes and/or in the form of adenosine tri-
phosphate (ATP) and other compounds with high-energy bonds.
Only small amounts of the partially reduced forms of O_2 are produced
in the metabolism of aerobic organisms. Also, these organisms contain
high levels of enzymes that rapidly eliminate O_2^- and H_2O_2, preventing
accumulation of these potentially toxic substances. However, production of O_2^- and H_2O_2 can become significant when the usual electron
flow to O_2 is disrupted by electron-transport inhibitors or other per-
turbants. Also, specialized cells of higher organisms produce large
amounts of O_2^- and/or H_2O_2 to accomplish specific purposes. Examples
are the O_2-dependent antimicrobial and antitumor activities of leukocytes and the synthesis of iodinated substances in the thyroid gland.

Although all living cells require energy, many anaerobic microorganisms do not use O_2 as an electron acceptor. Also, the facultative aerobes adopt an anaerobic type of metabolism in the absence of O_2. Some other substance may serve in place of O_2 as the acceptor for electron transport processes. Alternatively, these organisms may depend on O_2-independent pathways for synthesis of high-energy compounds. Nevertheless, when the anaerobically grown organisms are exposed to air, reduction of O_2 does occur.

Microorganisms classified as facultative anaerobes grow in the presence or absence of O_2, but their energy metabolism is of an anerobic type regardless of growth conditions. They depend on O_2-independent pathways such as glycolysis for ATP synthesis. Glycolysis yields little ATP compared with aerobic pathways of metabolism, so that these organisms must rapidly metabolize large amounts of carbohydrate to meet their energy requirements, and often produce extraordinary amounts of glycolytic end products such as lactate. This class of microorganisms includes the streptococci and lactobacilli. These bacteria are referred to as *lactic acid bacteria*, although this term may be applied more restrictively to bacteria that produce lactate and are unable to metabolize it. In the presence of O_2, some facultative anaerobes produce large amounts of H_2O_2 and release it to the extracellular medium.

The obligate anaerobes do not grow in the presence of O_2, and may be killed by prolonged exposure to O_2. For these microorganisms, reduction of O_2 is an unforeseen and inadvertent consequence of mixing O_2 with reduced substances. In part, O_2 may inhibit growth because reduction of O_2 diverts the flow of electrons from energy-conserving pathways into reactions that release energy as heat or other forms that are not useful. However, most studies on the O_2 sensitivity of obligate anaerobes have focused on the production of toxic O_2 metabolites, such as O_2^- and H_2O_2.

The toxicity of H_2O_2 and other activated O_2 metabolites depends on the presence of catalysts, the most important of which are free or chelated ions of transition metals such as iron and copper. Chelated forms of these ions also form the prosthetic groups of enzymes that mediate the toxicity of H_2O_2. For example, lactoperoxidase (LP) is an iron-containing catalyst that amplifies the toxicity of H_2O_2.

As indicated earlier, facultative anaerobes are the major class of microorganisms that produce and release large amounts of H_2O_2. Many of these organisms take up O_2 at rates similar to those of aerobic organisms, and a substantial portion of O_2 uptake goes into production of partially reduced forms of O_2. Another factor that contributes to H_2O_2 release is the absence of catalase, which eliminates H_2O_2 in aerobic organisms. Nevertheless, the facultative anaerobes have other enzymes that eliminate H_2O_2.

II. ENZYMES INVOLVED IN H_2O_2 PRODUCTION

A. Flavoprotein Oxidases

The principal class of enzymes that reduce O_2 to O_2^- and/or H_2O_2 are
the flavoprotein oxidases (12,65,86). Reducing equivalents required
for O_2 reduction come from NADH or NADPH, or from a wide variety of
other electron donors. One catalytic function of these enzymes is to
facilitate the transfer of electrons from the electron donor to the bound
flavin moiety. The second O_2-reducing function is also obtained with
free reduced FMN, FAD, or other flavin compounds, some of which
react with O_2 at rates similar to those of flavoproteins.

These enzymes are not inhibited by cyanide which does inhibit
hemoproteins such as the cytochrome oxidase enzymes of mitrochondria
and many aerobic microorganisms. The lack of inhibition by cyanide is
often used as a test to exclude participation of hemoproteins in O_2 uptake. However, cyanide can have other inhibitory effects, including
reactions with disulfide bonds, with bound metals such as copper, and
with NADH and NADPH.

Certain flavoprotein oxidases reduce O_2 to H_2O_2 without releasing
O_2^- as an intermediate. Familiar examples are glucose oxidase and the
amino acid oxidases. Other enzymes such as the metalloflavoprotein
xanthine oxidase release O_2^- and/or H_2O_2, depending on O_2 concentration (12,65,86). As described later, flavoprotein oxidases that reduce
O_2 to water without releasing O_2^- or H_2O_2 have also been reported.

Flavoprotein oxidases differ from flavoprotein dehydrogenases in
their biological role. For example, NADH-linked lactate dehydrogenase
transfers electrons from NADH to pyruvate to form NAD^+ and lactate,
so that pyruvate rather than O_2 is the electron acceptor. However,
many dehydrogenases transfer electrons to O_2 in place of the biologically relevant electron acceptor, particularly when the concentration of
O_2 is high, the concentration of the usual acceptor is low, or when the
enzyme is damaged and partially inactivated. For this reason, it is
often difficult to identify the oxidase activity that is responsible for
H_2O_2 production in a cell, cell extract, or subcellular organelle.

B. Copper-Containing Oxidases

Several copper-containing oxidases reduce O_2 to H_2O_2 without releasing
O_2^- (62). Examples are galactose oxidase and certain amine oxidases.
Also, a few copper-containing oxidases reduce O_2 directly to H_2O
without releasing O_2^- or H_2O_2. Such enzymes are rare and few have
been characterized, although one of them (cytochrome oxidase) is
ubiquitous in higher organisms. Such enzymes may contain flavins,
hemes, or other bound metals in addition to copper. It was proposed
that multiple interactions of O_2 with bound copper are required for
reduction of O_2 to H_2O (62,86). The copper-containing oxidases are
inhibited by cyanide.

C. Nonheme Iron Proteins

Proteins containing iron (Fe^{3+} or Fe^{2+}) chelated in forms other than hemes, usually in iron-sulfur linkages, play an important role in electron transport processes. Such proteins often participate in the flow of electrons from flavoprotein dehydrogenases to quinones or cytochromes. Also, nonheme iron centers may participate in O_2 reduction by certain flavoproteins or hemoproteins. The reduced form of certain nonheme iron proteins reduces O_2 to O_2^- (66,76). However, it is not clear that a direct interaction with O_2 is part of their biological role.

D. Hemoprotein Peroxidases

Hemoprotein peroxidases catalyze the oxidation of many substances by O_2, and small amounts of O_2^- and H_2O_2 are produced as intermediates. Compounds oxidized include NADH, NADPH, sulfhydryl compounds, and other readily oxidized substances (41,42). Horseradish peroxidase (HRP) has been studied most extensively, but similar O_2-dependent oxidations are obtained with catalase at low pH (39), and with LP and myeloperoxidase. These reactions are accelerated by manganese (Mn^{2+}).

Because these reactions generate H_2O_2, which can then be used in peroxidase-catalyzed reactions, the net effect is to make the peroxidase independent of an external source of H_2O_2. The biological significance is unclear, in that all peroxidase activity may be largely regulated by the H_2O_2 supply. Also, LP-catalyzed oxidation of NADH or sulfhydryl compounds by O_2 is suppressed by SCN^- (E. L. Thomas, unpublished results), so that these reactions probably do not occur under biologically relevant conditions. The phenomenon is of interest because it illustrates the versatility of Fe^{3+}-containing catalysts in reactions involving O_2. Also, it is responsible for reports of Mn^{2+}-stimulated NADH or sulfhydryl oxidation, O_2 uptake, and O_2^- or H_2O_2 production associated with peroxidases (e.g., Refs. 21,74,75).

III. ROLE OF ANTIBIOTICS AND OTHER PERTURBANTS

A number of antibiotics and other agents increase the production of activated forms of O_2 in biological systems (6,49). This effect may be due to at least 3 mechanisms of action, or to a combination of mechanisms. First, electron transport inhibitors block electron flow at a particular point in an electron transport chain, so that the low-potential components of the chain accumulate in the reduced state. Also, the O_2 concentration may rise as the flow of electrons to O_2 is interrupted. These effects increase the probability that O_2 will accept electrons from a low-potential component of the chain, rather than at the usual O_2 reduction site (e.g., cytochrome oxidase). Second, a number of these agents are redox active. That is, they have physical properties that permit an interaction with a reduced component in an electron transport chain, and an oxidation potential that permits them to accept electrons from the reduced component. The reduced agent may then react with O_2 to form O_2^- or H_2O_2. The inhibitory effects of these agents may be due to interference with energy metabolism, as well as to the O_2^- or H_2O_2 produced. A third class of agents is exemplified by the antibiotic and antitumor agent bleomycin (49). The active form of bleomycin contains Fe^{3+}, which can accept electrons, probably from sulfhydryl compounds or NADH. The reduced Fe^{2+} can react with O_2 to form a complex that may react directly with nucleic acids, or which may release activated forms of O_2. Therefore, the antibiotic has many of the properties of a peroxidase or oxidase enzyme.

IV. ENZYMES THAT ELIMINATE SUPEROXIDE (O_2^-) AND H_2O_2

A. Superoxide Dismutase

Although O_2 is reduced to O_2^- and H_2O_2 in all cells, these agents usually do not accumulate to high concentrations. The O_2^- anion is stable in strong base, but spontaneous dismutation is a rapid reaction at biologically relevant pH. In addition, all aerobic and most faculatative anaerobic bacteria contain SOD enzymes, which accelerate dismutation (35,38). Some microorganisms accumulate manganese (Mn^{2+}), which serves as a nonenzymatic catalyst of dismutation (6).

The O_2^- anion can act as an oxidizing or reducing agent, and acts as both in the dismutation reaction. Reduction of cytochrome C (cyt C) can be used to eliminate O_2^- and to measure O_2^- formation (34)

$$O_2^- + \text{cyt C (Fe}^{3+}) \longrightarrow O_2 + \text{cyt C (Fe}^{2+})$$

Similar reactions may contribute to eliminating O_2^- in biological systems. If so, the yield of H_2O_2 would be lower than when dismutation is the only pathway for eliminating O_2^- (37).

B. Catalase

Unlike O_2^-, H_2O_2 is a stable molecule that can accumulate to high concentrations. However, all aerobic organisms contain catalase, which eliminates H_2O_2 by catalyzing the dismutation of H_2O_2 (83).

$$2H_2O_2 \longrightarrow 2H_2O + O_2$$

Catalase is a hemoprotein, and the enzymatic mechanism is similar to that of peroxidases such as lactoperoxidase (LP). Catalase reacts with one H_2O_2 molecule to form the compound I (oxidized) state, then reacts with a second H_2O_2 molecule to return to the ground (reduced) state. A number of compounds can serve as the electron donor in place of the second (reducing) molecule of H_2O_2, and the oxidation of these compounds may be biologically significant.

Many anaerobic bacteria also contain catalase (70). In some bacteria, catalase is an inducible enzyme that is synthesized in response to O_2, H_2O_2, or some other substance formed when H_2O_2 is present (50). Lactic acid bacteria do not synthesize hemes, and therefore lack hemoproteins such as cytochrome oxidase and other respiratory cytochromes and catalase.

There have been a number of reports of catalase activity in lactic acid bacteria, but *catalase* has often been used as a vague term to describe the ability to eliminate H_2O_2. The term catalase should be reserved for enzymes that yield 0.5 mol O_2 per mole of H_2O_2, and preferably for the hemoprotein enzyme having the specific properties of catalase. Added Fe^{3+}, Mn^{2+}, or zinc (Zn^{2+}) results in formation of catalaselike activity in 2 unusual strains of *Streptococcus faecalis* (53). The activity yields 0.5 mol O_2 per mole H_2O_2, but is not associated with a hemoprotein. Many hemoproteins, hemes, and free Fe^{2+} have weak catalase activity (36). Also, certain chelated forms of Fe^{3+} catalyze a reaction that yields O_2 as one of the products (40,67) and that might be mistaken for catalase activity. Similarly, oxidation of Mn^{2+} to Mn^{3+} by O_2^- yields H_2O_2, and 2 Mn^{3+} can oxidize H_2O_2 to O_2 (6).

C. Nonhemoprotein Peroxidases

Peroxidase enzymes catalyze the oxidation of electron donors (AH_2) by peroxides:

$$AH_2 + H_2O_2 \longrightarrow A + 2H_2O$$

Reactions of this kind are catalyzed by several enzymes that do not contain heme. Although the reactions are formally identical to those catalyzed by hemoprotein peroxidases, the mechanism is different and does not involve compound I and II states. Also, the specificity for the electron donor is high, in contrast to the wide variety of oxidation reactions catalyzed by hemoprotein peroxidases.

The major nonhemoprotein peroxidase of mammalian cells is glutathione (GSH) peroxidase (33), which catalyzes the oxidation of 2GSH to glutathione disulfide (GSSG):

$$2GSH + H_2O_2 \longrightarrow GSSG + 2H_2O$$

This enzyme acts together with GSSG reductase (32), which catalyzes the regeneration of GSH at the expense of NADPH:

$$GSSG + NADPH + H^+ \longrightarrow 2GSH + NADP^+$$

Glutathione peroxidase is an effective scavenger for H_2O_2 at low
H_2O_2 concentrations, and can also eliminate alkyl hydroperoxides.
The combination of GSH peroxidase and GSSG reductase is more important than catalase in eliminating the small amounts of H_2O_2 that are
present in mammalian tissues (16,33).

There is little information on the occurrence of GSH- or other sul-
fhydryl-peroxidases in microorganisms. GSH does occur in bacteria
(30,61), and probably all bacteria have a pool of sulfhydryl compounds
composed of GSH, cysteine, or similar compounds. Some streptococci
were reported to lack GSH or GSSG (30), although *S. mutans* can take
up these compounds (104,106). No GSH- or cysteine-peroxidase was
detected in *S. mutans* (105).

Streptococci and lactobacilli contain a nonhemoprotein, NADH
peroxidase, that catalyzes reduction of H_2O_2 to water (26,69,95):

$$H_2O_2 + NADH + H^+ \longrightarrow 2H_2O + NAD^+$$

In some bacteria, synthesis of NADH peroxidase may be induced by
growth in the presence of O_2 (84). The NADH peroxidase, like GSH
peroxidase, depends on a continuing supply of reducing equivalents.
No H_2O_2 is eliminated at low temperature, in the presence of metabolic
inhibitors, or when the bacteria are deprived of metabolizable substrates.

D. Hemoprotein Peroxidases

Hemoprotein peroxidases such as LP are widely distributed in nature.
Their biological role is to catalyze oxidation of specific substances.
These reactions consume H_2O_2 and thus prevent the accumulation of
H_2O_2.

Such enzymes are not prevalent in bacteria. A peroxidase was
reported in *Escherichia coli*, but this activity is associated with catalase or a precursor in the synthesis of catalase (17). There are many
reports of bacterial peroxidases, based on oxidation of one of the
many phenols or aromatic amines that are oxidized by hemoprotein
peroxidases. However, hemoproteins including hemoglobin and catalase, other metalloproteins, free hemes, and free or chelated forms
of iron have a weak pseudo peroxidase activity.

Yeast mitochondria contain cyt C peroxidase, which catalyzes
oxidation of reduced cyt C (100). The probable role for this enzyme
is to protect the electron transport chain against H_2O_2 formed at the
flavoprotein or nonheme iron level. This protective role is accomplished
by oxidizing some of the cyt $C(Fe^{2+})$ produced in the usual operation
of the chain. Because O_2^- and H_2O_2 are often produced together, the
combination of cyt C and cyt C peroxidase could act to eliminate both
O_2^- and H_2O_2:

$$O_2^- + \text{cyt C } (Fe^{3+}) \xrightarrow{\text{nonenzymatic}} O_2 + \text{cyt C } (Fe^{2+})$$

$$H_2O_2 + 2 \text{ cyt C } (Fe^{2+}) \xrightarrow{\text{peroxidase}} 2H_2O + 2 \text{ cyt C } (Fe^{3+})$$

net:

$$2O_2^- + H_2O_2 \longrightarrow O_2 + 2H_2O$$

A cyt C peroxidase activity was reported in *Pseudomonas fluorescens* (60), and the activity is due to a hemoprotein peroxidase (107).

V. RELEASE OF O_2^- AND H_2O_2

Because O_2^- is short-lived, O_2^- production is measured by "trapping" O_2^-. Incubation of O_2^--releasing cells with cyt C results in reduction of cyt C, and the amount of O_2^- released is calculated from the accumulation of reduced cyt C. Release of O_2^- and H_2O_2 from *S. faecalis* was reported based on SOD- and catalase-inhibited chemiluminescence (2). However, the quantitative relation between chemiluminescence and release of O_2 metabolites is unknown.

Release of H_2O_2 is measured by incubating cells with an H_2O_2-trapping system consisting of a peroxidase and an oxidizable indicator substance (11,77,78). The amount of H_2O_2 released is calculated from accumulation of the oxidized indicator. Hydrogen peroxide is thought to diffuse readily through cell membranes. However, H_2O_2 produced intracellularly may be rapidly eliminated so that little appears in the medium. Depending on the site of H_2O_2 production and the activity of H_2O_2-consuming activities in the cell, the rate of H_2O_2 release (concentration of oxidized indicator per unit time) may be lower than the rate of H_2O_2 production.

If all of the O_2 uptake by cells is due to reduction of O_2 to O_2^- or H_2O_2, then rates of O_2^- or H_2O_2 production can be calculated from the rate of O_2 uptake. However, oxidation of O_2^- or dismutation of H_2O_2 will influence the observed rate of O_2 uptake so that the rate of O_2 uptake may be less than the true rate of O_2 reduction (12,37,93).

VI. TOXICITY OF H_2O_2

Although H_2O_2 is a powerful oxidizing agent, it is a stabilized molecule that reacts sluggishly with biological materials and, in itself, is not highly toxic. This kinetic barrier to the toxicity of H_2O_2 can be overcome in several ways. If the H_2O_2 concentration is high, the rate of reaction may become significant. In studies on washed cells of *S. mutans* strains at a cell density of 2-2.5 mg dry wt./ml, H_2O_2 concentrations of 2-3 mM are required for a 50% or greater inhibition of glucose metabolism (E. L. Thomas, unpublished data). It is doubtful that H_2O_2 occurs at these levels in vivo, except when H_2O_2 is used as an antiseptic agent.

The kinetic barrier to H_2O_2 toxicity can also be overcome with catalysts. The biologically significant catalysts are the hemoprotein peroxidases such as LP. The H_2O_2-dependent oxidation of I^- or SCN^- by LP yields agents that are not as powerful as H_2O_2 as oxidizing agents, but which have a lower kinetic barrier. In combination with LP and SCN^-, the amount of H_2O_2 required for inhibition of *S. mutans* cells is about 100 μM for the most resistant strains, and about 10 μM for the most sensitive. Therefore, LP-mediated toxicity is from 20 to 300 times greater than that of H_2O_2 alone. There are a number of reports in which H_2O_2 was proposed to be a toxic product of microbial metabolism. In many cases, the toxicity of H_2O_2 is probably due to peroxidase-catalyzed reactions.

Transition-metal ions also act as catalysts for H_2O_2 toxicity (80). Contamination by trace metals is a problem in evaluating toxicity of H_2O_2 or other O_2 metabolites. It is especially significant in studies on growing bacteria, because the usual microbiological media are heavily contaminated with Fe^{3+} and probably with other metals. Catalysis by trace metals probably accounts for widely varying estimates of the toxicity of the H_2O_2 produced by bacteria, or of added (exogenous) H_2O_2. It may be possible to block the action of metal ions with chelating agents, but some of the chelates are even better catalysts. Two chelating agents that deactivate Fe^{3+} have been identified (40), but they have not been used in studies with intact microorganisms. Many bacteria excrete chelating agents during growth, but the catalytic properties of the chelates have not been studied.

In some reports on the toxicity of bacterial H_2O_2 production, either O_2^- or the combination of O_2^- and H_2O_2 may account for the results. As one possible example, H_2O_2 was reported to be more toxic to *Peptostreptococcus anaerobius* when the cells were metabolizing than when metabolism was blocked (73). Toxicity may be due to the combined action of the added H_2O_2 and the O_2^- produced by the metabolizing cells.

As in the case of H_2O_2, the toxicity of O_2^- plus H_2O_2 requires catalysis, because O_2^- does not react with H_2O_2 at physiological pH. The reaction is catalyzed by free or chelated forms of transition-metal ions, such as the EDTA-Fe^{3+} and lactoferrin-Fe^{3+} chelates (39,67). The principal agent that is thought to be produced in this reaction is the HO (hydroxyl) radical.

VII. THE O_2 METABOLISM OF FACULTATIVE ANAEROBES

A. Flavoprotein Oxidases and Peroxidases

Flavoprotein NADH oxidases account for the major portion of O_2 uptake and H_2O_2 production by streptococci, lactobacilli, and other bacteria that lack cytochromes (26,89,90). These bacteria contain NADH oxidases that can produce O_2^-, H_2O_2, or water, and also contain an NADH peroxidase that can reduce H_2O_2 to water. One organism can express differing activities as the result of changes in growth conditions. The differing activities may be due to altered forms of one or two enzymes.

In cell-free extracts from *Clostridium perfringens*, O_2 uptake is due to a flavoprotein NADH oxidase that oxidizes 2 mol of NADH per mol of O_2 taken up (25,26,45). The enzyme reduces O_2 to water without releasing O_2^- or H_2O_2:

$$2NADH + 2H^+ + O_2 \longrightarrow 2NAD^+ + 2H_2O$$

A similar enzyme has been purified from *S. faecalis* (102). Such enzymes make a major contribution to O_2 uptake by other streptococci (101,103). The enzymes have not been characterized in sufficient detail to determine whether they contain copper or other metals, but they are not inhibited by cyanide.

In other studies on extracts from *S. faecalis*, 2NADH were oxidized per O_2 taken up, but this activity was attributed to the combination of a H_2O_2-producing NADH oxidase and a H_2O_2-reducing NADH peroxidase (24,26):

$$NADH + H^+ + O_2 \longrightarrow NAD^+ + H_2O_2$$

$$NADH + H^+ + H_2O_2 \longrightarrow NAD^+ + 2H_2O$$

The two activities reside in different proteins, though both are flavoproteins. Extracts from *Lactobacillus casei* also contain NADH oxidase and peroxidase activities, but the 2 activities reside in the same protein (84,95).

S. faecalis extracts also carry out NADH-dependent reduction of cyt C, and this activity resides in a protein distinct from the major oxidase and peroxidase (24,26). At the time of those studies, the ability of flavoproteins to produce O_2^- and the ability of O_2^- to reduce cyt C were unknown. The results may indicate that O_2^- was formed, but many agents can reduce cyt C (6,69,97). More recent studies indicate that O_2^- formation accounts for 17% of NADH-dependent O_2 uptake (13):

$$NADH + 2O_2 \longrightarrow NAD^+ + H^+ + 2O_2^-$$

Utilization of NADH for O_2 or H_2O_2 reduction in these organisms requires metabolic pathways other than glycolysis. Conversion of glucose to 2-pyruvate, followed by reduction of the 2-pyruvate to 2-lactate does not yield net NADH. Therefore, part of the pyruvate or other glycolytic intermediates must be diverted into other metabolic pathways, to spare NADH for O_2 metabolism. In *S. faecalis*, O_2 uptake is associated with a decreased yield of lactate (26).

Recent studies on *L. plantarum* indicate the presence of an O_2-inducible metabolic pathway that yields H_2O_2, but which does not involve NADH oxidase (71). Lactate accumulates during growth on glucose, and then lactate is metabolized when glucose is exhausted. Lactate is oxidized to pyruvate, and the electrons are transferred to an unidentified acceptor (not NAD^+). Pyruvate is oxidized in a reaction catalyzed by a H_2O_2-producing pyruvate oxidase, which requires thiamine pyrophosphate as a cofactor:

$$\text{Pyruvate} + \text{Pi} + O_2 \longrightarrow \text{acetyl-P} + CO_2 + H_2O_2$$

Similar pyruvate and lactate oxidases occur in other bacteria (26) and α-glycerol phosphate oxidase accounts for O_2-dependent metabolism of glycerol in *S. faecalis* (26,52):

$$\alpha\text{-Glycerol-P} + O_2 \longrightarrow \text{acetyl-P} + CO_2 + H_2O_2$$

The acetyl-phosphate produced in these oxidase reactions yields ATP in the reaction catalyzed by acetate kinase:

$$\text{Acetyl-P} + \text{ADP} \longrightarrow \text{acetate} + \text{ATP}$$

Therefore, these organisms have O_2-dependent metabolic pathways that yield high-energy compounds. The definition of facultative anaerobes may be too restrictive to apply to these organisms. The ability to metabolize lactate is not widely distributed among the lactobacilli and streptococci, but all produce pyruvate. Pyruvate may be oxidized without first being converted to lactate, particularly under conditions that suppress lactic dehydrogenase activity (98). Similarly, all of these organisms produce α-glycerol phosphate. The distribution of H_2O_2-producing pyruvate or α-glycerol phosphate oxidases among these bacteria is unknown.

A different sequence of reactions may be required to account for O_2-dependent metabolism of lactate in *L. brevis* (29). Metabolism of lactate is also obtained under anaerobic conditions when H_2O_2 is added. The apparent stoichiometry is oxidation of 1 mol lactate to acetate and CO_2, with reduction of 2 mol of H_2O_2. This stoichiometry appears consistent with a sequence of reactions catalyzed by NADH-linked lactic dehydrogenase, pyruvate dehydrogenase (14,26), and NADH peroxidase:

$$\text{Lactate} + NAD^+ \longrightarrow \text{pyruvate} + \text{NADH} + H^+$$

$$\text{Pyruvate} + \text{NAD}^+ + \text{CoA} \longrightarrow \text{acetyl CoA} + \text{CO}_2 + \text{NADH}$$

$$2\text{NADH} + \text{H}^+ + \text{H}_2\text{O}_2 \longrightarrow \text{NAD}^+ + 2\text{H}_2\text{O}$$

Net:

$$\text{Lactate} + 2\text{H}_2\text{O}_2 + \text{H}^+ \longrightarrow \text{acetyl CoA} + \text{CO}_2 + 4\text{H}_2\text{O}$$

In the absence of H_2O_2, all of the cellular content of NAD^+ is converted to NADH, and metabolism stops. Adding H_2O_2 oxidizes NADH to
NAD^+, allowing metabolism to continue. In the presence of O_2, NADH
oxidase or oxidase plus peroxidase can perform the function of reoxi-
dizing NADH.

B. Kinetics of O_2 Uptake

Measuring the disappearance of O_2 by manometric techniques or with a
polarographic O_2 electrode permits studies of the rate of O_2 uptake as
a function of O_2 concentration, $[O_2]$. When bacteria are well supplied
with metabolizable substrates, the enzymatic mechanism of O_2 uptake
may be saturated with respect to reducing equivalents, so that the rate
of O_2 uptake (V) depends only on the maximum rate (V_{max}), the apparent affinity for O_2, and the $[O_2]$. The rate may remain constant
over a wide range of $[O_2]$, if the affinity is high (the K_m is low), so
that $[O_2] > K_m$ and $V = V_{max}$. On the other hand, if the affinity is
low (high K_m), then the rate will decrease as $[O_2]$ decreases. A
number of flavoprotein oxidases exhibit mixed kinetics. This behavior
is probably associated with 2 types of electron transfer (13,34,66,86).
That is, the transfer of 2 electrons to O_2 may occur at low $[O_2]$,
whereas 1 electron may be transferred at high $[O_2]$.

Studies on streptococci indicate that some exhibit high-affinity O_2
uptake and others low-affinity uptake (3). The same kinetics of O_2
uptake are observed when cell-free extracts are incubated with NADH.
It was reported that the NADH oxidase from streptococci that released
large amounts of H_2O_2 can be distinguished from that of other strains
on the basis of plots of $[O_2]$ versus time. Linear plots are obtained
with the first class (e.g., *S. lactis*), whereas the slope decreases with
decreasing $[O_2]$ with the second class [e.g., *S. cremoris*). With the
first class, H_2O_2 accumulates in the medium during growth. The
validity of this classification system has not been widely tested.

A different approach was used in a study on extracts from *S.
faecalis* (72). The $[O_2]$ was varied, and the rate of oxidation of NADH
was measured. It was reported that the rate was nearly independent
of $[O_2]$, and a K_m for O_2 of 20 μM was calculated. However, NADH
oxidation may be due to 2 distinct enzymes, the H_2O_2-producing oxidase and the H_2O_2-reducing peroxidase. An apparent high affinity for

O_2 would be observed if the rate-limiting step in NADH oxidation was
the peroxidase-catalyzed reaction, so that the peroxidase is saturated
with respect to H_2O_2 at low $[O_2]$. Both the K_m for O_2 uptake and
the K_m for NADH oxidation should be measured in studies of this kind.

C. Utilization of Iron or Hemes

Although streptococci and lactobacilli do not synthesize hemes, some
may use performed hemes to assemble hemoproteins (96). However,
there is little evidence for formation of functional hemoprotein enzymes.
Some of the results are perhaps due to nonspecific association of hemes
or Fe^{3+} with cell-surface components, yielding pseudo peroxidase and
pseudo catalase activities. Spectrophotometric characterization of cytochromelike components in *S. faecalis* grown in the presence of hemes
suggests the presence of a b_2-type cytochrome (15), though some features of the spectrum can be attributed to absorbed hemes (81). These
cytochromelike substances were not shown to undergo cyclic oxidation
and reduction in O_2 reduction or other electron transport processes.

A number of studies suggest that growth in the presence of iron,
hemes, or porphyrin compounds confers cytochromelike respiration on
certain streptococci and similar bacteria (96). Such evidence is indirect
and based on several types of observations and assumptions. First,
uptake of O_2 without release of H_2O_2 is assumed to be due to an activity similar to that of cytochrome oxidase. Second, enhanced growth
rates in the presence of O_2 are assumed to be due to a form of oxidative phosphorylation (87). Third, cytochromelike respiration is inferred from membrane-associated NADH oxidation that can be inhibited
by cyanide (82).

However, uptake of O_2 can occur without release of H_2O_2 if H_2O_2
is rapidly eliminated by NADH peroxidase, or if O_2 is reduced by a
four-electron transferring NADH oxidase. The O_2-dependent ATP
synthesis may be due to the combination of oxidase and kinase activities (e.g., pyruvate oxidase and acetate kinase). Also, ATP synthesis may be coupled to reduction of metabolic products, rather than to
reduction of O_2. Finally, inhibition by cyanide can be due to a number
of mechanisms. Therefore, cytochromelike respiration does not indicate
or require the presence of cytochromes.

Some strains of streptococci that are clearly cytochrome-free do
contain a membrane-associated electron transport chain, probably composed of flavoproteins, quinones (10), and nonheme iron proteins
(27). Also, the streptococci contain a membrane-bound ATPase (or
ATP synthetase) similar to that of mitochondria and to that of many
aerobic bacteria (47). In the streptococci, the enzyme is thought to
act as a proton (H^+)-pumping ATPase, rather than as an ATP synthetase driven by the transmembrane H^+ gradient (46,48). Because these
bacteria rapidly convert neutral molecules such as glucose to strong
acids such as pyruvic, lactic, acetic, and formic acid, ATP-driven

expulsion of H^+ from the cell plays an important role in maintaining a neutral intracellular pH. Nevertheless, phosphorylation of ADP can be obtained when the electrochemical H^+ gradient across the membrane of cells or isolated membrane vesicles is reversed (54,63).

NADH-dependent synthesis of ATP was obtained in a membrane fraction from *S. faecalis*, with fumarate rather than O_2 as the electron acceptor (31). This result indicates that electron transport components are oriented in the membrane so as to expel H^+ and to obtain energy for this process from the flow of electrons from NADH to fumarate. It is not known whether O_2 can serve as the electron acceptor for this or a similar electron transport chain.

D. O_2 Metabolism of *Streptococcus mutans*

Several *S. mutans* strains release H_2O_2 (43), although according to one report, they do not contain NADH oxidase activity (82). These oral bacteria coexist with the LP antimicrobial system, so it is of interest to determine whether they release H_2O_2, and whether the amount of H_2O_2 released is sufficient to have an inhibitory effect in combination with LP and SCN^-. These bacteria are pathogens, and understanding their O_2 metabolism may lead to methods for their control or eradication.

Bacteria classified as *S. mutans* are heterogeneous, and can be subclassified according to serotype (i.e., the distinct antigens expressed on their cell surface), their ability to metabolize a number of sugars or amino acids, and possibly with respect to their host and the site that they colonize within the mouth (20,43,57,85). Therefore, it is difficult to generalize about characteristics of these bacteria. In our studies (105,106),11 different strains were used, with at least 1 representative of serotypes a through g (see Table 1).

When the washed cells were incubated with glucose, all strains took up O_2 at high rates. When $[O_2]$ was held constant at 0.2 mM (the solubility of O_2 in an air-saturated solution at 37°C), from 0.2 to 0.5 mol of O_2 was taken up per mole of glucose metabolized.

Reducing equivalents required for O_2 metabolism came at least partly at the expense of reduction of pyruvate to lactate. That is, the cells produced less lactate per mole of glucose metabolized under aerobic conditions. Also, those cells with the highest O_2 uptake rates had the lowest ratios of lactate produced to glucose metabolized. The decreased yield of lactate was associated with an increased yield of acetate and other volatile products.

Under anaerobic conditions, acetate and formate were the major volatile products. These bacteria contain pyruvate formate lyase activity (99), which yields acetyl CoA and formate:

$$\text{Pyruvate} + \text{CoA} \longrightarrow \text{acetyl CoA} + \text{formate}$$

Under aerobic conditions, the yield of acetate increased, but no formate was detected. These results may indicate the presence of pyruvate

Table 1   Release of O_2 Metabolites From *S. mutans* Strains

Class I: High levels of H_2O_2 release and accumulation

Strain	Serotype[a]	Subclassification[b]	Biotype[c]
FA-1	b	*S. rattus*	II
BHT	b	*S. rattus*	II
OMZ-176	d	*S. sobrinus*	IV

Class II: High levels of H_2O_2 release but low levels of H_2O_2 accumulation

B-13	d	*S. sobrinus*	IV
Ingbritt	c	*S. mutans*	I

Class III: Low levels of H_2O_2 release and no H_2O_2 accumulation

III-A: Measurable O_2^- release

AHT	a	*S. cricetus*	III
HS-6	a	*S. cricetus*	III

III-B: O_2^- release not measurable

6715-15	g	*S. sobrinus*	IV
GS-5	c	*S. mutans*	I
LM-7	e	*S. mutans*	I
OMZ-175	f	*S. mutans*	I

[a]From Refs. 43 and 57.
[b]From Ref. 20.
[c]From Ref. 85.

oxidase (26), pyruvate dehydrogenase (14,26), or formate dehydrogenase (88) activity:

$$\text{Pyruvate} + \text{Pi} + O_2 \longrightarrow \text{acetyl-P} + CO_2 + H_2O_2$$

$$\text{Pyruvate} + \text{CoA} + \text{NAD}^+ \longrightarrow \text{acetyl CoA} + CO_2 + \text{NADH}$$

$$\text{Formate} + \text{NAD}^+ \longrightarrow CO_2 + \text{NADH}$$

Any of these reactions could account for the decreased yield of formate, and each provides additional reducing equivalents for O_2 reduction.

Cells from growing cultures (or stationary-phase cells that were preincubated with glucose) took up O_2 in the absence of extracellular glucose. These bacteria store glucose as intracellular carbohydrate polymers (43) for later utilization. The cells obtained a higher yield of reducing equivalents (NADH) for O_2 uptake when stored glucose was the substrate for carbohydrate metabolism. Under these conditions, the cells produced acetate and other volatile products, but little or no lactate.

Kinetics of O_2 uptake were mixed. Over a wide range of $[O_2]$, the rate of O_2 uptake was proportional to $[O_2]$. This low-affinity process was the major mechanism of O_2 uptake except at very low $[O_2]$. At low $[O_2]$, O_2 uptake appeared saturable with a low V_{max} and a K_m of <5 μM. Cell-free extracts contained NADH oxidase activity, and the kinetics of O_2 uptake in the presence of excess NADH were the same as observed with whole cells. The O_2 uptake by cells or extracts was not inhibited by cyanide.

As indicated in Table 1, the 11 strains could be divided into 3 classes, according to the amount of H_2O_2 that accumulated in the incubation medium when the washed cells were incubated with glucose. The largest amount of H_2O_2 accumulation was observed with class I, less with class II, and no H_2O_2 accumulated with class III. The class III strains could be further subclassified. In class III-A, two strains released measurable amount of O_2^-.

With cells of class I strains from stationary phase, about 0.1 mol of H_2O_2 was released per mole of glucose metabolized, when $[O_2]$ was held constant at 0.2 mM. The rate of H_2O_2 accumulation was only slightly lower than the rate of H_2O_2 release, and H_2O_2 accumulated to 1-2 mM in the incubation medium. With cells of class II strains, about 0.05 mol of H_2O_2 was released per mole glucose metabolized, but H_2O_2 accumulation stopped when the H_2O_2 concentration was 0.05-0.1 mM. With cells of class III-A strains, H_2O_2 release was measurable, but it is likely that all of the H_2O_2 detected was due to release of O_2^-, followed by dismutation of O_2^- in the medium. As a minimum estimate, released O_2^- accounted for 6% of total O_2 uptake. With cells of class III-B strains, a very low level of H_2O_2 release was detected, but release of O_2^- was below measurable levels. It is likely that all strains released at least small amounts of O_2^- and H_2O_2. Adding SOD, catalase, or SOD plus catalase to the incubation medium slightly stimulated the rate of aerobic glucose metabolism with all strains, presumably by relieving an inhibitory effect of O_2 metabolites.

Little or no H_2O_2 accumulated in the growth medium during the active (logarithmic) growth phase of any of the strains. Instead, H_2O_2 accumulation was characteristic of stationary-phase cells. However, if class I strains were allowed to grow to stationary phase (16-24 hr) and then glucose was added, H_2O_2 accumulated in the growth medium.

The change in behavior as these bacteria entered stationary phase was not associated with increased O_2 uptake. With all strains, O_2 uptake by intact cells and NADH oxidase activity in extracts were higher with growing cells. However, the ability of cells of class I strains to reduce H_2O_2 to water did decrease sharply in stationary phase. The loss of H_2O_2-reducing activity was demonstrated by incubating cells with H_2O_2 and glucose under anaerobic conditions, and measuring the rate at which H_2O_2 was eliminated from the medium. Also, the NADH peroxidase activity of extracts was low. When the extracts were incubated aerobically with NADH, H_2O_2 accumulated to high levels.

With class III strains, the ability to reduce H_2O_2 decreased in stationary-phase cells, but the ability to take up O_2 also decreased. When extracts were incubated aerobically with NADH, about 2 mol of NADH was oxidized per mole of O_2 taken up and little or no H_2O_2 accumulated.

These results suggested that O_2 metabolism consisted of NADH-dependent reduction of O_2 to H_2O_2 and NADH-dependent reduction of H_2O_2 to water. Presumably, the rate at which H_2O_2 was released to the medium was the difference in the rates of these 2 reactions. However, this interpretation was not adequate to explain the observations. With all strains, the rate of O_2 uptake by intact cells was faster than the rate of H_2O_2 reduction under anaerobic conditions. Also, the rates of NADH-dependent O_2 uptake and O_2-dependent oxidation of NADH by cell-free extracts were much faster than the rate of NADH-dependent reduction of H_2O_2 under anaerobic conditions. Therefore, cells of all strains appeared to contain NADH oxidase activity that could use 2 mol of NADH to reduce 1 mol of O_2, without releasing H_2O_2 as an intermediate.

The results suggested that there are qualitative differences in NADH oxidase activity among the different strains, or even in a culture of a single strain at different phases of growth. That is, some cells contained higher levels of the H_2O_2-producing oxidase activity, relative to the oxidase that did not produce H_2O_2. Despite these differences, all strains had similar kinetics of O_2 uptake. Therefore, it was not possible to distinguish between the different oxidase activities on the basis of their apparent affinity for O_2. Also, in contrast to results obtained with *S. lactis* and *S. cremoris* (3), it was possible to obtain high levels of H_2O_2 release and accumulation from cells with low-affinity O_2 uptake.

As a final complication, qualitative differences in peroxidase activity were also observed. That is, the H_2O_2-reducing activity of the class II strains had a low affinity for H_2O_2. As H_2O_2 was released and the H_2O_2 concentration in the medium increased, eventually a concentration was reached at which the rate of H_2O_2 reduction equaled the rate of H_2O_2 release. When the rates were equal, the H_2O_2 concentration remained constant. This steady-state level of H_2O_2 accumulation was about 0.1 mM with B-13 cells and about 0.05 mM with Ingbritt cells.

Extracts from all strains carried out NADH- and O_2-dependent reduction of cyt C, which could be blocked by SOD. Therefore, all cells could produce at least small amounts of O_2^-. It has not been determined whether O_2^- production is due to either of the major types of NADH

oxidase activity described above. Extracts from cells of class III-A
strains did not produce more O_2^- than those from other cells, but had
low SOD activity. Therefore, release of O_2^- from these cells appeared
to be due to the low rate of dismutation.

The class III-A strains were also the only strains that were clearly
O_2-sensitive. These strains grew slowly in continuously aerated cultures, and the metabolic activity of cells harvested from aerated cultures was low under anaerobic or aerobic conditions. Therefore, low
SOD activity may account for the O_2 sensitivity of these strains. The
SOD activity measured in extracts from all strains was due to SOD
enzymes, and was not lost upon dialysis or inhibited by EDTA. The
S. mutans 6715 strain (94) and *S. faecalis* (13) contain SOD enzymes
with bound Mn^{2+}, whereas many lactobacilli accumulate free Mn^{2+} (4-6).

Some of the techniques used in these studies have been applied
to measuring H_2O_2 release from the mixed microbial flora of human saliva (E. L. Thomas, unpublished results; 92). In most samples, high
levels of H_2O_2 release were observed when metabolizable carbohydrate
was provided. The mean rate with added glucose was 0.1 mM H_2O_2/hr
from the microorganisms obtained from 1 ml of saliva Considerable
differences in the rate of H_2O_2 release were observed, depending on
the sugar provided. The highest levels of H_2O_2 release were obtained
with the amino sugars glucosamine and N-acetylglucosamine.

VIII. H_2O_2 AND OTHER O_2 METABOLITES IN MICROBIAL ECOLOGY AND DISEASE PROCESSES

Uptake of O_2 and release of O_2 metabolites by lactic acid bacteria and
other facultative anaerobes may be of significance in microbial ecology.
The presence of O_2 influences the metabolic products released from
these microorganisms, and O_2 or H_2O_2 confer the ability to metabolize
certain substances that are not metabolized under anaerobic conditions.
Also, O_2 uptake enables these organisms to create an anaerobic environment when they are present at high cell densities, or in regions
of slow O_2 diffusion. Although this anaerobic environment does not
necessarily provide a direct advantage, it could prevent the growth of
O_2-requiring microorganisms, or slow the growth of the many microorganisms that grow faster when O_2 is available.

Also, release of O_2^- or H_2O_2 may damage other microorganisms
(22,51,79). Released H_2O_2 has been proposed to be a bacteriocin or
antagonism factor. On the other hand, the O_2 metabolites may damage
the microorganisms that produce them (3,19,23,28,51,59). Also, the
host tissues may be damaged, as in the destruction of oral tissues
observed in acatalasemia (1). Damage to other host tissues has been
proposed to be involved in disease processes associated with many
microorganisms (7,18,19).

Release of O_2^- or H_2O_2 may also activate host-defense systems. For example, catalase-negative bacteria are more susceptible to the O_2-dependent antimicrobial activities of phagocytic leukocytes (8,9,55, 56,64). Release of H_2O_2 may also activate the LP antimicrobial system (44,92). On the other hand, the prevalence of H_2O_2-releasing bacteria in the oral environment (58) suggests that these organisms have developed resistance to the LP system, and may have subverted this host-defense system to their advantage (91,92). Bacterial resistance to the LP system is discussed in detail in Chap. 8. Further study of the relation between bacterial O_2 metabolism and the LP antimicrobial system will be required to understand this complex interaction.

ACKNOWLEDGMENTS

Supported by Research Grants DE 04235 and AI 16795 from the National Institutes of Health, by Cancer Center Support Grants CA 08480 and CA 21765 from the National Cancer Institute and by ALSAC. I thank my collaborators K. Pera, K. Smith, A. Chwang, and H. Rao, and P. Nicholas for manuscript preparation.

REFERENCES

1. Aebi, H., and Suter, H., in *The Metabolic Basis of Inherited Disease*, Stanberry, J. B., Wyngaarden, J. B., and Fredickson, D. S. (Eds.), McGraw-Hill, New York, p. 1792 (1972).
2. Allen, R. C., in *Developments in Biology*, Bannister, W. H., and Bannister, J. V. (Eds.), vol. 2A, Elsevier/North-Holland, New York, p. 116 (1980).
3. Anders, R. F., Hogg, D. M., and Jago, G. R., *Appl. Microbiol. 19:* 608 (1970).
4. Archibald, F. S., and Fridovich, I., *J. Bacteriol. 145:* 442 (1981).
5. Archibald, F. S., and Fridovich, I., *J. Bacteriol. 146:* 928 (1981).
6. Archibald, F. S., and Fridovich, I., *J. Bacteriol. 214:* 452 (1982).
7. Avery, O. T., and Morgan, H. J., *J. Exp. Med. 39:* 275 (1924).
8. Babior, B. M., *N. Engl. J. Med. 298:* 659, 721 (1978).
9. Badwey, J. A., and Karnovsky, M. L., *Ann. Rev. Biochem. 49:* 695 (1980).
10. Baum, R. H., and Dolin, M. I., *J. Biol. Chem. 240:* 3425 (1965).
11. Boveris, A., Martino, E., and Stoppiani, A. O. M., *Anal. Biochem. 80:* 145 (1977).
12. Bright, H. J., and Porter, D. J. T., in *The Enzymes*, Boyer, P. D. (Eds.), vol. 12, Academic Press, New York, p. 421 (1975).

13. Britton, L., Malinowski, D. P., and Fridovich, I., *J. Bacteriol.* *134*: 229 (1978).

14. Broome, M. C., Thomas, M. P., Hillier, A. J., and Jago, G. R., *Aust. J. Biol. Sci.* *33*: 15 (1980).

15. Bryan-Jones, D. C., and Whittenbury, R., *J. Gen. Microbiol.* *58*: 247 (1969).

16. Chance, B., Sies, H., and Boveris, A., *Physiol. Rev.* *59*: 527 (1979).

17. Claiborne, A., Malinowski, D. P., and Fridovich, I., *J. Biol. Chem.* *254*: 11664 (1979).

18. Cohen, G., Somerson, N. L., *J. Bacteriol.* *98*: 547 (1969).

19. Cook , F. D., and Quadling, C., *Can. J. Microbiol.* *8*: 933 (1962).

20. Coykendall, A. L., *Int. J. Syst. Bacteriol.* *27*: 26 (1977).

21. Curutte, J. T., Karnovsky, M. L., and Babior, B. M., *J. Clin. Invest.* *57*: 1059 (1976).

22. Dahiya, R. S., and Speck, M. L., *J. Dairy Sci.* *51*: 1568 (1968).

23. deVries, W., Donkers, C., Boellaard, M., and Srouthamer, A. H., *Arch. Microbiol.* *119*: 167 (1978).

24. Dolin, M. I., *Arch. Biochem. Biophys.* *55*: 415 (1955).

25. Dolin, M. I., *J. Bacteriol.* *77*: 383 (1959).

26. Dolin, M. I., in *The Bacteria*, Gunsalus, I. C., and Stanier, R. Y. (Eds.), vol. 2, Academic Press, New York, p. 425 (1961).

27. Dolin, M. I., and Baum, R. H., *Bacteriol. Proc.* *65*: 96 (1965).

28. Donoghue, H. D., and Tyler, J. E., *Arch. Oral Biol.* *20*: 381 (1975).

29. Douglas, H. C., *J. Bacteriol.* *54*: 272 (1947).

30. Fahey, R. C., Brown, W. C., Adams, W. B., and Worsham, M. B., *J. Bacteriol.* *133*: 1126 (1978).

31. Faust, P. J., and Vandemark, P. J., *Arch. Biochem. Biophys.* *137*: 392 (1970).

32. Flohe, L., and Gunzler, W. A., in *Glutathione: Metabolism and Function*, Arias, I. M., and Jakoby, W. B. (Eds.), Raven Press, New York, p. 17 (1976).

33. Flohe, L., Gunzler, W. A., and Ladenstein, R., in *Glutathione: Metabolism and Function*, Arias, I. M., and Jakoby, W. B. (Eds.), Raven Press, New York, p. 115 (1976).

34. Fridovich, I., *J. Biol. Chem.* *245*: 4053 (1970).

35. Fridovich, I., *Ann. Rev. Biochem.* *44*: 147 (1975).

36. George, P., *Biochem. J.* *43*: 287 (1948).

37. Green, T. R., Schaefer, R. E., and Makler, M. T., *Biochem. Biophys. Res. Commun.* *94*: 12 13 (1980).

38. Gregory, E. M., and Dapper, C. H., *J. Bacteriol.* *144*: 967 (1980).

39. Halliwell, B., *FEBS Lett.* *80*: 291 (1977).

40. Halliwell, B., *FEBS Lett. 92*: 321 (1978).
41. Halliwell, B., *Planta 140*: 81 (1978).
42. Halliwell, B., and DeRycker, J., *Photochem. Photobiol. 28*: 757 (1978).
43. Hamada, S., and Slade, H. D., *Microbiol. Rev. 44*: 331 (1980).
44. Hamon, C. B., and Klebanoff, S. J., *J. Exp. Med. 137*: 438 (1973).
45. Harding, G. L., and Britton, L. N., Abstr. D22, *Am. Soc. Microbiol.* (1982).
46. Harold, F. M., *Curr. Top. Bioenerg. 6*: 83 (1976).
47. Harold, F. M., Baarda, J. R., Baron, C., and Abrams, A., *J. Biol. Chem. 244*: 2261 (1969).
48. Harold, F. M., and Papineau, D., *J. Memb. Biol. 8*: 45 (1972).
49. Hassan, H. M., and Fridovich, I., *Arch. Biochem. Biophys. 196*: 385 (1979).
50. Hassan, H. M., and Fridovich, I., *Rev. Infect. Dis. 1*: 357 (1979).
51. Holmberg, K., and Hallander, H. O., *Arch. Oral Biol. 18*: 423 (1973).
52. Jacobs, N. J., and VanDemark, P. J., *J. Bacteriol. 79*: 532 (1960).
53. Jones, D., Deibel, R. H., and Niven, C. F., Jr., *J. Bacteriol. 88*: 602 (1964).
54. Kaback, H. R., *N. Y. Acad. Sci. 339*: 53 (1980).
55. Kaplan, E. L., Laxdal, T., and Quie, P. G., *Pediatrics 41*: 591 (1968).
56. Klebanoff, S. J., and White, L. R., *N. Engl. J. Med. 280*: 460 (1969).
57. Kral, T. A., and Daneo-Moore, L., *J. Dent. Res. 60*: 1713 (1981).
58. Kraus, F. W., Nickerson, J. F., Perry, W. I., and Walker, A. P., *J. Bacteriol. 73*: 727 (1957).
59. Lee, I. H., Fredrickson, A. G., and Tsuchiya, H. M., *J. Gen. Microbiol. 93*: 204 (1976).
60. Lenhoff, H. M., and Kaplan, N. O., *Nature* (Lond.) *172*: 739 (1953).
61. Loewen, P. C., *Can. J. Biochem. 57*: 107 (1979).
62. Malkin, R., and Malmstrom, B. G., *Adv. Enzymol. 33*: 177 (1970).
63. Maloney, P. C., Kashket, E. R., and Wilson, T. H., *Proc. Natl. Acad. Sci. USA 71*: 3896 (1974).
64. Mandel, G. L., and Hook, E. W., *J. Bacteriol. 100*: 531 (1969).
65. Massey, V., Palmer, G., and Ballou, D., in *Flavins and Flavoproteins*, Kamin, H. (Ed.), University Park Press, Baltimore, p. 349 (1971).
66. McCord, J. M., Beauchamp, C. O., Goscin, S., Misra, H. P., and Fridovich, I., in *Oxidases and Related Redox Systems*,

King, T. E., Mason, H. S., and Morrison, M. (Eds.), vol. 1, University Park Press, Baltimore, p. 51 (1973).

67. McCord, J. M., and Day, E. D., Jr., *FEBS Lett. 86:* 139 (1978).

68. Michelson, A. M., in *Superoxide and Superoxide Dismutases,* Michelson, A. M., McCord, J. M., and Fridovich, I. (Eds.), Academic Press, London, p. 87 (1977).

69. Mizushima, S., and Kitihara, K., *J. Gen. Appl. Microbiol. 8:* 56 (1962).

70. Molland, J., *Acta Pathol. Microbiol. Scand. (Suppl.) 66:* 1 (1947).

71. Murphy, G., and Condon, S., Abstr. 136, Am. Soc. Microbiol. (1982).

72. Niederpruem, D. J., and Hacket, D. P., *Plant Physiol. 33:* 113 (1958).

73. Nyberg, G. K., and Carlsson, J., *Antimicrob. Agents Chemother. 20:* 726 (1981).

74. Olsen, J., and Davis, L., *Biochim. Biophys. Acta 445:* 324 (1976).

75. Oram, J. D., and Reiter, B., *Biochem. J. 100:* 382 (1966).

76. Orme-Johnson, W. H., and Beinert, H., *Biochem. Biophys. Res. Commun. 36:* 905 (1969).

77. Perschke, H., and Broda, E., *Nature (Lond.) 190:* 257 (1961).

78. Pick, E., and Keisari, Y., *J. Immunol. Methods 38:* 161 (1980).

79. Price, R. J., and Lee, J. S., *J. Milk Food Technol. 33:* 13 (1970).

80. Repine, J. E., Fox, R. B., Berger, E. M., and Harada, R. N., *Infect. Immun. 32:* 407 (1981).

81. Ritchey, T. W., and Seeley, H. W., Jr., *J. Gen. Microbiol. 85:* 220 (1974).

82. Ritchey, T. W., and Seeley, H. W., Jr., *J. Gen. Microbiol. 93:* 195 (1976).

83. Schonbaum, G. R., and Chance, B., in *The Enzymes,* Boyer, P. D. (Ed.), vol. 13, Academic Press, New York, p. 363 (1976).

84. Seeley, H. W., and Vandemark, P. J., *J. Bacteriol. 61:* 27 (1951).

85. Shklair, I. L., and Keene, H. J., in *Proceedings, Microbial Aspects of Dental Caries,* Stiles, H. M., Loesche, W. J., and O'Brien, T. C. (Eds.), Sp. Supp. Microbiol. Abstr., vol. 1, Washington, D.C., p. 201 (1976).

86. Singer, T. P., and Edmonson, D. E., in *Molecular Oxygen in Biology: Topics in Molecular Oxygen Research,* Hayaishi, O. (Ed.), North-Holland, Amsterdam, p. 315 (1974).

87. Smalley, A. J., Jahrling, P., and VanDemark, P. J., *J. Bacteriol. 96:* 1595 (1968).

88. Stadtman, T., *Adv. Enzymol.* *48*: 1 (1979).
89. Strittmatter, C. F., *J. Biol. Chem.* *234*: 2789 (1959).
90. Strittmatter, C. F., *J. Biol. Chem.* *234*: 2794 (1959).
91. Thomas, E. L., Bates, K. P., and Jefferson, M. M., *J. Dent. Res.* *59*: 1466 (1980).
92. Thomas, E. L., Bates, K. P., and Jefferson, M. M., *J. Dent. Res.* *60*: 785 (1981).
93. Thomas, E. L., and Fishman, M., *Arch. Biochem. Biophys.* *215*: 355 (1982).
94. Vance, P. G., Keele, B. B., Jr., and Rajagopalan, K. V., *J. Biol. Chem.* *247*: 4782 (1972).
95. Walker, G. A., and Kilgour, G. L., *Arch. Biochem. Biophys.* *111*: 534 (1965).
96. Whittenberg, R., in *Streptococci*, Skinner, F. A., and Quesnel L. B. (Eds.), Academic Press, New York, p. 51 (1978).
97. Winterbourn, C. C., *Arch. Biochem. Biophys.* *209*: 159 (1981).
98. Yamada, T., and Carlsson, J., *J. Bacteriol.* *124*: 55 (1975).
99. Yamada, T., and Carlsson, J., in *Proceedings, Microbial Aspects of Dental Caries*, Stiles, H. M., Loesche, W. J., and O'Brien, T. C. (Eds.), Sp. Supp. Microbiol. Abstr., vol. 3, Washington, D.C., p. 809 (1976).
100. Yonetani, T., in *The Enzymes*, Boyer, P. D. (Ed.), vol. 13, Academic Press, New York, p, 345 (1976).
101. Bruhn, J. C., and Collins, E. B., *J. Dairy Sci.* *53*: 857-860 (1970).
102. Hoskins, D. D., Whiteley, H. R., and Mackler, B., *J. Biol. Chem.* *237*: 2647-2651 (1962).
103. Pugh, S. Y. R., and Knowles, C. J., *J. Gen. Microbiol.* *128*: 1009-1017 (1982).
104. Thomas, E. L., *J. Bacteriol.* *157*: 240-246 (1984).
105. Thomas, E. L., and Pera, K. A., *J. Bacteriol.* *154*: 1236-1244 (1983).
106. Thomas, E. L., Pera, K. A., Smith, K. W., and Chwang, A. K., *Infect. Immun.* *39*: 767-778 (1983).
107. Ronnberg, M., Araiso, T., Ellfolk, N., and Dunford, H. B., *Arch. Biochem. Biophys.* *207*: 197-204 (1981).

10

Effect of Sugars and Sugar Alcohols on Salivary Peroxidase

KAUKO K. MÄKINEN* / *Institute of Dentistry, University of Turku, Turku, Finland*

Current affiliation:
*School of Dentistry, The University of Michigan, Ann Arbor, Michigan

I. INTRODUCTION

The activity and concentrations of several salivary enzymes are selec-
tively affected by the diet. The activities of many salivary enzymes
may fluctuate from day to day and from hour to hour within a relatively broad range. Such fluctuations are usually associated with the
normal physiological functions of the salivary glands. The effects of
dietary sugars on the activity of the salivary peroxidase are particularly interesting, because of the participation of the peroxidase system
in host-defense mechanisms. The first evidence of diet-dependent
changes in salivary peroxidase activities were obtained in the Turku
sugar studies. These studies consisted of a 2-year human feeding
trial that demonstrated the non- and anticariogenic effects of xylitol
(23). Because of the proposed antimicrobial role of salivary peroxidase
in oral biology, it was at first believed that the xylitol-induced increase in peroxidase levels would partially explain the advantageous
dental effects of xylitol (17,18). The current view is, however, that
the non- and anticariogenic properties of xylitol are chiefly based on
the low or nil fermentability of xylitol by cariogenic microorganisms,
and on the direct and indirect effects of xylitol on the chemistry of
saliva (5,6,9). The effects of sugars and sugar alcohols on salivary
peroxidase, nevertheless, have an intrinsic interest, since these effects may be selective. This review summarizes the work so far carried
out in this field.

II. EFFECT OF CARBOHYDRATE DIET ON SALIVARY
PEROXIDASE LEVELS

A. Turku Sugar Studies

A detailed description of these long-term human feeding trials has been
given previously (23). This trial involved almost complete substitution
of sucrose by fructose or xylitol during a period of 2 years. Most of
the subjects were young adults (mean age 27.5 years), and they were
assigned to the experimental groups as follows: 35 subjects in the
sucrose group, 38 in the fructose group, and 52 in the xylitol group.
The mean individual monthly intake of sucrose, fructose, and xylitol
was 2.2, 2.1, and 1.5 kg, respectively. All subjects were found to
be healthy during the trial, and no delayed pathological changes were
detected in the blood and urine chemistry of these subjects several
years after completing the study (19,20).

Biochemical analyses of peroxidases in whole saliva, dental plaque,
and gingival exudate samples were carried out several times during
the feeding schedule (17). Preliminary experiments showed that the
peroxidase activity of centrifuged, pooled whole saliva was consistently
higher in the xylitol group than in other feeding groups. Salivary
sediment and plaque aqueous extracts also displayed high peroxidase
activity, but no consistent differences between feeding groups were

found in these cases. Detailed chromatographic experiments on CM-cellulose (18) and Sephadex G-100 suggested that the peroxidase activity that was increased in the saliva of the xylitol-consuming subjects could be attributed to the involvement of the salivary peroxidase and not to enzymes of plaque or leukocyte origin (17). The results were similar whether the peroxidase activity was expressed in terms of seconds according to the assay method of Chance and Maehly (2), or in terms of specific activities. The molecular weight of the peroxidase component whose activity was increased in the saliva of the xylitol-consuming subjects was estimated to be 73,500 (17), which is in fairly good agreement with the values previously given for salivary peroxidase (see the discussion in Ref. 17). The total inactivation of the enzyme by 10^{-4} M CN^- and its fractionation characteristics provide further evidence that it was the salivary peroxidase whose activity levels were increased in the whole saliva of subjects fed substantial amounts of xylitol. Xylitol, fructose, and sucrose had no detectable effect on the peroxidase-catalyzed oxidation of guaiacol (the electron donor used in the peroxidase assays).

B. The Effect of a Carbohydrate Diet on Peroxidase Levels of Cannulated Monkey Saliva

The long-term feeding studies on human whole saliva discussed earlier suggested a further investigation using monkeys. Five monkeys (*Macaca mulatta*) were fed either a sucrose or xylitol diet for 3 days (crossover design). An estimated total of 15-20 g/day of sucrose or xylitol was consumed ad libitum by each monkey, from drinking water or in solid form. In this study both parotid and submandibular saliva samples were collected using a cannulation technique (10) on the second and third test days. Salivary flow was stimulated by a subcutaneous injection of pilocarpine under anesthesia (using thiamylal intravenously and maintained on a fluotane-oxygen mixture). Ingestion of xylitol was associated with a significant increase in the activity of the salivary peroxidase (Fig. 1). The concentrations of protein were also increased. The relative increases were the same whether the enzyme activities were expressed as units per milliliter of saliva, units per milligram of protein, or units excreted per minute—xylitol feeding was always associated with increased peroxidase levels. These results indicated that at the moment when the collection of saliva was started the acinar units of the salivary glands were filled with fluid containing proteins and enzymes, the concentrations of which depended on whether monkeys were fed xylitol or sucrose. The activity of salivary amylase was also increased during xylitol ingestion (1). The specific enzyme activities did not differ between sucrose and xylitol diets. The effect of xylitol and sorbitol on the salivary peroxidase levels was also studied with *M. fascicularis* (10). In this case the individual variations were considerable, and no statistically significant differences in the peroxidase activity were seen between xylitol and sorbitol.

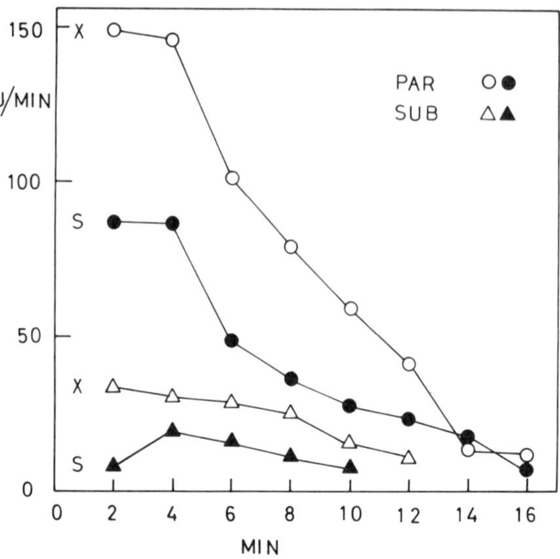

Figure 1 Secretion of peroxidase in parotid (PAR) and submandibular (SUB) saliva of monkeys (*Macaca mulatta*) fed xylitol (X) or sucrose (S) for 2-3 days. Salivary flow was stimulated by a subcutaneous injection of pilocarpine (at 0 min). Cannulated saliva samples were collected as 2-min aliquots for chemical assays. Peroxidase was assayed by the guaiacol method. (From Ref. 10.)

C. The Effect of a Carbohydrate Diet on Peroxidase Levels of Human Parotid Saliva

At the next stage it was thought that, if peroral xylitol had a specific effect on the salivary peroxidase levels, the manifestation of such effects should also be studied with more rational doses of xylitol. Therefore, the following study was performed in the author's laboratory. Human subjects of both sexes (11 females, 6 males, age 19-35 years) participated in a two-phase experiment involving single dosage of xylitol or sucrose pastils. The daily xylitol dose was 5 g per subject, whereas in the sucrose pastils the total dose of hexose-based carbohydrates was 9.9 g/day per subject, of which 5 g was sucrose. At the first phase, the subjects chewed 15 sucrose-sweetened fruit pastils in the morning (8 a.m.). Four to five pastils were chewed at a time, and the whole chewing period was completed in 15 min. Samples of citric acid-stimulated parotid saliva were collected during the subsequent 15-min period, which started approximately 60 sec after chewing was finished. Other samples were obtained 1, 2, and 4 hr later. The collection of the samples was performed in three groups: 0-5, 5-10, and 10-15 min. The flow rates were recorded. The first sample was thus obtained 16-21 min after the start of stimulation. For practical reasons, the first 15-min collection was considered to represent the 0-hr phase (Fig. 2). The subjects did not eat anything during the 4-hr experiment; otherwise they were asked to maintain their normal oral hygiene and dietary habits during the entire study (except that the consumption of commercial xylitol- and sorbitol-containing products was

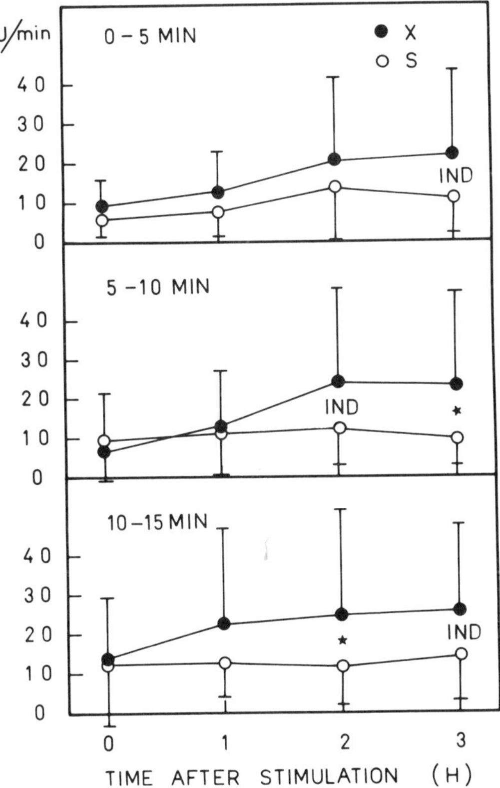

Figure 2 Secretion of peroxidase in human parotid saliva after stimulation with fruit pastils sweetened with sucrose (S) or xylitol (X). The enzyme activity is given in guaiacol units per minute. Saliva samples were collected as three 5-min aliquots starting collection 1 min after finishing stimulation (0 hr), and 1, 2, and 3 hr later. The arithmetic means and the standard deviations are indicated. The 0-hr samples were obtained immediately following the 15-min stimulation of saliva with fruit pastils. Number of samples studied was 34. Analysis of variance revealed the following significance levels for the differences between means: *, $p < 0.05$; IND, $p < 0.1$ (denoting indicative difference). Other details are mentioned in text.

forbidden during a 1-week period preceding the experiments). During the second phase, 1 week later, the previous experiment was repeated with the same subjects replacing the sucrose-sweetened pastils with those sweetened with xylitol. The saliva samples were analyzed for peroxidase, protein, amylase, carbonic anhydrase, and Sakaguchi-positive compounds (chiefly comprising free and bound arginine). Figure 2 shows the secretion of peroxidase in parotid saliva. In this case the consumption of xylitol pastils was associated with higher peroxidase activity, and secretion compared with the consumption of sucrose pastils. The activities of amylase, but not those of carbonic anhydrase, behaved similarly to peroxidase. These elevated enzyme levels were considered to result from increased flow rates and protein concentrations of saliva after stimulation with xylitol.

D. Peroxidase Levels of Whole Saliva in a Human Formula Diet Study

As indicated above, the first report on the xylitol-associated increased salivary peroxidase levels was based on the Turku sugar studies involving 2-year regular consumption of food sweetened with either sucrose, fructose, or xylitol (17,18). Following the completion of this study in October 1974, a group of nine volunteers continued to substitute dietary sucrose partially with xylitol. In spring 1978, these subjects were examined thoroughly within the framework of a formula diet study involving four periods as indicated later and in Fig. 3 (20). This continuation study was designed to provide information on general health and other effects of prolonged regular consumption of xylitol. During this formula diet study, the nine volunteers also provided whole saliva samples that were analyzed for several biochemical parameters including peroxidase activity. The study design and the subjects were previously described in detail (13,20). It may be mentioned, however, that in this formula diet study, period I lasted 3 days (with normal diet); period II lasted 7 days [with a defined formula diet; Biosorbin MCT, supplemented with 70 g (females) or 100 g (males) of sucrose daily]; period III lasted 14 days [with formula diet supplemented with 70 g (females) or 100 g (males) of xylitol daily]; period IV lasted 7 days (with normal diet). These periods comprised a continuous sequence without pause. Sucrose and xylitol were taken in 10-g portions evenly distributed throughout the day. Whole saliva samples (3 ml) were collected during these periods from Mondays to Fridays, by paraffin stimulation, at 7:30-8:30 a.m. following regular oral hygiene (13).

Figure 3 shows that the activity of peroxidase displayed two maxima, both of which occurred at the end of the two subsequent formula diet periods. The values attained during consumption of xylitol were slightly higher than those determined during sucrose consumption. Figure 3 shows the result in enzyme units per milligram of protein, but essentially similar results were obtained by expressing the activity in

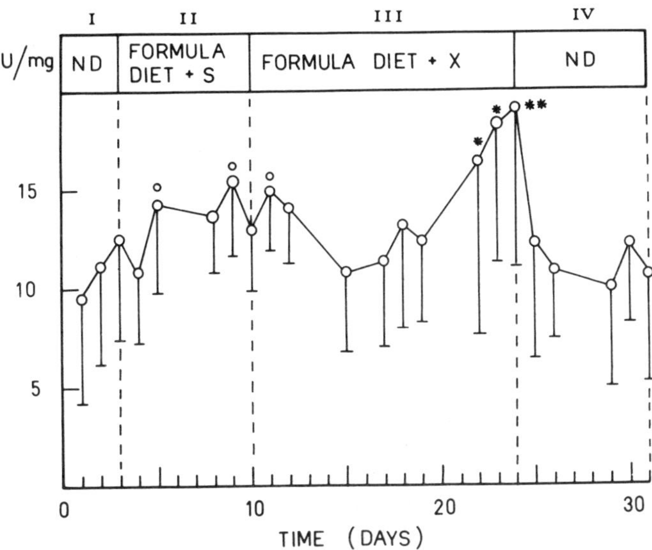

Figure 3 Specific activity of human whole saliva peroxidase (in enzyme units per milligram protein) of nine chronic xylitol users. The values shown are the mean ± SD (n = 9). The significance levels of the differences between the first 3-day normal diet period (combined starting values) and other test days are marked as follows (t-test): **, p < 0.01; *, p < 0.05; o, p < 0.1. ND = normal diet; S = sucrose; X = xylitol. Other details are mentioned in text and elsewhere. (From Ref. 13.)

enzyme units per milliliter of saliva. In this study the flow rates of saliva were not recorded.

The design of this study differed in an essential way from that involved in all previous xylitol feeding studies, since the subjects studied were chronic xylitol users. Furthermore, the Biosorbin MCT contained 60% of carbohydrates (mono-, oligo-, and polysaccharides) (20), a fact that may have masked more pronounced xylitol effects. Figure 3 indicates that the salivary peroxidase levels showed an increasing trend during the last experimental days involving xylitol consumption, whereas the peroxidase activity measured in the tenth day (last day involving sucrose intake) was smaller than that determined on the preceding days, suggesting that a maximum in the peroxidase levels had been reached in the sucrose period.

E. Studies on Human Saliva Showing Little or No Correlation Between Xylitol Administration and Peroxidase Levels

In connection with the 2-year human feeding trial mentioned previously, a 1-year chewing gum study was also carried out (24). In this experiment the daily xylitol dosage was 6.7 g per subject. As a control, a sucrose-containing chewing gum was used. The daily frequency of intake of xylitol and sucrose gums was 4.5 and 4, respectively. Whole saliva samples were collected in the mornings with paraffin stimulation in the beginning and in the end of the 1-year experimental period. The experimental groups did not differ in the activity levels of peroxidase and amylase, or in the concentrations of whole saliva proteins.

In another chewing gum study, 33 young adults were divided into three groups (14,22). In one group the chewing gums were sweetened with sorbitol (56% of dry weight), in the second with a mixture of sorbitol (49%) and xylitol (7%), and in the third group with another mixture of sorbitol (10%) and xylitol (63%). The subjects consumed 7.8 sticks of chewing gum per day. The chewing period lasted 4 weeks, and the daily intakes of sorbitol and xylitol amounted to 4-6 g per subject. In the beginning of the schedule stimulation was performed with paraffin, but in the end of the study the experimental chewing gums were used as stimulators. Stimulation of saliva with chewing gums containing xylitol increased the peroxidase activity (in enzyme units per milliliter of saliva) more than the sorbitol gums, but the differences were not statistically significant (14).

In another study, 7 human volunteers participated in a two-phase loading experiment involving 2 days. In the first 24-hr phase the subjects consumed 200 g of sucrose in the form of normal food and candies, including a 100-ml dose of sucrose-sweetened water containing 36 g of sucrose. On day 2 the subjects consumed a similar amount of xylitol. Parotid saliva samples were collected 2 and 4 hr following the last intake of the tested carbohydrates. The stimulation of parotid saliva was accomplished with a diluted citric acid solution. This study suffered from the lack of crossover design, and the peroxidase activities showed considerable variation. The peroxidase levels did not differ between sucrose and xylitol consumption.

In 1977, Harper et al. carried out a study on salivary peroxidase that, according to the information available, has been published in an abstract form only (3). In this experiment, 7-16 fruit pastils sweetened with a mixture of xylitol and sorbitol, or sucrose, were used to stimulate the flow of parotid saliva. Single dosage of the xylitol-sorbitol pastils (30% xylitol, 20% sorbitol) was associated with elevated peroxidase levels, but the difference between the polyol- and sucrose-sweetened pastils was not statistically significant.

In another study, 4 human volunteers (age 22-38 years) participated in a two-phase experiment involving single administration of glucose or xylitol (0.6 g/kg body weight) (16). The interval between the intakes of glucose and xylitol was 1 week. Whole saliva samples were collected with paraffin stimulation 1, 2, and 6 hr following the intake of the carbohydrate solutions. The specific peroxidase activity, but not the activity in enzyme units per milliliter, increased steeply after intake of xylitol. The increase was less pronounced after glucose administration. As a result of large individual variations, the differences between glucose and xylitol were not statistically significant (16).

In an experiment with mentally retarded children from a special day school, the subjects were given xylitol in the form of chewable tablets for a period of 2 months. The daily xylitol dosage was 16-20 g. Children from the same school who did not receive these tablets were used as controls. At the 30-day stage of the study, the specific salivary peroxidase activity was higher than before the commencement of the intake of xylitol pastils. This difference, however, was not seen at the 60-day stage of the experiment (21).

F. Experiments with Animals Other Than Monkeys

Rats were given xylitol or sorbitol (2.0 g/kg body weight per day) perorally during a period of 150 days in drinking water. At the end of the feeding schedule, the parotid, submandibular, and lacrimal glands were collected, homogenized, and analyzed for peroxidase activity. There were no significant differences between the feeding groups (12). When the effect of polyol feeding on the composition of sow milk was studied (15), the milk samples did not show any detectable peroxidase activity 12 hr after farrowing when the standard guaiacol method was used (2). The samples collected 1 and 3 weeks later showed peroxidase activity, but the polyol and control groups did not differ significantly. The term *polyol* used here stands for a residual polyol mixture (RPM) resulting from xylitol manufacturing. RPM contains chiefly natural pentitols and hexitols (11,15). The use of RPM in the diet of dairy cows was investigated with special reference to milk peroxidase levels (11), but xylitol consumption was not found to increase the enzyme activity significantly.

G. Effect of Carbohydrates on Salivary Gland Peroxidase Secretion in Vitro

Mäkinen, Söderling, and Kölling (unpublished data) studied the effect of some simple carbohydrates on the peroxidase activity secreted by slices of bovine and human submandibular and parotid glands. The homogenized tissue slices (200 mg each) were incubated with various carbohydrates (6-10 mM) for 48 hr at 37°C in a gas mixture containing 5% CO_2 and 95% air. The rates of transport of U[^{14}C]xylitol, -sorbitol, and -glucose into these gland slices did not differ significantly. In repeated long-term incubations (24 or 48 hr), the secretion rates of peroxidase from the submandibular gland slices and that of amylase from the parotid gland slices were, without exception, higher in the presence of xylitol as compared with sorbitol, myo-inositol, or glucose.

III. EFFECT OF CARBOHYDRATE DIET ON SALIVARY THIOCYANATE (SCN⁻) LEVELS

It is interesting that except for one (16) experiment, all feeding studies so far carried out have shown xylitol administration to increase slightly the salivary SCN^- concentrations. The first experiment dealing with this aspect was performed in connection with the Turku sugar studies (17). No increase in the salivary SCN^- levels was found when the three feeding groups as such were compared with each other. However, when the subjects consuming the highest quantities of the three carbohydrates tested were separately compared, the highest SCN^- concentrations were discovered in the whole saliva of subjects fed xylitol (7). Table 1 lists most feeding experiments in which salivary SCN^- concentrations have been analyzed. It is necessary to emphasize that the increase of the SCN^- concentration by xylitol administration in the cases described earlier is not statistically significant.

Thiocyanate ions have been reported to interfere with the quaiacol assay (4) that has been used in most experiments reported in this review. However, this interference does not explain the observed differences between various sugars because the interference caused by increased SCN^- levels in saliva should result in a decrease in the measured enzyme activities (4).

IV. POSSIBLE MECHANISMS

The mechanism of the xylitol-dependent increase of salivary peroxidase in unknown. Clearly, the increase is dependent on the method of xylitol consumption and possibly also on the dose. The effect seems to require systemic administration. Local activation of peroxidase in the mouth is unlikely. Although nonenzymatic macromolecules, such as keratin, gelatin, and various polysaccharides, can enhance phenol (e.g., guaiacol) oxidation by horseradish peroxidase and H_2O_2 (25), this is an unlikely explanation for the xylitol effect since xylitol does not affect guaiacol oxidation by salivary peroxidase in vitro. Furthermore, increased peroxidase activity has been demonstrated in saliva fractions purified by column chromatography. Small molecular activators or stabilizers of peroxidase (e.g., SCN^-) would be effectively separated from the enzyme during these procedures.

The most likely explanation for increased peroxidase levels is the increased de novo synthesis of the enzyme. The formation of peroxidase from constituent amino acids, or conversion of an inactive precursor to active peroxidase, and simultaneous stimulation of emptying

Table 1 Concentration of Salivary SCN^- (in mM) in Feeding Studies Involving Administration of Xylitol or Other Simple Carbohydrates[a]

Species	Feeding group			Notes	Ref.
	Xylitol	Sucrose	Fructose		
Human	2.14 ± 1.21 (17)	1.60 ± 0.98 (15)	1.72 ± 1.12 (16)	After 2-year full substitution of sucrose with xylitol or fructose	7
Human	1.16 ± 0.43 (9)	0.95 ± 0.42 (9)	b	After loading with sucrose or xylitol in a formula diet study	13
Human	0.51 (1 month) 1.02 (2 months) (Pooled samples)	0.26 (Normal diet)	b	After using xylitol pastils for 2 months	21
Monkey					
M. mulatta	0.09	0.03	b	Parotid saliva after 2-day consumption	10

[a]In the human studies indicated the stimulation of whole saliva was performed with paraffin. In the monkey study the stimulation was accomplished with a subcutaneous injection of pilocarpine under anesthesia (10). Unless otherwise indicated, the values shown are the mean ± SD, number of samples studied in parentheses.
[b]Not studied.

of acinar cells may be causes of the observed increased peroxidase
levels in saliva. In fact, the study with salivary gland slices suggested selective effects of carbohydrates on the rate of synthesis and/or
secretion of enzymes in these glands despite similar transport rates of
various carbohydrates into the glands.

V. CONCLUSIONS AND RESEARCH NEEDS

Diet composition has been recognized, for a long time, as a factor
affecting the composition of salivary secretions. The studies so far
carried out as described in this chapter have approached this problem
from the point of view of diverse dietary carbohydrates in eliciting
changes in the activities of specific enzymes, especially salivary peroxidase. Such an approach may be of some interest since the autonomic
innervation to the salivary glands has been considered to regulate the
composition of saliva. Several human feeding studies and one monkey
experiment suggest that the salivary enzyme levels may, under certain experimental conditions, respond not only to the presence of
proteins and carbohydrates in the diet, but that simple carbohydrates
may exert independent selective effects as well. In most cases the
differences observed between peroxidase levels after consumption of
different carbohydrates have been marginal. These observed differences probably have no physiological significance. The mechanism of
these effects has not been elucidated. The present information about
the selective effects of simple carbohydrates on the levels of peroxidase and other salivary proteins is thus too scant to allow final conclusions to be drawn regarding the significance and biochemical mechanisms of these effects. Our understanding of these effects would be
aided by future research in the following areas:

1. Confirmation of the studies in which xylitol-associated changes
    in the activity of salivary peroxidase have been detected, and
    extension of these studies to the effects of other carbohydrates.
2. Elucidation of the mechanisms of peroxidase elevation and of its
    possible physiological significance.
3. Study of the concentrations of H_2O_2, SCN^-, and $OSCN^-$ in saliva
    following carbohydrate administration. The effects of various
    sugars on the concentrations of $OSCN^-$ and H_2O_2 of the dental
    plaque should also be investigated. Initial steps in this direction
    have been taken (26,27).

REFERENCES

1. Bird, J. L. Baum, B. J., Mäkinen, K. K., Bowen, W. H., and
    Longton, R., W., *J. Nutr. 108*: 779 (1977).

2. Chance, B., and Maehly, A. C., *Methods Enzymol.* 2: 764 (1955).

3. Harper, L. R., Poole, A. E., and Wolf, S. I., *Int. Assoc. Dent. Res. 55th Session*, Abstract No. 78 (1977).

4. Hoogendoorn, H., *The Effect of Lactoperoxidase-Thiocyanate-Hydrogen Peroxide on the Metabolism of Cariogenic Microorganisms In Vitro and In the Oral Cavity.* Mouton, Den Haag, The Netherlands (1974).

5. Mäkinen, K. K., *Experientia (Suppl.) 30:* 1 (1978).

6. Mäkinen, K. K., *Adv. Food Res. 25:* 137 (1979).

7. Mäkinen, K. K., and Scheinin, A., *Acta Odontol. Scand. 33 (Suppl. 70):* 129 (1975).

8. Mäkinen, K. K., and Scheinin, A., *Acta Odontol. Scand. 33 (Suppl. 70):* 317 (1975).

9. Mäkinen, K. K., and Scheinin, A., *Ann. Rev. Nutr. 2:* 133 (1982).

10. Mäkinen, K. K., Bowen, W. H., Dalgard, D., and Fitzgerald, G., *J. Nutr. 108:* 779 (1978).

11. Mäkinen, K. K., Hämäläinen, M., Tuori, M., and Poutiainen, E., *Nutr. Rep. Int. 23:* 1077 (1981).

12. Mäkinen, K. K., Kölling, D., and Mäkinen, P.-L., *Int. J. Vit. Nutr. Res. 50:* 79 (1980).

13. Mäkinen, K. K., Kölling, D., and Mäkinen, P.-L., *Proc. Finn. Dent. Soc. 77:* 262 (1981).

14. Mäkinen, K. K., Läikkö, I., Rekola, M., and Scheinin, A., *Kariesprophylaze 3:* 103 (1980).

15. Mäkinen, K. K., Näsi, M., and Alaviuhkola, T., *Nutr. Rep. Int. 23:* 793 (1981).

16. Mäkinen, K. K., Söderling, E., Mäkinen, P.-L., and Tenovuo, J., *Int. J. Vit. Nutr. Res. 48:* 405 (1978).

17. Mäkinen, K. K., Tenovuo, J., and Scheinin, A., *Acta Odontol. Scand. 33 (Suppl. 70):* 247 (1975).

18. Mäkinen, K. K., Tenovuo, J., and Scheinin, A., *J. Dent. Res. 55:* 652 (1976).

19. Mäkinen, K. K., Ylikahri, R., Söderling, E., Scheinin, A., and Mäkinen, P.-L., *Int. J. Vit. Nutr. Res. (Suppl.) 22:* 9 (1981).

20. Mäkinen, K. K., Ylikahri, R., Mäkinen, P.-L., Söderling, E., and Hämäläinen, M., *Int. J. Vit. Nutr. Res. (Suppl.) 22:* 29 (1981).

21. Pakkala, U., Liesmaa, H., and Mäkinen, K. K., *Proc. Finn. Dent. Soc. 77:* 271 (1981).

22. Rekola, M., Läikkö, I., Anttinen, H., Scheinin, A., and Mäkinen, K. K., *Kariesprophylaxe 2:* 21 (1980).

23. Scheinin, A., and Mäkinen, K. K., *Acta Odontol. Scand. 33 (Suppl. 79):* 1 (1975).

24. Scheinin, A., Mäkinen, K. K., Tammisalo, E., and Rekola, M.,
    Acta Odontol. Scand. 33 (Suppl. 70): 307 (1975).
25. Siegel, S. M., in *Biology of the Mouth*, P. Person (Ed.),
    American Association for the Advancement of Science, Washing-
    ton, D.C., pp. 111 (1968).
26. Thomas, E. L., Bates, K. P., and Jefferson, M. M., *J. Dent.
    Res. 59*: 1466 (1980).
27. Thomas, E. L., Bates, K. P., and Jefferson, M. M., *J. Dent.
    Res. 60*: 785 (1981).

11

Activation of the Salivary Peroxidase Antimicrobial System: Clinical Studies

HENK HOOGENDOORN / *Akzo Consumenten Produkten bv, The Hague, The Netherlands*

I. INTRODUCTION

The components of the salivary peroxidase system and the interactions of this system with oral microorganisms have been discussed at length in other chapters in this book. There is little doubt that the system plays an important part in the defense mechanisms operating in the human mouth and that the availability of hydrogen peroxide is a limiting factor for the effective antimicrobial action of the system. Safe and effective methods for generating appropriate quantities of hydrogen peroxide in the human mouth have been developed. These methods are based upon the use of peroxidogenic enzymes either in form of mouth rinses or toothpaste. The results of several clinical trials of these preparations will be discussed in this chapter.

II. ACTIVATION OF THE SALIVARY PEROXIDASE SYSTEM

A. The Effect on Tooth Surface pH

Since in vitro studies have shown that acid formation by many strains
of oral microorganisms is inhibited by the activated peroxidase system,
the effect of the activated system on tooth surface pH was investigated
(1). When sugar is consumed, bacteria on the tooth surface are stimulated and produce acid that results in a lower tooth surface pH. Activation of the peroxidase system should prevent this pH drop. The
study was carried out in two phases. First, a test group of children
(approximately 12 years of age) rinsed their mouths with a solution containing peroxidogenic enzymes (amyloglucosidase and glucose oxidase)
on 2 successive days (once a day, 3 hr after the initial pH measurement). Second, another test group of children (12-18 years) brushed
their teeth for 4 weeks with a toothpaste also containing these enzymes.
The two control groups used rinses without the enzymes or used commercial toothpastes. At the beginning and at the end of the test
periods, pH measurements were made on specifically selected molar
surfaces using antimony electrodes. On the days of measurement, pH
was observed at the same sites on the tooth surfaces before and after
sugar consumption.

The results of this study indicated that activation of the salivary
peroxidase system by peroxidogenic enzymes used either as mouth
rinse or in toothpaste reduces the fall in tooth surface pH produced by
sugar consumption. A further result of these studies was the discov-
ery that the foaming agents normally present in commercial toothpastes
inactivate the salivary peroxidase system.

B. The Effect on Plaque Accumulation

This study (4) was carried out to test the hypothesis that activation
of the salivary peroxidase system would reduce the growth of oral
microorganisms and thus decrease the buildup of dental plaque.

Plaque accumulation was measured in 15 subjects over a period of
5 days. The subjects were divided into three groups of 5 subjects each
and were assigned to one of the following regimens:

Regimen I: One lump of sugar consumed every hour; no measures of
              oral hygiene except for three daily mouth rinses with a
              placebo solution

Regimen II: One lump of sugar consumed every hour; no measures of
              oral hygiene except for three daily mouth rinses with a
              solution containing amyloglucosidase and glucose oxidase

Regimen III: No additional sugar consumption; no measures of oral
              hygiene

The results show (Table 1) that the additional consumption of sucrose clearly increased the development of dental plaque. Rinses with the enzyme solution not only prevented this increased plaque accumulation but even reduced the plaque index below those of the subjects who did not consume additional sugar. The same results were obtained for all subjects tested.

Plaque development was also studied by analysis of photographs taken of each subject after the plaque had been stained with fuchsin. Analysis of these photographs showed that the plaque accumulated during regimen II was smoother, thinner, and less easily stained than the plaque formed during regimens I and III. However, there were some areas of plaque development on tooth surfaces of the regimen II subjects that were similar to those of subjects on the other regimens. These observations suggest that bacterial growth is strongly retarded by the activated peroxidase system, but the antibacterial effectiveness of the system varies from site to site in the mouth.

C. The Effect on Dental Caries

Since activation of the peroxidase system has been shown to inhibit bacterial acid production and to decrease plaque buildup, a study was undertaken to determine the effect of activating the system on the development of early dental caries (3). Bacterial growth was stimulated by mouth rinses with sucrose solutions, and the salivary peroxidase system was activated by mouth rinses containing peroxidogenic enzymes. At the end of the test period, the test group using enzyme rinses had a much larger number of intact buccal surfaces than did the control group using placebo rinses (Table 2). The test group also had a significantly lower number of new carious lesions than did the control group. However, there was no significant difference in the plaque index recorded for the test and the control groups in this study. This result seems to be in contrast to what was observed (Sec. II. B) earlier. However, the test conditions and scoring periods were different for these two studies, and the results cannot be strictly compared.

The significant differences in these two studies are the length of the test periods and the method of administering sucrose. The sucrose rinses may dilute the salivary peroxidase system to a greater extent than does the eating of sugar lumps, and this dilution may reduce the inhibition of the plaque bacteria by the peroxidase system. This reduction in inhibition over an extended period might produce the observed accumulation of plaque. It should be pointed out that in spite of the accumulation of plaque in the test subjects, the cariogenicity was low compared with controls (Table 2). Thus, activation of the peroxidase system may result in a less cariogenic plaque even though, under some conditions, the quantity of plaque accumulated may not be reduced.

Table 1 The Effect of Three Regimens[a] on Plaque Accumulation

| Tooth surfaces | Plaque index at the end of regimen | | | | | |
| | I (one lump of sugar every hour, 3 daily mouth rinses with placebo solution) | | II (one lump of sugar every hour, 3 daily mouth rinses with enzyme[b] solution) | | III (no sugar, no rinsing) | |
	Mean (n = 5)	SE	Mean (n = 5)	SE	Mean (n = 5)	SE
Proximal	2.1	0.14	1.5	0.16	1.7	0.15
Lingual	1.6	0.16	0.7	0.10	1.2	0.12
Buccal	2.1	0.15	1.4	0.16	1.6	0.16
All surfaces	2	0.14	1.3	0.30	1.6	0.14

[a]All teeth were thoroughly cleaned at the beginning of each regimen. During each regimen subjects refrained from all measures of oral hygiene except as indicated. After 5 days, plaque was scored according to Ref. 10.
[b]Mixture of amyloglucosidase and glucose oxidase.

Table 2 Number of New Carious Surfaces and Surface Segments After a 21-Day Cariogenic[a] Regimen

		Intact surfaces (caries index[b] = 0)		New caries	
		Day 0	Day 21	Lesions[b]	Reversals[c]
Buccal surfaces	Test[b]	63	41	28	6
	Control[b]	63	27	38	2
Buccal surface Segments (distal, central, mesial)	Test	290	246	55	11
	Control	283	192	100	9

[a]Subjects were divided into two groups of 11 each. Caries index was scored on day 0 after all teeth were cleaned. All subjects refrained from measures of oral hygiene for 21 days and rinsed their mouths 10 times a day with 65% sucrose solution. In addition, the control group rinsed three times daily with a placebo solution, and the test group rinsed with a solution containing amyloglucosidase and glucose oxidase. On day 21 all teeth were cleaned and the caries index recorded.

[b]Caries index scored by a modification (3) of the von der Fehr system. Severity of lesions varies from 0 (intact surface) to 3 (pronounced decalcification). A new lesion was scored on a surface when the index changed from 0 to a higher value.

[c]Caries index changed from a higher value to 0.

The effect on development of new carious lesions of incorporating peroxidogenic enzymes into toothpaste was studied by Koch and Strand (5). Three large groups (250 students each) of Swedish school children participated in this study. At the intial clinical examination, the children in the three groups were given either a monofluorophosphate (MFP)-containing toothpaste, one containing amyloglucosidase and glucose oxidase together with NaF, or an identical formulation containing NaF but no enzymes. (In Scandinavia and in other European countries, clinical trials on children are not permitted unless all tested dentifrices contain protective fluoride components.)

Subsequently, it was discovered that the enzyme-containing toothpaste did not generate sufficient hydrogen peroxide to activate effectively the salivary peroxidase system during the short (40 sec) period of brushing that children use. Therefore, it was not surprising that at the end of the first year there were no significant differences in the mean number of new carious lesions developed by these three groups.

During a second 9-month period of the study, the enzyme formulation was changed to ensure the generation of an adequate amount of hydrogen peroxide. At the end of this 9-month period, the group using the enzyme-NaF toothpaste developed significantly fewer lesions than the group using the formulation with NaF but without enzymes. However, there was no significant difference between the group using the MFP toothpaste and the group using the enzyme-NaF preparation. Since the amount of fluoride was lower in the NaF preparation than in the MFP toothpaste, the fluoride effect makes the separate evaluation of the effectiveness of peroxidogenic enzymes impossible. Therefore, a study using rats was carried out by Rotgans and Hoogendoorn (9).

In their rat study, Rotgans and Hoogendoorn treated three groups of rats with toothpaste that contained either enzymes with fluoride (350 ppm), fluoride only (350 ppm), or no enzymes and no fluoride. The rats were not inoculated with a cariogenic strain of bacteria. The subsequent development of caries due to the normal oral flora in these animals was studied after the animals had been fed a cariogenic diet. Treatment with the paste containing the peroxidogenic enzymes produced an impressive and statistically significant reduction in caries when compared with treatment with either of the other preparations tested. These results show that in the rat, activation of the salivary peroxidase system by peroxidogenic enzymes substantially reduces the cariogenicity of the normal oral flora.

Mühlemann et al. (7) used the rat model in a different experimental design. In their studies, the animals were inoculated with *Streptococcus mutans* and *Actinomyces viscosus*. These strains are important contributors to dental caries in human beings, and they are commonly used as inocula in animal experiments designed to test the effectiveness of agents having a direct antimicrobial action. The results of this study did not show any significant difference in caries development between groups of animals treated with toothpastes containing amyloglucosidase and glucose oxidase and those treated with preparations lacking the peroxidogenic enzymes. It is important to note that the strain of *A. viscosus* used in these studies is catalase positive and would therefore block the effectiveness of the salivary peroxidase system by decomposing the hydrogen peroxide generated by the peroxidogenic enzymes. Also, the diet fed the animals in this study contains components that destroy the antibacterial products of the peroxidase system. Finally, it must be remembered that the peroxidogenic enzymes function by activating the natural salivary peroxidase system that depends, for its effectiveness, upon the regulation of the natural flora in the mouth. Thus, results obtained from rats inoculated with human pathogens are not strictly comparable with results obtained in experiments where caries activity is due to the natural flora in the test animal.

D. The Effect on Gingivitis

Since activation of the salivary peroxidase system may reduce both the quantity and the cariogenicity of dental plaque and since the severity of gingivitis is correlated with plaque accumulation, activation of the peroxidase system should cause a reduction in gingivitis.

However, changes in gingivitis are difficult to quantitate by controlled clinical tests. Variations in the efficiency of the removal of gingivitis-inducing plaque deposits by individual tooth-brushing produce wide variations in gingival indices. Furthermore, there is a strong tendency for subjects participating in a clinical trial to exercise greater than normal care in their tooth-brushing routines prior to examination. In order to minimize these variations, Rotgans and Hoogendoorn (8) required their test subjects to report to the clinic for evaluation of oral health three times a week during a 50-day test period. The frequency of examination over such a long period of time minimized the incentive of the subjects to be overly conscientious in their tooth-brushing habits. They were also instructed not to brush on the examination days. There were three test periods for each subject. During the initial period each subject used his own favorite toothpaste. During the second period a placebo paste that did not contain enzymes was used, and during the third period a paste containing amyloglucosidase and glucose oxidase, but otherwise identical to the placebo paste, was used. There was a significant increase in gingivitis during the period when the placebo paste was used and a significant reduction when the subjects used the paste containing the peroxidogenic enzymes. Thus, activation of the salivary peroxidase system causes a reduction in gingivitis even under conditions where tooth-brushing is restricted to only 4 days/week.

E. The Effect on Aphthous Lesions

A relationship between activation of the salivary peroxidase system and the occurrence of aphthous lesions (oral ulcers or canker sores) was discovered by accident. A Dutch dentist, Van Meel, who had been involved in the early clinical investigations of the toothpastes containing peroxidogenic enzymes, found that one of his patients who had suffered from recurrent oral ulcerations remained free of these lesions as long as he used the enzyme-containing paste. Subsequently, Van Meel found five other patients who reacted in the same way. These experiments provided the impetus for a detailed clinical study (2). Local physicians and dentists in a Dutch town selected 120 patients who suffered frequently from aphthous lesions. These patients participated in a double-blind, crossover study. One group started with an enzyme-containing paste and the other group with a placebo. Weighed quantities of the pastes were given to the patients by the pharmacist, but they were given no instructions about the paste or about measures

of oral hygiene. In order to monitor the extent of use of the paste,
the patients had to ask for new tubes when the supplied tubes were
empty. Some patients were eliminated from the study because their use
of the paste was too infrequent or too limited in quantity. A total of
26 patients dropped out of the study or were removed for various
reasons. At the end of the test period (130 days), the patients filled
out a questionnaire regarding their aphthous lesion experiences.
Analysis of the results from these questionnaires showed that more
patients using the enzyme toothpaste reported reduction in lesion experience than did those using the placebo. The difference was statistically significant.

After the initial test period, all patients continued with the enzyme-containing toothpaste for 130 days. At the end of this period 33%
reported no ulcers, 27% reported minor spots that did not develop into
ulcers, and 15% reported a reduction (compared with their individual
normal experience) in size, pain, and healing time of the ulcers that
did occur. These positive results prompted a further study.

A large population of subjects was selected on the basis of a detailed survey and subdivided into several different treatment groups.
Over 80% of this population had been suffering from aphthous lesions
for more than 5 years. Only 34% had experienced sporadic ulcer-free
periods of more than 8 weeks. Each subject was assigned to one of the
following treatment groups (35 subjects per group):

I: A toothpaste containing standard quantities of the enzymes
     amyloglucosidase and glucose oxidase was used.
II: Subjects used the same toothpaste as group I, but they were in-
     structed not to use water during brushing, to brush for 2 min,
     and to use a stripe of toothpaste over the whole brush.
III: Subjects used a toothpaste containing twice the amount of enzymes
     as the preparation used by group I.
IV: A standard commercial toothpaste (repacked in blank tubes) was
     used.
V: Subjects used the same toothpaste as in group I, without any
     special instructions. This group was not involved in the 8-week
     test period but had to report after 9 months.

At the end of a test period of 8 weeks, the subjects reported their
aphthous lesion experiences in detail on a standard form. There was
no significant difference between the results for group I compared
either with group II or group III. However, the number of ulcers in
group I decreased by 55% over the test period, whereas the number of
ulcers in the control group (IV) decreased only 9%. There was a
steady and significant decline (Fig. 1) in ulcer frequency in the group
(I) using enzymes compared with the control group (IV).

Following this 8-week test period, all subjects used the enzyme-
containing paste for 9 months. At the conclusion of this long-term test,
60% of the subjects reported that they were free or nearly free of les-

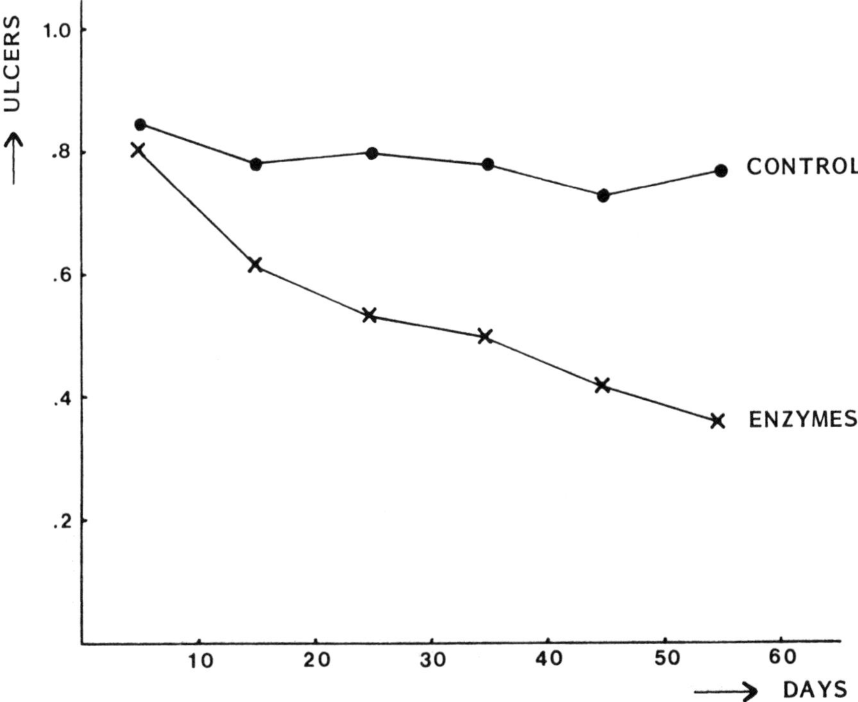

Figure 1 Average number of aphthous lesions present per individual in patients using toothpaste with amyloglucosidase and glucose oxidase or a control paste.

ions, 22% reported an improved condition, and only 18% of the 203 subjects reported that their aphthous lesion experience was unchanged.

Another clinical trial of the enzyme-containing toothpaste was reported by Koch (6). The results of this study (Table 3) offer strong support for the effectiveness of the peroxidogenic enzymes in controlling aphthous lesions. In this study, more than 90% of the patients reported either no ulcers or an improved condition after using the enzyme-containing toothpaste for 6 months. This improved condition deteriorated when the subjects returned to their previously used toothpaste (which contained no enzymes). Donatsky et al. reported a double-blind clinical trial with crossover on recurrent aphthous ulcers (11). In this well-controlled study in which 25 patients were involved, 72% of the patients responded positively when using toothpaste with enzymes. When using the control, the positive responses were 40%. The difference between both treatments was statistically significant (0.025 > p > 0.01).

Table 3 The Effect of a Toothpaste Containing Peroxidogenic Enzymes[a] on the Frequency of Aphthous Lesions (Ulcers)[b]

	No ulcers (%)	Improved (%)	Unchanged (%)
Use of enzyme[a] toothpaste			
For 3 months	37	49	14
For 6 months	49	42	9
Use of subject's own toothpaste			
For 3 months	17	25	58

[a]Amyloglucosidase and glucose oxidase.
[b]A total of 207 patients suffering from recurrent aphthous lesions were selected by 80 dentists distributed throughout Sweden. For the first 6 months of the test period, patients used the enzyme-containing toothpaste. Their aphthous lesion experience was evaluated at 3 and 6 months. After 6 months, all patients returned to their usual toothpaste, and the aphthous lesion experience was evaluated 3 months later.

The control paste without enzymes was identical with respect to the other components. This basic composition of the paste was selected in such a way that no components would interfere with the peroxidase system and no bactericidal action could hamper the natural flora. Whether or not the positive responses observed when using the control paste are caused by this selection of ingredients must be determined by additional trials.

The various studies summarized show clearly that the activation of the salivary peroxidase system by an appropriate combination of peroxidogenic enzymes provides an effective treatment for aphthous lesions. The mechanism by which the treatment works is unknown. This lack of understanding is due, in part, to the lack of knowledge about the etiology of aphthae. However, the following hypothesis may be suggested.

If aphthous lesions are the direct result of microorganisms, then there are indications that aphthous lesions are caused by autoimmune reactions, triggered by microorganisms, and initiated by a trauma. Certain microbial strains that proteolytically break down the IgA-barrier are considered suspect. The inhibitory action of the salivary peroxidase system could result in a low activity of these microbial strains, rendering them in this respect less pathogenic.

Some concluding observations may help in the formulation of better hypotheses. The peroxidogenic enzymes are equally effective on men and women. Patients who have remained free of ulcers because of a long period of use of the enzyme-containing toothpaste may, in some cases, remain free of ulcers even though they stop using the paste. However, in most instances, the aphthous lesions return when use of the enzyme-containing toothpaste is abandoned.

III. SUMMARY

Activation of the salivary peroxidase system by peroxidogenic enzyme preparations (amyloglucosidase and glucose oxidase either in a mouth rinse or in a toothpaste) reduces acid formation by oral microorganisms. Clinical studies have shown that plaque accumulation, gingivitis, early carious lesions, and aphthous lesions may all be reduced by appropriate applications of these enzyme preparations. However, because of the complexity of the salivary peroxidase system the design of clinical and animal studies is critical and must be taken into account in the evaluation of the results.

REFERENCES

1. Hoogendoorn, H., *The Effect of Lactoperoxidase-Thiocyanate-Hydrogen Peroxide on the Metabolism of Cariogenic Microorganisms In Vitro and in the Oral Cavity*. Mouton, Den Haag, The Netherlands (1974).
2. Hoogendoorn, H., and Scholtes, W., *Ned. Tijdschr. Tandheelk.* *86*: 36 (1979).
3. Hugoson, A., Koch, G., Thilander, H., and Hoogendoorn, H., *Odontol. Revy 25*: 69 (1974).
4. Koch, G., Edlund, K., and Hoogendoorn, H., *Odontol. Revy 24*: 367 (1973).
5. Koch, G., and Strand, G., *Swed. Dent. J. 3*: 9 (1979).
6. Koch, G., *Tandlak. Tidn. 73*: 264 (1981).
7. Mühlemann, H. R., Schmid, R., and Firestone, A. R., *Caries Res. 15*: 46 (1981).
8. Rotgans, J., and Hoogendoorn, H., *Caries Res. 13*: 144 (1979).
9. Rotgans, J., and Hoogendoorn, H., *Caries Res. 13*: 150 (1979).
10. Silness, J., and Löe, H., *Acta Odontol. Scand. 22*: 121 (1964).
11. Donatsky, O., Worsaae, N., Schiödt, M., and Johnsen, T., *Scand. J. Dent. Res. 92*: 376 (1983).

12

Antibody Targeting of the Antimicrobial and Antitumor Activity of the Peroxidases

ROLAND R. ARNOLD / *Emory University School of Dentistry, Atlanta, Georgia*

I. INTRODUCTION

The preceding chapters have dealt primarily with the structure, characteristics, and biological function of lactoperoxidase as it relates to microbial viability and metabolism. In addition to lactoperoxidase, the myeloperoxidase (MPO) of the azurophilic granules of polymorphonuclear leukocytes (PMN) and blood monocytes and the peroxidase of eosinophils (EPO) have been shown to play a role in the host defense against a variety of microorganisms. Relatively recent studies have also extended the spectrum of peroxidase activity to include several mammalian cell types, including tumor cells.

Both the tumoricidal effects and the antibacterial activities of
the peroxidases are dependent upon the presence of H_2O_2 and electron donors, such as thiocyanate or halides. Availability of H_2O_2 is
usually the limiting factor for the system. Peroxide is generated
either as a product of bacterial metabolism or in the course of the oxidative burst of the phagocyte. The host tissues contain effective
peroxide-reducing systems that minimize the detrimental effects of
H_2O_2 on host tissues. These enzymes, such as catalase, may limit the
effectiveness of the antibacterial and antitumor activity of the peroxidases. Selective delivery of H_2O_2 in relatively high concentrations
to the target cell could act to focus the peroxidase activity. Thus,
antibodies to tumor and bacterial antigens covalently linked to enzymes
that generate H_2O_2 offer the potential for manipulation of the specificity
of the peroxidase system.

A. Lactoperoxidase, Myeloperoxidase, and Eosinophilic Peroxidase

Due to the sequestered nature of the mucosal sites with which lactoperoxidase (LP) is associated, it is unlikely that systemically applied
antibody conjugates could reach target cells at mucosal surfaces.
There may be potential under special circumstances for local application of conjugates for enhancement of LP activity. In general, however, studies with conjugates utilizing LP as the effector system have
been used as in vitro models to test the feasibility and specificity of
such a system.

Extensive studies have been done on the functional role of peroxidase in the neutrophil (5,38,42,44,47,48,52,62), and more recent
studies have investigated the nature of human eosinophilic peroxidase
(10,44,48,54). Both enzymes are inhibited or destroyed by excess
H_2O_2, azide, or cyanide, and both show a pH optimum near 6 (55).
MPO in combination with H_2O_2 and a halide (either iodide, chloride,
or bromide) has been shown to be lethal to bacteria, viruses, fungi,
and mycoplasma (5,38,42,43,47,48,52,62).

B. Tumoricidal Activity of Polymorphonuclear Leukocytes

The traditionally accepted role of the PMN is the ingestion and killing
of invading organisms. A number of recent studies have also implicated PMN in the destruction of tumor cells (14,17,18,27,34,40,58,59,64,
72), suggesting that the neutrophil may be involved in protection of
the host against neoplasia, as well as microbial infection.

Several mechanisms may be operational in the antimicrobial system
and at least three of these have potent cytotoxic activity against mammalian tumor cells. Considerable effort has been directed toward defining the cellular and biochemical mechanisms operative in such cell-
mediated cytotoxicity. From the varied reports in the literature, it is
apparent that either the MPO-H_2O_2-halide system, oxygen-dependent

but peroxidase-independent or nonoxidative systems may each pre-
dominante under different experimental conditions. PMN may exert
cytotoxic effects in vitro in several model systems—during phagocytosis of inert particles (14,19), in the presence of antitarget cell antibody (17,27,34,41), and in the presence of certain soluble activating
agents such as complement fragments, phorbol esters, and lectins (18,
34,40,58,59,67,72,76). Depending on the model chosen, cytotoxicity
appears to be mediated by different mechanisms.

When PMN are exposed to bacteria, inert particles, or soluble
activating factors, there is a large increase in oxygen uptake (13,36,
52,68) that is not related to mitochondrial electron transport, since
chemical inhibitors of mitochondria, such as cyanide and azide, do not
inhibit this respiratory burst (13,68,75). There is also a concomitant
stimulation of the hexose monophosphate shunt and the release of
superoxide anion (O_2^-) into the medium (45,75). The spontaneous
dismutation products of O_2^-, including H_2O_2, singlet oxygen, and hy-
droxyradical ($\cdot OH$), can also be detected (45,75). The phagocytic
process can occur in the absence of a respiratory burst (68,69). However, with many systems oxygen is required for postphagocytic killing
(50,69).

The respiratory burst in PMN presumably involves the activation
of a membrane-bound oxidase that catalyzes the transfer of single
electrons from reduced nicotnamide adenine dinucleotide phosphate
(NADPH) to oxygen (13). Most evidence suggests that this enzyme
resides on the outer surface of the PMN plasma membrane (23,32,33).
It is postulated that activation of the PMN activates the plasma membrane-bound oxidase that produces extracellular O_2^- from cytosolic
NADPH via transmembrane electron transport. The O_2^- dismutates to
yield H_2O_2 and singlet oxygen ($^1O_2$). The H_2O_2 can, in turn, react
with the MPO system to produce oxidized halide or with more O_2^- to
produce $\cdot OH$ radicals (44,53).

As mentioned previously, the method used for stimulating the
PMN may result in different mechanisms for tumoricidal activity.
Clark and Klebanoff (14) reported that ingestion of preopsonized zy-
mosan by human PMN resulted in the killing of cocultured tumor target
cells and ascitic, Maloney virus-induced lymphoma (LSRTA). These
studies clearly implicated the involvement of the MPO system in extracellular cytotoxicity. This cytotoxicity required intact PMN, ingestible
particles, and halides, and was blocked by the addition of MPO (heme)
inhibitors (azide and cyanide) and by degradation of H_2O_2 (catalase).
PMN from patients with MPO deficiency or with chronic granulomatous
disease (CGD, defective in normal postphagocytic metabolic burst) were
not cytotoxic, but activity was restored by the addition of purified
MPO and H_2O_2, respectively. Both MPO (3,35) and H_2O_2 (4) have
been shown to be released by PMN in the extracellular fluid during
phagocytosis, and it was proposed that the cytotoxicity of PMN during
phagocytosis of inert particles was due to excreted MPO-H_2O_2 (14).

Experimental evidence also indicates that the lectin, concanavalin A (Con A), is capable of mediating tumor cell cytotoxicity by the MPO system (18). Lectin-stimulated PMN-mediated cytotoxicity can be blocked by glycolytic inhibitors and agents that interfere with microtubules and microfilaments (71). Con A-induced cytotoxicity of LSTRA cells by human PMN was rapid with an effector to target cell ratio as low as 1 PMN to 20 tumor cells (18). Cytotoxicity required halide, was markedly reduced by agents that inhibit heme enzymes or degrade H_2O_2, and was impaired in neutrophils deficient in MPO or defective in respiratory burst (18). Con A initiated the MPO-dependent iodination by PMN, and both cytotoxicity and iodination could be inhibited by α-methyl-D mannoside in a dose-related fashion. These data suggest that lectin binding results in surface stimulation of PMN, resulting in secretion of MPO and H_2O_2, which in combination with halide are at least in part responsible for cytotoxicity of mammalian tumor cells.

Phorbol myristate acetate (PMA) is a nonbiological substance that is a potent stimulus for PMN metabolic activation and enzyme secretion (6,22,31,60,65,66). PMA-stimulated cytotoxic activity by PMN involves mechanisms mediated by H_2O_2 alone (58,59,76) or in combination with MPO and halide (20,40,72). The involvement of the MPO system is indicated by the inhibitory effect of azide and cyanide, by the failure of MPO-deficient PMN to kill unless supplemented with MPO, by the inhibition of cytotoxicity with catalase, and the lack of activity with PMN from CGD patients (20). Superoxide dismutase (SOD) had no effect on cytotoxicity, suggesting the lack of involvement of O_2^- or ·OH. In contrast to these studies, the data of Nathan et al. (58,59) indicated that PMA-stimulated mouse peritoneal granulocytes and macrophages killed tumor target cells by H_2O_2 activity independent of peroxidase. Similarly, Weiss and LoBuglio (76) reported that destruction of autologous erythrocytes by PMN-activated human PMN was inhibited by catalase, SOD, and azide but not by cyanide or putative ·OH or $^1O_2$ scavengers. The destruction of endothelial cells by PMN-activated PMN required H_2O_2, but not MPO, O_2^-, $^1O_2$, or ·OH (77).

Several laboratories have presented evidence for PMN-mediated antibody-dependent cellular cytotoxicity (ADCC) with convincing evidence for the involvement of oxygen-dependent mechanisms (9,12,17, 34,41) that are dependent on MPO (9,12,17). This is an immunologically specific system requiring viable PMN (17). The requirement for respiratory burst was indicated by the minimal activity observed with PMN from patients with CGD. In contrast, activity was normal with MPO-deficient cells and was maintained in the presence of azide, cyanide, and catalase. Granular cationic proteins were apparently not responsible for the activity because there was no inhibition by heparin. There was also a requirement for glycolysis, divalent cations, and microtubular function (17). The target cells, LSTRA, used in these experiments have been previously shown to be sensitive to the MPO system (15) and to granular cationic proteins (16), yet neither of these appear to be operational in PMN-ADCC.

II. ANTIBODY CARRIERS OF ENZYMES AND TOXINS

A major problem with therapy for neoplasia and eukaryotic pathogens is that the toxic systems employed also often have adverse effects on the host tissues, especially at concentrations necessary to kill the invasive cells. A number of laboratories have attempted to deliver a variety of toxic substances specifically to target cells by coupling to target-specific antibodies. The concept of using the specificity of antibody to focus activity on a specific target goes as far back as Ehrlich (25). Several studies have coupled diphtheria toxin to tumor-specific antibodies (30,56,57). Moolten et al. (56) demonstrated cytotoxicity of hapten-coated tumor cells by antihapten-diphtheria toxin conjugates. In a later study they employed tumor-specific antibody-diphtheria toxin conjugates in the immunotherapy against tumor induced by Simian virus 40 (57). Methotrexate-antibody conjugates are effective in the experimental chemotherapy of murine ovarian carcinoma (11). Antibody-phospholipase C conjugates have specific cytotoxic activity for Friend leukemia cells (26). The tumoricidal effects of chlorambucil (28), daunomycin (37,49), and adriamycin (37) have been successfully focused using tumor-specific antibody to deliver the drugs (29). This method has also been employed to deliver H_2O_2-generating enzymes in the vicinity of microbial and tumor targets (2,7,8,46,61,63,70).

III. ANTIBODY FOCUSING OF PEROXIDASE ACTIVITY

A. Antibacterial

Knowles et al. (46) produced rabbit IgG with antibacterial antibody opsonic activity to several test strains including pneumococci, group A streptococci, *Staphylococcus aureus*, *Proteus mirabilis*, *Pseudomonas aeruginosa*, and *Escherichia coli*. The H_2O_2-generating enzyme, glucose oxidase, was coupled to these antibacterial antibody preparations and to opsonic human IgG using diethyl malonimidate. These antibody-enzyme conjugates were tested in vitro for bactericidal activity in the presence of LP and potassium iodide (KI). There was potent bactericidal killing of all strains tested, except for *P. aeruginosa*, only with the complete system (glucose, iodide ions, and peroxidase, either LP or horseradish peroxidase). There was significant killing within 60 min at antibody-enzyme concentrations as low as 10 µg/ml. These investigators suggested that such antibody-enzyme conjugates may prove of practical value in the treatment of patients with fulminate bacteremia or leukocyte dysfunctions.

A potential problem of clinical application suggested by Knowles et al. (46) is the requirement for multiple factors—antibody enzyme, enzyme substrate, peroxidase, and halide. Okuda and colleagues (61) conjugated both LP and xanthine oxidase (H_2O_2-generating enzyme) to antibody specific for *Candida albicans*. This antibody-enzyme conjugate was fungicidal in vitro in the presence of xanthine and KI (see page 233), and provided partial protection to candidal-infected mice when simultaneously injected with xanthine and KI. This system causes H_2O_2 production in the vincinity of the target and in proximity to the fungicidal mediator, lactoperoxidase. If it is necessary to provide exogenous peroxidase (perhaps in MPO deficiency), then such dual-enzyme conjugates may prove most efficient as long as sufficient halide can be maintained to prevent peroxidase destruction by H_2O_2.

Preliminary studies by Arnold et al. (2) investigated the effects of glucose oxidase-conjugated serotype-specific antibodies on metabolism of *Streptococcus mutans* in the presence of LP and thiocyanate ion (SCN^-). Washed exponential-phase *S. mutans* serotype c (ATCC 10449) and serotype d, g (NCTC 6715) were incubated for 10 min at 37°C with a 1:5000 dilution of either d-specific or c-specific antibody-enzyme conjugate. The cells were washed free of unreacted antibody, and resuspended in a stirred pH stat chamber with 2.5 mM KSCN. Glucose was added to 1%, and the rate of acid production was recorded as the volume of 1 mM NaOH necessary to maintain a pH 6.5. LP was added at 4 min after glucose addition. Metabolism was inhibited within minutes when bacteria were pretreated with the homologous enzyme-antibody preparation. However, there was no effect with the heterologous system (Fig. 1). Enzyme activity could be detected in association with those cells treated with the homologous antibody system, but not those of the heterologous system. The concentration of H_2O_2 generated by cell-associated enzyme was well below the concentration of exogenous H_2O_2 necessary to result in equivalent inhibition in nontreated cells. These data suggest that generation of H_2O_2 in the vicinity of the target cell enhances the efficiency of the LP system and an antibody conjugate may provide a specific mechanism for focusing LP activity (Fig. 2).

B. Antitumor

In studies by Philpott et al. (63), antibodies to the 2,4,6-trinitrophenyl (TNP)-lysyl derivative conjugated to glucose oxidase were used in combination with LP (50 μg/ml) and iodide (20 μM) to obtain selective cytotoxicity of TNP-substituted HeLa and HEP-2 cells. The cytotoxic activity of the antibody-enzyme conjugate was correlated with 98% killing at 57 μg/ml of conjugate and 41% killing at 1.1 μg/ml. These data suggest the H_2O_2 limitation of the cytotoxic activity of the LP system. Free hapten (ε-DNP lysine) significantly reduced cytotoxicity, and

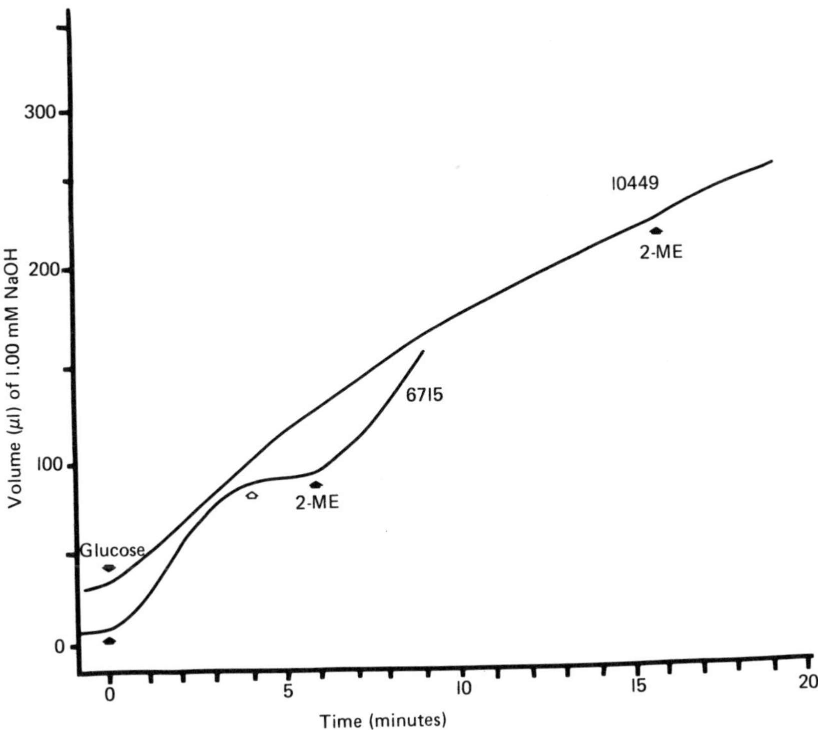

Figure 1 Glucose metabolism as NaOH-titratable acid production by *Streptococcus mutans* strains 10449 and 6715 (serotype c and g, respectively). Both bacterial suspensions were preincubated with serotype g-specific antibody conjugated to glucose oxidase (GO) and washed free of unbound antibody conjugate. Glucose was added to 1% after 5-min preincubation of bacteria suspended in 1 mM KSCN in a pH stat chamber. Bovine lactoperoxidase (10 µg/ml) was added to both suspensions 4 min after glucose addition, as indicated by the open arrow. Only strain 6715 was inhibited by the anti-6715-GO conjugate and inhibition was reversible with 2-mercaptoethanol. Experiments using anti-10449-GO conjugate also showed only homologous inhibition.

minimal killing was seen with unsubstituted cells, suggesting the specificity of the activity.

These artificial antigen studies were extended to a system in which natural membrane antigens served as tumor-specific antigens. Rabbit or goat antisera to carcinoembryonic antigen (CEA) and to a human colonic cancer cell line (HT-29) served as a source of globulin for conjugation to glucose oxidase. These Ig-GO conjugate preparations were

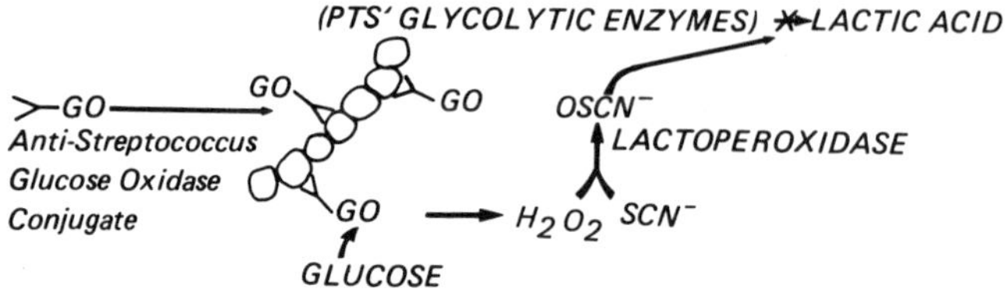

Figure 2 Model of the antibacterial-GO conjugate targeting of inhibition of streptococcal glycosis metabolism by the lactoperoxidase system.

tested for cytotoxicity against several different tumor cell types. The anti-HT-29 antibody conjugate was considerably more effective than the anti-CEA, though coupling of GO to the anti-CEA significantly increased its cytotoxicity over its complement-mediated activity. It is likely that the broader specificity of the anti-HT-29 antibodies permits a greater number of antibody-enzyme molecules on the target cell surface. Beyerle and Arnold (7,8, unpublished results) have utilized a human choriocarcinoma cell line (JEG-3) as target for antibody-focused peroxidase activity. These cells synthesize human choriogonadotropin (HCG) as a tumor-specific marker and anti-HCG IgG-GO was employed as the H_2O_2 delivery system. In preliminary experiments attempts were made to kill this cell line by the LP system using various concentrations of exogenous H_2O_2 or glucose-glucose oxidase as an H_2O_2 source. These systems had no effect on the viability of the tumor. The cells were able to survive even large concentrations of exogenous H_2O_2. The activity of the anti-HCG-GO conjugate preparations was assessed by microagglutination of HCG-coated latex beads ($\geq \log_2 9$) and by quantitating rates of H_2O_2 generation as a measure of enzyme activity bound to the HCG-coated beads. Significant enzyme activity could be detected on the surface of antibody-GO JEG-3 cells despite their apparent capacity for H_2O_2 reduction.

In in vitro experiments (Table 1) 10 μg of antibody conjugate in 2 ml of Dulbecco's PBS was incubated with a monolayer or with a cell suspension at 37°C for 30 min and washed free of unbound conjugate. The cells were then incubated for 1 hr at 37°C with LP and KI. Cytotoxicity was assessed by trypan blue permeability and by the inability of treated cells to reestablish in culture. The anti-HCG-CO-treated cells were killed only in the presence of both LP and KI. Unconjugated anti-HCG IgG had no significant effect on viability or the ability of these cells to establish in culture. Preincubation of the cells with anti-HCG blocked the ability of anti-HCG-GO to attach to the cells (no detectable bound enzyme activity) and inhibited the cytotoxic effects of the antibody conjugate (control D, Table 1). These data suggest the stability of the cell-associated HCG as a tumor marker after antibody binding.

Table 1 Viability of a Choriocarcinoma Tumor Cell Line with Tumor-Specific Antibody-Enzyme Conjugate, Lactoperoxidase (LP) and KI

Group	Anti-HCG-GO[a]	Anti-HCG[a]	LPO (50 μg/ml)	KI (20 μM)	Cell death
Experimental	+	−	+	+	+[b]
Control A	−	+	+	+	−
Control B	−	−	+	+	−
Control C	+	−	−	−	−
Control D	+	+[c]	+	+	−

[a]Washed (Dulbecco's PBS) monolayer incubated at 37°C/30 min with 10 μg bovine antihuman choriocarcinoma conjugated to glucose oxidase in 2 ml of Dulbecco's PBS and washed free of unbound conjugate.
[b]100% killing as determined by uptake of trypan blue. Cells sloughed in 30 min and did not reattach in Ham's F-12.
[c]Cells preincubated with anti-HCG, washed, and incubated with anti-HCG-GO.

The capacity of this antibody-enzyme preparation to function in vivo with host cofactors was assessed in a congenitally athymic (nude) mouse system (Table 2). Washed cells harvested from monolayer were incubated with either anti-HCG-GO, anti-HCG, or PBS, at 37°C for 30 min, washed, and injected subcutaneously in nu/nu mice on a Swiss-Webster background (8). Within 10 days there were 100% takes as detected by visible tumor in both the PBS and antibody control groups. In contrast, after 45 days there were no detectable tumors in the animals injected with anti-HCG-GO-treated cells, although tumors did develop in two animals by 60 days. It is important to emphasize that all cells were viable at the time of injection, as they had not been exposed to peroxidase or halide in vitro. These data suggest that the enzyme antibody is activating the mouse host-defense system (Fig. 3). It is possible that PMN or macrophages serve as a source of MPO in response to the tumor challenge and that halide cofactor (Cl^- or I^-) is available for the generation of tumoricidal products.

IV. CONCLUSIONS

The concept of activating the host's natural defense systems by natural enzymes (as opposed to toxic products) focused at the target by antibody carriers is especially attractive, particularly in an immuno-compromised host. The potent biological system of the peroxidases is particularly amenable to such manipulation. Hydrogen peroxide is generally the limiting component for the antimicrobial and antitumor activity of the peroxidases, and a number of enzymes are available that are capable of generating H_2O_2. In addition to glucose oxidase and

Table 2 Effects of Anti-HCG-GO on Tumor Growth in Athymic Mice

Pretreatment[a]	Tumor take	Serum HCG[b]	In vitro viability[c]
A. AB-GO	0/4 (>45 days)	Negative	Positive
B. AB	4/4 (10 days)	Positive	Positive
C. Dulbecco's PBS	10/10 (10 days)	Positive	Positive

[a]Washed cell suspensions incubated with 1 µg AB-GO, 10 µg or PBS at 37°C/30 min, washed and 10^5 cells in PBS injected sq. in nu/nu mice.
[b]Determined by microagglutination with anti-HCG-coated latex beads or by indirect ELISA with anti-HCG-GO.
[c]Growth in vitro after treatment. Viability of cells treated with anti-HCG-GO was lost only after LPO and KI addition.

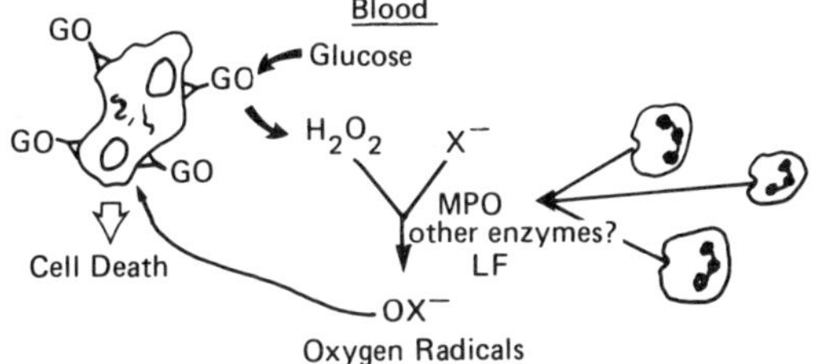

Figure 3 Proposed model of in vivo tumor inhibition by anti-tumor IgG-glucose oxidase preparations in athymic mice. Inhibition of tumor growth was affected only by the antibody-enzyme conjugates. Unmodified antibody had no effect on tumor takes. No exogenous co-factors were required for inhibition, suggesting that host factors were necessary for inhibition. It is possible that myeloperoxidase provided by neutrophils and/or macrophages catalyzes halide (X^-) that result in the tumoricidal event. In addition, the H_2O_2 generated by the localized enzyme may be converted to more reactive oxygen radicals, possibly by lactoferrin (LF)-associated iron.

xanthine oxidase, there are other enzymes (e.g., D-amino acid oxidase, L-amino acid oxidase, galactose oxidase, and SOD) that may prove more appropriate depending on pH optima required and substrate availability. These efforts will be enhanced by the rapidly advancing monoclonal antibody technology. It may also be possible to take advantage of the host's own antibodies that may normally prove to be protective for the tumor (blocking antibodies) but may be tumoricidal when appropriately conjugated to enzyme. With refinement in identifying the defining tumor and microbe-specific antigens and with improvement in conjugate preparations, such an approach could prove highly effective and exquisitely specific in the immunotherapy of neoplasia, as well as of fulminating microbial infections.

ACKNOWLEDGMENTS

The work presented here was supported in part by Grants NIH/NIDR DE 05722, ACS #IN-111E and by the University of Louisville Graduate Research Support Program. The author wishes to thank Drs. Pruitt, Adamson, and Beyerle for their contributions and criticisms.

REFERENCES

1. Allen, R. C., and Steele, R. H., *Fed. Proc.* 32: 478 (1973).
2. Arnold, R. R., Adamson, M., and Pruitt, K. M., *J. Dent. Res.* 59B: 961 (1980).

3. Baehner, R. L., Karnovsky, M. J., and Karnovsky, M. L.,
    J. Clin. Invest. 48: 187 (1969).
4. Baehner, R. L., Nathan, D. G., and Castle, W. B., *J. Clin.
    Invest. 50*: 2466 (1971).
5. Belding, M. E., and Klebanoff, S. J., *Science 167*: 195 (1970).
6. Bentwood, B. J., and Henson, P. M., *J. Immunol. 124*: 855
    (1980).
7. Beyerle, M. P., and Arnold, R. R., *Fed. Proc. 40*: 2409 (1981).
8. Beyerle, M. P., and Arnold, R. R., *Fed. Proc. 41*: 3115 (1982).
9. Borregard, N., and Kargballe, K., *J. Clin. Invest. 66*: 676
    (1980).
10. Bujak, S. J., and Root, R. K., *Blood, 43*: 727 (1974).
11. Burstein, S., and Knapp, R., *J. Med. Chem. 20*: 950 (1977).
12. Capsone, F., Meroni, P. L., Ciboddo, G. F., and Colombo,
    G., *N. Engl. J. Med. 300*: 44 (1979).
13. Cheson, B. D., Curnutte, J. T., and Babior, B. M., in *Pro-
    gress in Clinical Immunology,* vol. 3, Schwartz, R. S. (Ed.),
    Grune & Stratton, New York, pp. 1-65 (1977).
14. Clark, R. A., and Klebanoff, S. J., *J. Exp. Med. 141*: 1442
    (1975).
15. Clark, R. A., Klebanoff, S. J., Einstein, A. B., and Fefer, A.,
    Blood 45: 161 (1975).
16. Clark, R. A., Olsson, I., and Klebanoff, S. J., *J. Cell. Biol.
    70*: 719 (1976).
17. Clark, R. A., and Klebanoff, S. J., *J. Immunol. 119*: 1413
    (1977).
18. Clark, R. A., and Klebanoff, S. J., *J. Immunol. 122*: 2605
    (1979).
19. Clark, R. A., and Klebanoff, S. J., *J. Immunol. 124*: 399
    (1980).
20. Clark, R. A., and Szot, S., *J. Immunol. 126*: 1295 (1981).
21. Cohn, Z. A., and Morse, S. I., *J. Exp. Med. 111*: 667 (1960).
22. DeChatelet, L. R., Shirley, P. S., and Johnston, R. B., Jr.,
    Blood 47: 545 (1976).
23. Dewald, B., Baggiolini, M., Curnutte, J. T., and Babior,
    B. M., *J. Clin. Invest. 63*: 21 (1979).
24. Domanski, J., and Ostrowski, W., *Biochim. Biophys. Acta
    235*: 419 (1971).
25. Ehrlich, P., in *Collective Studies on Immunities,* Boldman, C.,
    (translator), Wiley, New York, pp. 441-442 (1906).
26. Flickinger, R. A., and Frost, S. R., *Eur. J. Cancer 12*: 159
    (1976).
27. Gale, R. P., and Zighelboim, J., *J. Immunol. 114*: 1047 (1975).
28. Ghose, T., Norvell, S. T., Guclu, A., Cameron, D., Bodurtha,
    A., and MacDonald, A. S., *Br. Med. J. 3*: 495 (1972).
29. Ghose, T., Guclu, A., Tai, J., MacDonald, A. S., Norvell,
    S. T., and Aquino, J., *Cancer 36*: 1646 (1975).

30. Gilliland, D. G., and Collier, R. J., *Cancer Res. 40*: 3564 (1980).

31. Goldstein, I. M., Hoffstein, S T., and Weissmann, G., *J. Cell. Biol. 66*: 647 (1975).

32. Goldstein, I. M., Roos, D., Kaplan, H. B., and Weissmann, G., *J. Clin. Invest. 56*: 1155 (1975).

33. Goldstein, I. M., Gerqueira, M., Lind, S., and Kaplan, H. B., *J. Clin. Invest. 59*: 249 (1977).

34. Hafeman, D. G., and Lucas, Z. J., *J. Immunol. 123*: 55 (1979).

35. Henson, P. M., *J. Immunol. 107*: 1535 (1971).

36. Holmes, B., and Good, R. A., *J. Reticuloendothel. Soc. 12*: 216 (1972).

37. Hurwitz, E., Levy, R., Maron, R., Wilchek, M., Arnon, R., and Sela, M., *Cancer Res. 35*: 1175 (1975).

38. Jacobs, A. A., Low, I. E., Paul, B. B., Strauss, R. R., and Sbarra, A. J., *Infect. Immun. 5*: 127 (1972).

39. Johnston, R. B., Jr., Keele, B. B., Misra, H. P., Lehmeyer, J. E., Webb, L. S., Baehner, R. L., and Bajagopalan, K. V., *J. Clin. Invest. 55*: 1357 (1975).

40. Jong, E. C., and Klebanoff, S. J., *J. Immunol. 124*: 1949 (1980).

41. Katz, P., Simone, C. B., Henkart, P. A., and Fauci, A. S., *J. Clin. Invest. 65*: 55 (1980).

42. Klebanoff, S. J., and Hamon, C. B., *J. Reticuloendothel. Soc. 12*: 170 (1969).

43. Klebanoff, S. J., *Science 169*: 1095 (1970).

44. Klebanoff, S. J., *Semin. Hematol. 12*: 117 (1975).

45. Klebanoff, S. J., and Rosen, H., *J. Exp. Med. 148*: 490 (1978).

46. Knowles, D. M., Sullivan, T. J., Parker, C. W., and Williams, R. C., *J. Clin. Invest. 52*: 1443 (1973).

47. Lehrer, R. I., *J. Bacteriol. 99*: 361 (1969).

48. Lehrer, R. I., and Cline, M. J., *J. Bacteriol. 98*: 996 (1969).

49. Levy, R., Hurwitz, E., Maron, R., Arnon, R., and Sela, M., *Cancer Res. 35*: 1182 (1975).

50. Mandell, G. L., *Infect. Immun. 9*: 337 (1974).

51. McCay, P. B., Fong, K. L., Lai, E. K., and King, M. M., in *Tocopherol, Oxygen and Biomembranes,* deDuve, C. and Hayaishi, O. (Eds.), Elsevier/North Holland, New York, pp. 41-57 (1978).

52. McRipley, R. J., and Sbarra, A. J., *J. Bacteriol. 94*: 1425 (1967).

53. Michelson, A. M., in *Toxic Effects of Active Oxygen,* Hayaishi, O., and Asada, K. (Eds.), University Park Press, Baltimore, Md., pp. 155-170 (1977).

54. Migler, R., DeChatelet, L. R., and Bass, D. A., *Blood 51*: 445 (1978).

55. Migler, R., and DeChatelet, L. R., *Biochem. Med. 19*: 26 (1978).

56. Moolten, F. L., Capparell, N. J., and Cooperband, S. R., *J. Natl. Cancer Inst. 49*: 1057 (1972).

57. Moolten, F. L., Capparell, N. J., Zajdel, S. H., and Cooperband, S. R., *J. Natl. Cancer Inst. 55*: 473 (1975).

58. Nathan, C. F., Brukner, L. H., Silverstein, S. C., and Cohn, Z. A., *J. Exp. Med. 149*: 84 (1979).

59. Nathan, C. F., Silverstein, S. C., Brunker, L. H., and Cohn, Z. A., *J. Exp. Med. 149*: 100 (1979).

60. Newburger, P. E., Chovaniec, M. E., and Cohen, H. J., *Blood 55*: 85 (1980).

61. Okuda, K., Ishiwara, K., Noguchi, Y., Takahashi, T., and Tadokoro, I., *Infect. Immun. 27*: 690 (1980).

62. Paul, B. B., Jacobs, A. A., Strauss, R. R., and Sbarra, A. J., *Infect. Immun. 2*: 414 (1970).

63. Philpott, G. W., Shearer, W. T., and Bower, R. J., and Parker, C. W., *J. Immunol. 111*: 921 (1973).

64. Pickaver, A. H., Ratcliffe, N. A., WIlliams, A. E., and Smith, H., *Nature (New Biol.) 235*: 186 (1972).

65. Repine, J. E., White, J. G., Clawson, C. C., and Holmes, B. M., *J. Clin. Invest. 54*: 83 (1974).

66. Repine, J. E., White, J. G., Clawson, C. C., and Holmes, B. M., *J. Lab. Clin. Med. 83*: 911 (1974).

67. Sacks, T., Moldow, C. F., Craddock, P. R., Bowers, T. K., and Jacob, H. S., *J, Clin. Invest. 61*: 1161 (1978).

68. Sbarra, A. J., and Karnovsky, M. L., *J. Biol. Chem. 234*: 1355 (1959).

69. Selvaraj, R. J., and Sbarra, A. J., *Nature 211*: 1272 (1966).

70. Shearer, W. T., Turnbaugh, T. R., Coleman, W. E., Aach, R. D., Philpott, G. W., and Parker, C. W., *Int. J. Cancer 14*: 539 (1974).

71. Simchowitz, L., and Schur, P. H., *Immunology 31*: 313 (1976).

72. Slivka, A., LoBuglio, A. F., and Weiss, S. J., *Blood 55*: 347 (1980).

73. Strauss, R. R., Paul, B. B., Jacobs, A. A., and Sbarra, A. J., *J. Reticuloendothel. Soc. 7*: 754 (1970).

74. Strauss, R. R., Paul, B. B. Jacobs, A. A., and Sbarra, A. J., *Infect. Immun. 3*: 595 (1971).

75. Weiss, S. J., Rustagi, P. K., and LoBuglio, A. F., *J. Exp. Med. 147*: 316 (1978).

76. Weiss, S. J., and LoBuglio, A. F., *Blood 55*: 1020 (1980).

77. Weiss, S. J., Young, J. LoBuglio, A. F., Slivka, A., and Nimeh, N., F., *J. Clin. Invest. 68*: 714 (1981).

78. Woeber, K. A., Doherty, G. F., and Ingbar, S. H., *Science 176*: 1039 (1972).

Index